Pharmacology case studies
for nurse prescribers

Second edition, revised and updated

Contents

Acknowledgements   x
List of contributors   xi
List of reviewers   xii
Introduction   xiv

1 How the body affects drugs   1
Case study: Statin toxicity 15
Answers to activities 23

2 How drugs affect the body   27
Answers to activities 42

3 Types of adverse drug reactions and interactions   45
Case study: Warfarin–amiodarone interaction 57
Answers to activities 57

4 Understanding and using the British National Formulary   61
Answers to activities 77

5 Adherence   81
Case study: Choosing a combined pill 84
Case study: Barriers to adherence 89
Answers to activities 90

6 Pharmacological case studies: Pregnancy and breastfeeding   95
Case study: Pregnancy with diabetes 109
Case study: Pain relief while pregnant or breastfeeding 112
Case study: Blood pressure treatment while breastfeeding 113
Answers to activities 113

7 Pharmacological case studies: Children   119
Case study: Paracetamol 124
Case study: NSAIDs 125
Case study: Prescribing small doses 127
Case study: Multimodal analgesia 127
Answers to activities 128

8 **Pharmacological case studies: Sexual health and contraception**   133
    Case study: Choosing a combined pill 141
    Case study: Off-label contraceptive prescribing 142
    Case study: Prescribing for gonorrhoea 143
    Case study: Not prescribing for vaginal infection 144
    Answers to activities 147

9 **Pharmacological case studies: Stable angina**   151
    Case study: Atypical presentation of coronary artery disease 1 156
    Case study: Atypical presentation of coronary artery disease 2 157
    Case study: Chest pain 165
    Answers to activities 167

10 **Pharmacological case studies: Hypertension**   173
    Case study: Hypertension 1 184
    Case study: Hypertension 2 186
    Answers to activities 188

11 **Pharmacological case studies: Heart failure**   197
    Case study: Heart failure 1 212
    Case study: Heart failure 2 213
    Answers to activities 215

12 **Pharmacological case studies: Chronic obstructive pulmonary disease (COPD)**   221
    Case study: Breathlessness 230
    Case study: COPD 231
    Case study: Smoking 231
    Answers to activities 232

13 **Pharmacological case studies: Neurological disorders**   239
    Case study: Seizure 241
    Case study: Parkinson's disease 247
    Answers to activities 251

14 Pharmacological case studies: Gastrointestinal disorders 257
Case study: Use of antacids 265
Case study: Constipation and pharmacological management of peptic ulcer 269
Case study: Gastrointestinal conditions affecting drug absorption 275
Answers to activities 277

15 Pharmacological case studies: Urinary incontinence in adults 283
Case study: Mixed urinary incontinence 296
Answers to activities 298

16 Pharmacological case studies: Diabetes 305
Case study: Type 2 diabetes 313
Case study: Diabetic drug adherence 319
Answers to activities 320

17 Pharmacological case studies: Mental health illness 327
Case study: Medication management 332
Case study: Depression 1 342
Case study: Depression 2 345
Answers to activities 351

18 Pharmacological case studies: Eye problems 361
Case study: Contact lens hypersensitivity 372
Case study: Blepharitis 373
Case study: Glaucoma 378
Case study: Conjunctivitis 380
Answers to activities 384

19 Pharmacological case studies: Complex health needs and polypharmacy 389
Case study: Complex health needs 392
Answers to activities 397

20 Pharmacological case studies: Frailty — 403
Case study: Adjusting a frail patient's medication 406
Answers to activities 407

21 Pharmacological case studies: Palliative care — 409
Case study: Gastric cancer 419
Case study: Motor neurone disease 420
Answers to activities 423

22 Insights into professional prescribing — 435
Answers to activities 440

Glossary — 441
List of abbreviations — 447
Index — 453

Acknowledgements

This book would not have been completed without the contributions of all the authors.

I would like to give a special mention to my husband David Scholefield for his unfailing support and encouragement throughout the process.

I am also very indebted to my co-editors, Alan Sebti and Alison Harris, who helped to make it all possible.

The graphics used throughout the book were created by Janette Earney and David Scholefield.

List of contributors

Kola Akinlabi
BSc (Hons), MSc Advanced Cardiorespiratory (UCL)

Beverley Bostock
MSc, MA, QA, RGN
Educational Lead/Clinical Specialist, Education for Health

Siobhan Corbett
BSc Hons, ENP, MSc in Advanced Clinical Practice. RN (Adult)
Nurse Consultant/Trauma Lead/ACP Lead in ED at Darent Valley Hospital.

Jennie Craske
PhD, RN (child)
Clinical Nurse Specialist, Pain and Sedation Service, Alder Hey Children's NHS Foundation Trust

Kirstie Dye
MPhil, BSc (Hons), RN
Senior Lecturer, Health and Education, Middlesex University, London

Su Everett
MSc, BSc (Hons), RN V300 Independent Prescriber.
Senior Lecturer, Senior Teaching Fellow Health and Education, Middlesex University, London

Andrea Gill
MSc, MRPharmS
Clinical Pharmacy Services Manager and Chair of Medication Safety Committee, Alder Hey Children's NHS Foundation Trust

Elizabeth Haidar
MSc, Bsc (Hons), RN Cert T/L

Alison Harris
MSc, BSc (Hons), RN, DipDN, PGCertHE. V100/150 Community Prescriber.
Senior Lecturer, Health and Education, Middlesex University, Lead Non-Medical Prescriber's Course

Hiba Yusuf
BSc (Hons), RN,
Clinical Nurse Specialist in Heart Failure, Harefield Hospital

Iram Husain
BPharm, MScAPP, MFRPSII
Regional Medicines Information Manager (Governance and Training), Specialist Pharmacy Services

Sophie Molloy
BSc (Hons), RN. V300 Independent Prescriber.
Module Leader for Contraception and Sexual Health, Lecturer in Adult Nursing, Health and Education, Middlesex University, London

Julie Moody
MSc, BSc (Hons), RN, DMS, PGCHE.
Registered Practice Educator. Lecturer, Health and Education, Middlesex University, London

Herbert Mwebe
MSc, Mprof. BSc, AdvDip, PGCert HE, Independent Prescriber CPPD.
Programme Lead, Senior Lecturer in Mental Health, Department of Mental Health and Social Work, Middlesex University, London

Anne Preece
MSc, BSc (Hons) Nursing Studies, BSc (Hons) Clinical Nursing Studies with RN, RM ENB 148 and Specialist Practitioner Award, ENB 100
Head Injury Clinical Nurse Specialist, University Hospitals Birmingham NHS Foundation Trust

Reviewers

Dr Melanie Romain
Consultant Physician and Geriatrician, Royal Free NHS Foundation Trust, London

Raquel Rosales
MSc, BSc (Hons), RN
Lecturer, Health and Education, Middlesex University, London

Donna Scholefield
MSc, BSc (Hons), RN, PGDip HE
Senior Lecturer, Health and Education, Middlesex University, London

Alan Sebti
BPharm, DipPharmPrac
Principal Pharmacist – Pharmacy Procurement, Royal Free London NHS Foundation Trust, London

Mahesh Seewoodhary
BSc (Hons), OND (Hons), RN, DN, FETC 730, ENB 100, RCNT, RNT, Cert Ed.
Senior Lecturer in Ophthalmic Nursing and Adult Nursing, University of West London, London

Jo Wilson
PhD, BSc (Hons), BA (Hons) Dip HSM, RGN
Macmillan Consultant Nurse Palliative Care, Royal Free London NHS Foundation Trust, London

Maria Yousif
MRPharmS, MPharm, PGDipGPP, PgCert
Pharmacist Specialist, Medicines Optimisation Team. Quality Care Commission

Dr Kaicun Zhao
PhD, MSc, MB, Clinical Pharmacology

List of reviewers

Elizabeth Denver
Hypertension Clinical Nurse Specialist. Department of Diabetes, Whittington Health NHS Trust, London

Albert B. Odro
RMN, RGN, Dip CPN, RNT, Cert Ed, BA(Hons), MEd.
Senior Lecturer, Middlesex University.

Jilly Pride
Senior Midwifery Lecturer. Programme Leader, Midwifery Short Programme. Middlesex University

Michelle Smith
Cardiac Nurse Specialist, Whittington Health NHS Trust, London

Introduction

Alison Harris and Donna Scholefield

All nurse prescribers are aware that, if they are to maintain their competence and be effective and safe prescribers, they must follow the most up-to-date advice on the prescribing of medicines and appliances. The safe prescribing, administration and evaluation of medicines is an essential skill for all nurses, as reflected in the NMC's *Standards of Proficiency for Registered Nurses* (NMC 2018). The *Standards* makes it explicit that all registered nurses must understand the principles of safe and effective medicines usage and have knowledge of drug allergies, adverse drug reactions, contraindications, polypharmacy, drug errors and prescribing practices.

With the continued expansion in non-medical prescribing, the different professional and regulatory bodies have acknowledged the need for a single set of competencies for all medical and non-medical prescribers. In 2016 the Royal Pharmaceutical Society (RPS) published *A Competency Framework for all Prescribers*. The Nursing and Midwifery Council (NMC 2018) has directed all nurses to abide by the RPS *Competency Framework*. In 2019 the Royal Pharmacological Society and Royal College of Nursing co-published *Professional Guidance on the Administration of Medicines in Healthcare Settings* (RPS & RCN 2019), offering further guidance for all healthcare professionals involved in drug administration. Nurse prescribers need to ensure that they are familiar with all statutory guidance and reflect on how it can be applied to their own sphere of clinical practice. Within higher education, the *Competency Framework* can be used to structure prescribing modules and programmes. Nurses can use the *Framework* for their NMC revalidation to demonstrate how they maintain their prescribing competencies. These standards should be read in conjunction with this text to support professional, ethical and accountable prescribing practice.

This second edition reflects those many changes and brings together the latest advice from NICE, the BNF, professional associations, primary research and clinical algorithms. All chapters are written by healthcare professionals with specialist knowledge. While the first edition was aimed at students undertaking the non-medical prescribing modules, this updated text has broadened its scope and is relevant to all trainee and qualified nurse prescribers.

The main aim of this book is to provide nurses with an introduction to pharmacological concepts, embedded in specific conditions, through case studies and self-assessment questions. By utilising a case study approach, we aim to help readers link pharmacological concepts with clinical practice and many of the conditions presented here will be commonly seen across all healthcare settings. In addition, the book will help students to understand some of the more technical pharmacology terms and may also provide a useful teaching resource for lecturers teaching the non-medical prescribing programme as well as those teaching pharmacology to undergraduate nursing students.

Introduction

The second edition has a new chapter on using the British National Formulary (BNF), reflecting the major changes in the structure of the Formulary that have occurred since the first edition. Other additions include chapters on pregnancy and breastfeeding and sexual health and contraception. Furthermore, with a growing elderly population leading to a greater emphasis on frailty syndrome, there is a new chapter dedicated to prescribing for frailty – recognising its association with a higher incidence of polypharmacy and adverse drug reactions. Finally, new developments in pharmacology (such as the emergence of biosimilar drugs) are also reflected within the text. All the other chapters from the first edition have also been revised and updated.

Finally, we would like to take this opportunity to remind both the trainee and the experienced nurse prescriber, often working autonomously and in complex and uncertain situations, that (in line with the NMC *Standards* and RPS *Competency Framework*) prescribers should only prescribe within their own scope or specialist area of practice and competence.

Objectives

The authors' objectives are to:

- Provide an overview of common conditions and their pharmacological management
- Demonstrate how to use the British National Formulary effectively
- Utilise a case study approach so that practitioners can apply pharmacological principles to real-life events
- Use self-assessment exercises to further challenge and engage the reader
- Give nurses an understanding of the fundamental pharmacological and physiological principles required for practical prescribing
- Support nurses in the pharmacological component of the non-medical prescribing programme.

How to use the text

It is not the authors' intention that this book should be used as a stand-alone text. Rather, it should be read in combination with other pharmacological and pathophysiological texts so that the questions may be fully addressed. A list of 'References and further reading', including key texts, national guidelines and frameworks, is provided for each chapter.

There are also sample answers, which can be developed further, for the activities found at the end of each section. Readers will gain greater knowledge and understanding of pharmacology if they consider the questions and then carry out some independent study (using the information in the 'References and further reading' list) before viewing the answers. The case studies presented focus on the practical realities of applied pharmacological concepts. A glossary and a list of abbreviations are also provided.

It is hoped that this book will give the reader an appreciation of the value of having a sound pharmacological knowledge base in order to deliver safe practice, effective prescribing and ultimately improved patient care.

References and further reading

The Nursing and Midwifery Council (NMC) (2018). *Standards of Proficiency for Registered Nurses.* https://www.nmc.org.uk/standards/standards-for-nurses/standards-of-proficiency-for-registered-nurses/ (Last accessed 15 July 2020).

Royal Pharmaceutical Society (RPS) (2016). *A Competency Framework for all Prescribers.* https://www.rpharms.com/Portals/0/RPS%20document%20library/Open%20access/Professional%20standards/Prescribing%20competency%20framework/prescribing-competency-framework.pdf (Last accessed 15 July 2020).

Royal Pharmaceutical Society (RPS) and Royal College of Nursing (RCN) (2019). *Professional Guidance on the Administration of Medicines in Healthcare Settings.* https://www.rpharms.com/Portals/0/RPS%20document%20library/Open%20access/Professional%20standards/SSHM%20and%20Admin/Admin%20of%20Meds%20prof%20guidance.pdf?ver=2019-01-23-145026-567 (Last accessed 15 July 2020).

How the body affects drugs

Dr Kaicun Zhao
PhD, MSc, MB, Clinical Pharmacology

Alan Sebti
BPharm, DipPharmPrac, Principal Pharmacist – Pharmacy Procurement, Royal Free London NHS Foundation Trust, London

This chapter:
- Discusses the advantages and disadvantages of different routes of drug administration
- Explains the main principles of drug absorption and the importance of these processes to the prescriber
- Explores how drugs are metabolised and excreted, as well as factors influencing these processes
- Demonstrates the importance of understanding the pharmacokinetics of a drug and how this knowledge assists safe and effective prescribing.

Introduction

Pharmacology includes the pharmacodynamic and pharmacokinetic study of drugs. Pharmacodynamics refers to the actions of drugs on different organs, tissues and biological systems, mediated through various mechanisms of action. The drug actions lead to effective correction of pathological conditions. Pharmacokinetics refers to the kinetic behaviour and disposition of drugs in the body – in other words, how the body affects the drug, either chemically or physically. The drug actions and their underlying mechanisms will be addressed in subsequent chapters. This chapter will focus specifically on pharmacokinetics.

For a drug to exert its therapeutic effects, it must reach its target site in an appropriate concentration. From a pharmaceutical formulation to a molecule acting on the target site, a drug must travel through various physical barriers. As drugs are foreign compounds, they have to enter the body and are eventually excreted by it. During this journey through the body, the drug will be affected by various biochemical environments. Generally, the journey involves several processes, namely absorption, distribution, metabolism and excretion (ADME). Figure 1.1 (below) is a schematic representation of a drug's progress through a biological body.

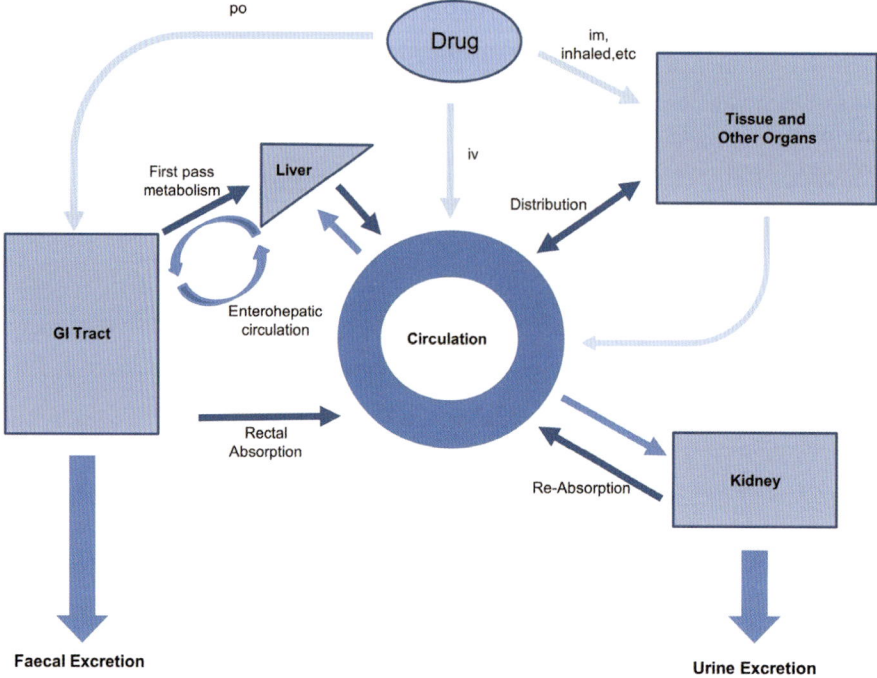

Figure 1.1: The processes undergone by a drug as it travels through a biological body; po (oral), im (intramuscular), GI (gastrointestinal), iv (intravenous)

Blood drug concentration

In clinical practice, it is difficult or impossible to measure or monitor drug concentration in tissues. However, the tissue concentration of the drug is proportional to the blood level of the drug. Since the blood level is generally easier to measure, it is commonly used as a proxy marker for the tissue concentration. Blood drug concentration is therefore an important indicator for studying and monitoring drug pharmacokinetic properties.

Pharmacokinetic parameters

To obtain effective drug concentration whilst minimising toxicity, it is essential to give the right dose. Designing an appropriate dosage regimen for a drug requires a basic understanding of the drug's fate in the body, including the way it is absorbed, distributed, metabolised and excreted. The fate of a drug in a biological body is described by its pharmacokinetic parameters. Generally, these parameters are derived from studies involving serial measurements of plasma concentration at various periods after administration of the drug. It is not within the scope of this book to discuss the calculation of the pharmacokinetic parameters. Instead, we will focus on the clinical applications of these parameters. Some key pharmacokinetic parameters and definitions are listed in Table 1.1 below.

Table 1.1: Commonly used pharmacokinetic parameters

Pharmacokinetic parameter	Definition
C_{max}	Maximum drug concentration after absorption
T_{max}	Time needed to achieve maximum drug concentration
K_e	Drug elimination rate constant
Cl	Systemic clearance of drug from the body
$t_{1/2}$	Half-life of drug – time taken for 50% of drug to be eliminated from the body
F	Bioavailability of a drug – a measure of both the rate and extent of drug absorption into blood circulation. In day-to-day use, bioavailability is generally used to describe the extent, i.e. the proportion (or percentage) of drug absorbed into blood circulation.
V_d	Volume of distribution – an indicator of the extent of drug distribution into tissues. This is the theoretical volume that would contain the total amount of drug in the body at the same concentration as it is in the blood.

Drug formulations and administration routes

Drugs can be delivered in different ways and in different forms. The administration route and formulation of a drug will influence its fate in the body. In clinical practice, administration route and drug formulation choices are primarily determined by both the physical and chemical properties of the drug, and by the therapeutic demands. Table 1.2 (page 4) lists the most frequently used administration routes and the relevant formulations, with their advantages and disadvantages.

Drug absorption

When a drug is delivered into the body, it will immediately go through absorption. Absorption is the process whereby a drug passes through biological membranes and is transported through tissues to reach the systemic circulation. All administration routes (except the intravenous route) require the drug to go through absorption in order to be transported from the delivery site to the systemic circulation. Intravenous injection will bring a drug directly into the systemic circulation, without the need to go through absorption.

Table 1.2: Drug administration routes and characteristics

Class	Administration route	Formulation	Advantages		Disadvantages
Enteral	Oral	Tablet, Pill, Capsule, Syrup, Tincture	• Easy and convenient for self-administration • Non-invasive		• Lag-time required to achieve effective blood concentration, due to absorption process • First-pass effect may reduce drug bioavailability • Various factors may affect drug absorption, such as food, other drugs, gastric emptying, etc.
	Sublingual	Tablet, Film	• Rapid absorption and onset of action • Avoids first-pass effect		• Not all drugs are suitable to be delivered in this way
Parenteral	Intravenous injection	Injections, Infusion	• Not subject to first-pass metabolism • Used in unconscious cases or patients who are nil by mouth • Used for drugs that are poorly absorbed or unstable in the GI tract	• Rapid action • Directly delivered into systemic circulation (bioavailability is 100%) • Easy dose control	• Not suitable for self-administration • Invasive • Risk of infection
	Intramuscular injection	Injections		• Absorption is relatively fast and complete	• Not often suitable for self-administration • Invasive and often painful
	Subcutaneous	Injections, Infusion		• Absorption is relatively slow • Infusion avoids the need for repeated injections	• Invasive • Risk of inflammation at the infusion site
Others	Inhalation	Pressurised metered-dose inhalers, Dry powder inhalers, Medical gases	• Rapid absorption • Used for local and systemic actions		• Only appropriate for drugs that can be made into gas form or those that can be dispersed in an aerosol
	Topical	Cream, Spray, Gel, Paste, Powder	• Easy to self-administer • Used for local actions		• Not always convenient
	Transdermal	Spray, Patch, Cream, Ointment or Gel	• Easy to self-administer • Used for continued slow drug delivery		• Not always convenient • Potential for irritation of skin • Significant lag-time to achieve effect
	Rectal	Suppository, Enema	• Avoids first-pass effect and destruction by intestinal enzymes or by low pH in the stomach • Useful for drugs that induce vomiting • Used in unconscious cases or patients who are vomiting or nil by mouth • Used for local and systemic actions		• Absorption is varied and often incomplete • Not convenient • Less acceptable to patients

Transportation of drugs

Passive diffusion

For a drug to be transported in the biological system, it has to cross the lipid bilayer of cell membranes. Passive diffusion is the most common way in which substances move across the phospholipid bilayer membranes. The vast majority of drugs can be absorbed through this mechanism. In passive diffusion, a drug moves from a high concentration site to a low concentration site without requiring any energy input.

Some relatively large molecule drugs cross cell membranes by passive diffusion via transmembrane proteins that act as carriers, thus facilitating their passage. The drugs still move from the side of high concentration to the side of low concentration without the need for energy. This type of passive diffusion is called facilitated diffusion. As the number of membrane carrier proteins is limited, facilitated diffusion can be subject to saturation and thus inhibited. Some of the cephalosporin antibiotics (such as cephalexin) are absorbed across the intestinal epithelial cells using facilitated diffusion.

Active transport

Some drugs, such as levodopa (used to treat Parkinson's disease), fluorouracil (anti-cancer drug) and iron salts, are absorbed by active transport. In contrast to passive diffusion, active transport needs specific membrane proteins to act as carriers. As there is a limited number of carrier proteins, the process of active transport can be saturated when the drug concentration reaches a certain level. This absorption process needs energy and can move drugs against a concentration gradient, from lower to higher concentration.

Endocytosis

Endocytosis is another way for drugs to be absorbed. In this process, drugs are engulfed by invaginated cell membrane to form a drug-filled vesicle. They are then transported into the cell, or across epithelial or enterocytic cells, by pinching off the drug-filled vesicle. Endocytosis is an energy-consuming process.

This absorption mechanism only plays a minor role in the transportation of drugs generally, but it is important for some large molecules, particularly for those with high polarity, that cannot pass through the hydrophobic plasma or cell membrane by passive diffusion, such as proteins. Vitamin B12 is an example of a drug that is absorbed across the gut wall, through endocytosis.

Factors affecting drug absorption and drug bioavailability

Many factors can affect the absorption process. It is important to understand these effects, as changes in a drug's absorption will also cause changes in its bioavailability, and consequently influence its effectiveness or even cause toxicity. Table 1.3 lists some of the most common factors that can significantly affect the absorption of drugs.

Table 1.3: Factors influencing drug absorption

Factors	Influence on drug absorption	Example
Blood flow to the absorption site	• Abundant blood flow to the absorption site will facilitate drug absorption.	• Digoxin bioavailability is increased when gastrointestinal blood flow is increased. Another example is that increased skin temperature increases the rate of absorption of drug from transdermal patches. Case reports indicate that this can be significant enough to cause toxicity.
Total surface area available for absorption	• The larger the surface area for absorption, the higher the rate and extent of absorption.	• Although aspirin is more easily absorbed from the stomach, the major absorption of aspirin is from the intestine, as the total surface area is much larger than that of the stomach.
Contact time at the absorption surface	• The longer the contact time at the absorption site, the greater the extent of the absorption.	• Plasma digoxin concentrations are increased by increased contact time in the intestine, due to decreased gastrointestinal motility.
Effect of pH on drug absorption	• The pH at the absorption site affects the ionisation of weak acid or weak base drugs, and influences absorption. The un-ionised form is usually more easily absorbed.	• Aspirin, as a weak acid, is un-ionised at the low pH of the stomach and better absorbed from the stomach than the small intestine. Note: See above comments on total surface area.
Physico-chemical properties of drugs	• Chemical instability: Some drugs may be sensitive to the environment of the gastrointestinal tract. • Hydrophobic drugs cross the lipid layer of the membranes more easily. But extreme hydrophobicity will reduce the drug's solubility. • Particle size: The smaller the drug particle size, the more easily the drug is absorbed.	• Benzylpenicillin is unstable in the low pH of the stomach. • Proteins, such as insulin, are normally destroyed by degradative enzymes.
First-pass hepatic metabolism	• Some drugs may experience extensive first-pass metabolism when given orally, significantly reducing the amount of drug that enters the systemic circulation.	• Propranolol undergoes significant biotransformation in the liver before entering the systemic circulation. Therefore the oral dose of propranolol is much higher than the intravenous dose.

Pharmacology case studies for nurse prescribers

Second edition, revised and updated

Edited by Donna Scholefield, Alan Sebti and Alison Harris

Pharmacology case studies for nurse prescribers
Donna Scholefield
Alan Sebti
Alison Harris

ISBN: 978-1-910451-25-0

First published 2015
Revised, updated second edition published 2021

All rights reserved. No part of this publication may be reproduced, stored in a retrieval system, or transmitted in any form or by any means, electronic, mechanical, photocopying, recording or otherwise, without either the prior permission of the publishers or a licence permitting restricted copying in the United Kingdom issued by the Copyright Licensing Agency, 90 Tottenham Court Road, London, W1T 4LP. Permissions may be sought directly from M&K Publishing, phone: 01768 773030, fax: 01768 781099 or email: publishing@mkupdate.co.uk

Any person who does any unauthorised act in relation to this publication may be liable to criminal prosecution and civil claims for damages.

British Library Cataloguing in Publication Data

A catalogue record for this book is available from the British Library

Notice

Clinical practice and medical knowledge constantly evolve. Standard safety precautions must be followed, but, as knowledge is broadened by research, changes in practice, treatment and drug therapy may become necessary or appropriate. Readers must check the most current product information provided by the manufacturer of each drug to be administered and verify the dosages and correct administration, as well as contraindications. It is the responsibility of the practitioner, utilising the experience and knowledge of the patient, to determine dosages and the best treatment for each individual patient. Any brands mentioned in this book are as examples only and are not endorsed by the Publisher. Neither the publisher nor the authors assume any liability for any injury and/or damage to persons or property arising from this publication.

Disclaimer

M&K Publishing cannot accept responsibility for the contents of any linked website or online resource. The existence of a link does not imply any endorsement or recommendation of the organisation or the information or views which may be expressed in any linked website or online resource. We cannot guarantee that these links will operate consistently and we have no control over the availability of linked pages.

Printed by Bell & Bain Ltd - www.bell-bain.com
Typeset by Jeremy Fisher - www.processcreative.co.uk

To contact M&K Publishing write to:
M&K Update Ltd · The Old Bakery · St. John's Street
Keswick · Cumbria CA12 5AS
Tel: 01768 773030 · Fax: 01768 781099
publishing@mkupdate.co.uk
www.mkupdate.co.uk

Formulation and drug interactions	• Various new formulation techniques, such as enteric coating and controlled release formulations, are applied in order to alter the rate of absorption or the site of delivery. • Drugs may influence each other's absorption. This influence can take various forms.	• Sustained-release nifedipine tablets extend the administration interval from 8-hourly to 12- or even 24-hourly. • Proton-pump inhibitor preparations are enteric-coated to prevent inactivation by low gastric pH. • Antacids bind to tetracyclines, reducing their absorption due to chelation and pH changes. • Administering iron with ascorbic acid (vitamin C) increases iron absorption.

First-pass effect

The special feature of oral administration is that drugs absorbed from the gastrointestinal tract enter the liver via the hepatic portal vein and are subjected to metabolism by the liver before reaching the main circulation. This process is called first-pass metabolism or pre-systemic metabolism. Some drugs can be severely affected by the first-pass effect. For instance, more than 90% of the anti-anginal drug glyceryl trinitrate (GTN) is eliminated by first-pass metabolism. For this reason, a simple tablet formulation of this drug, administered orally, will be almost completely ineffective.

To avoid first-pass effect, glyceryl trinitrate is usually administered by the sublingual route, as blood vessels are richly distributed under the tongue. Drugs placed sublingually will be absorbed by the capillary blood vessels, entering the systemic circulation directly, and avoiding first-pass metabolism. Although first-pass metabolism occurs mainly in the liver, some breakdown of drugs also occurs elsewhere, such as the intestinal mucosa, skeletal muscles and lungs.

Activity 1.1

1. List the main factors that can affect drug absorption.
2. Explain the term 'first-pass effect' and give examples of two drugs that undergo significant first-pass effect.
3. Identify at least three routes of drug administration that avoid first-pass hepatic effects.

Bioavailability

Bioavailability is a parameter used to measure the extent to which a drug is absorbed and made available, to be distributed for actions in the body. It is usually expressed as a fraction or percentage of the administered dose that reaches the systemic circulation. Different drugs show different bioavailability. Usually, intravenous injection is deemed to have the highest bioavailability (100%). Due to incomplete absorption, degradation or metabolism, all other drug delivery routes may have reduced bioavailability. The same drug may also show different bioavailability depending on its formulation.

Bioequivalence and therapeutic equivalence

When comparing related drug products, the concept of bioequivalence is used to reflect the similarity in pharmacokinetic behaviour; and therapeutic equivalence is used to reflect the similarity in pharmacodynamic activities of drug products.

Bioequivalence

If two or more related drug products show similar rate and extent of absorption (similar peak blood drug concentration, Cmax, and similar time required to achieve this maximum concentration, tmax), then they are said to be bioequivalent. Bioequivalent drug products display comparable bioavailability.

Therapeutic equivalence

If drug products possess similar efficacy and safety in clinical application, they are therapeutically equivalent. Therapeutic equivalent drug products may or may not be bioequivalent.

Drug distribution

Once a drug enters the main circulation system through an absorption process, it is distributed into the body fluids, various tissues and organs via the blood. Drug distribution is normally rapid, and a moving equilibrium is quickly achieved where a drug can reversibly move between the bloodstream and the interstitial tissues, extracellular body fluid and the organs. Drug distribution varies significantly from drug to drug.

The extent of drug distribution is usually described by the volume of distribution. This volume is calculated according to the plasma concentration of the drug and its dose. As the body is not homogeneous, the volume measured may not reflect the anatomical compartment. This is called apparent distribution volume (Vd), as it is a theoretical volume (see Table 1.1, p. 3). The larger the Vd, the more extensively the drug is distributed into the tissues. For example, warfarin is 99% bound to plasma proteins. Because of this, it remains largely in the plasma and therefore has a low volume of distribution. In contrast, digoxin is largely bound to myocardial tissue, meaning that relatively little remains in the plasma and therefore digoxin has a relatively high volume of distribution of the order of 500–600 litres (note that this volume is larger than the sum of all body compartments).

Factors affecting drug distribution

A number of factors determine or affect drug distribution in the body. Table 1.4 (below) lists some factors that influence the distribution of drugs to various tissues.

Table 1.4: Factors affecting drug distribution in the human body

Factors	Influence on drug distribution	Examples
Blood flow	Normally, the richer the blood supply to a tissue/organ, the more a drug is distributed to that tissue/organ.	The brain, liver and kidney have a greater blood flow rate and drugs tend to be distributed more to these organs.
Capillary permeability	The walls of capillary blood vessels in different tissues have varying structures, leading to different levels of permeability. For example, the capillary structure in the brain is formed with continuously arranged endothelial cells, forming a barrier that prevents many drugs from entering the brain. This is commonly referred to as the blood–brain barrier.	Dopamine does not readily cross the blood–brain barrier and has to be administered as levodopa – a prodrug – for the treatment of Parkinson's disease.
Chemical properties	Lipid solubility: Hydrophobic (lipophilic) drugs normally distribute into tissues more readily, because they can easily penetrate across the phospholipid bilayer membrane. Lipophilic drugs also tend to distribute more in lipid-rich tissues.	Due to its high lipophilic property, chloroquine shows a distribution volume of more than 100 L/kg, with a half-life of 1–2 months.
pH	Similar to the influences on drug absorption, pH conditions also affect the distribution of weak acid or base drugs. Changes in pH will affect the ratio of ionised over un-ionised forms of a drug, leading to changes in distribution, due to differing ability to penetrate across phospholipid bilayer membranes. Un-ionised forms of weak acid or base are more lipophilic and move more easily across membranes.	Un-ionised drugs cross cell membranes more readily, to distribute to the action site. Changes in environmental pH may therefore alter distribution, due to changes in ionisation of a drug. For example, lidocaine may be less effective in the acidic environment of infected tissue.

Protein binding	Drugs can bind to various proteins, including plasma and tissue proteins, either specifically or non-specifically. This can affect drug distribution, as the drug may be trapped in particular tissues.	The distribution volume of theophylline increases, due to reduction of its plasma protein binding in patients with hepatic cirrhosis.
Liver disease	This affects the extent of plasma protein binding of drugs.	Phenytoin distribution is significantly altered in hypoalbuminaemia – observed plasma concentrations therefore need to be corrected for this.

The blood–brain barrier

Due to the specific structure of the capillary blood vessel walls, with tight junctions between cells, there is an effective barrier between the blood and brain tissues. This is referred to as the blood–brain barrier (BBB), which only readily allows lipid-soluble drugs or those that can be actively transported by a carrier protein to enter the brain. Drugs with significant polarity, or with a positive or negative charge, cannot easily pass across the BBB – limiting the distribution of these drugs to the brain. A common example of this is dopamine, which does not cross the BBB and therefore cannot be used directly to treat the dopamine deficiency seen in Parkinson's disease. Instead, the prodrug levodopa is given. This is non-polar, and readily crosses the BBB. Once the levodopa reaches the brain, it is converted to dopamine by the enzyme dopa-decarboxylase.

Plasma protein binding of drugs and its clinical implications

Following absorption, a drug may bind to plasma proteins. The extent and affinity of this binding varies widely from one drug to another. The major binding protein in the plasma is albumin, which accounts for about 60% of all plasma proteins. Weak acids and hydrophobic drugs tend to bind to plasma albumin. Weak bases are more likely to bind to globulin or glycoproteins.

The binding of a drug to plasma proteins is normally reversible and non-specific. Equilibrium will be achieved and maintained between the bound and free forms of a drug. When the free drug is eliminated, the bound drug dissociates from the plasma protein to maintain the equilibrium; and the free-drug level remains at a constant proportion to the bound drug. Bound drugs are not diffusible and they are pharmacologically inactive. Only a drug in its free form can distribute to its site of action and exert a pharmacological effect. High plasma protein binding may reduce or slow the distribution of a drug into interstitial tissues or other organs.

When binding to plasma proteins is extremely high (>90%), it becomes clinically significant. In this case, only a relatively small portion of the drug is in its free form and therefore pharmacologically active and able to exert a therapeutic effect. This means that a relatively small change in the level of the bound drug may result in a relatively large change in the level of the free drug, leading to a significant increase in activity and/or potential for toxicity. This is particularly important for drugs with a small apparent volume of distribution and narrow therapeutic index. Warfarin is a typical example, and shows about 99% binding to plasma albumin. If any factor changes the degree of plasma protein binding, such as hypoalbuminaemia or the co-administration of a drug with a high affinity for albumin (such as tolterodine, aspirin or paracetamol), warfarin may be displaced from plasma proteins and the level of free warfarin will be increased. This may lead to toxicity, in the form of an enhanced anticoagulant effect and bleeding.

Activity 1.2
1. Briefly explain what is meant by the term 'drug distribution'.
2. If a drug's distribution volume is significantly larger than normal human body volume, what does that mean?

Drug metabolism

When a drug enters the body, the body's homeostatic mechanisms start to eliminate it. There are two ways through which the body eliminates a foreign compound. One way is metabolism and another is excretion. The process of metabolism, often referred to as biotransformation, transforms a drug into a chemically different compound or metabolite, usually converting lipophilic drugs into more polar hydrophilic metabolites and facilitating the excretion of the drug and its metabolites into the urine.

Drug metabolism is traditionally recognised as an inactivation process. After metabolism, the metabolites of a drug will commonly lose the pharmacological activities of the parent compound. However, this is not always the case. Some metabolites are as active as their parent drug (and sometimes even more active).

In some cases, the parent drug is administered as an inactive prodrug and must be metabolised to form a pharmacologically active compound before it exerts a therapeutic effect. For example, the cancer chemotherapy agent cyclophosphamide is a prodrug that is converted by liver cytochrome P450 (CYP) to form the pharmacologically active 4-hydroxycyclophosphamide.

Drugs can be metabolised in various different organs and tissues. However, the liver is the major organ responsible for drug metabolism. Other organs or tissues frequently involved in biotransformation of drugs include the kidney, lung and the gut wall. Drug metabolism is normally mediated by specific enzymes. In general, there are two kinds of biotransformation reaction, identified as phase I and phase II metabolism respectively.

Phase I metabolism

Phase I metabolism introduces polar functional group(s), such as hydroxyl (-OH), amide ($-NH_2$), sulfhydryl (-SH) and carboxyl (-COOH) chemical groups through oxidation, reduction or hydrolysis of a drug compound. These chemical functional groups generally facilitate the elimination of the drug from the system.

Oxidation is the most important metabolic pathway for a foreign compound in the human body. The oxidation reactions in phase I drug metabolism are commonly catalysed by the CYP monooxygenase system, which is located in the microsomes of cell endoplasmic reticulum. They are often referred to as microsomal mixed function oxidases.

The cytochrome P450 system

Cytochrome P450 is a super family of heme-containing enzymes containing a number of sub-families. The naming convention used for this family of enzymes is usually a number to indicate the CYP family, followed by a capital letter to indicate the sub-family and another number at the end to represent the specific isoenzyme, for example CYP1A1, CYP2E1 and CYP3A4. CYP enzymes exist in most cells but are found primarily in the liver and GI tract. The liver and the GI tract therefore play an important role in drug metabolism.

In humans, 57 CYP families have been identified and amongst these families CYP1, CYP2 and CYP3 have been identified as the main enzymes responsible for the metabolism of foreign compounds. Other families may be involved in the metabolism or synthesis of endogenous materials such as hormones, lipids, vitamins and cholesterol.

CYP3A4, CYP2D6, CYP2C9/10, CYP2C19, CYP2E1 and CYP1A2 are most commonly involved in drug metabolism, covering the vast majority of P450-catalysed reactions. Statistics have shown that these CYP isozymes (also known as isoenzymes) are responsible for more than 60% of the metabolism of xenobiotics in humans.

Phase II conjugation

Phase II metabolism is a form of conjugation reaction. Drugs and/or their metabolites from phase I metabolism are conjugated with an endogenous substrate, such as glucuronic acid, sulphuric acid, acetic acid, or an amino acid. Similar to phase I reactions, phase II metabolism also occurs mainly in the liver and to a lesser extent in the kidney and intestinal wall. The most common conjugation reaction is glucuronidation, in which a drug or its phase I metabolites are combined with glucuronic acid. Other conjugation reactions are listed in Table 1.5 (below). Various transferases are involved in conjugation reactions, such as glucuronyl transferase for glucuronidation.

Phase II conjugation reactions usually convert drugs into more polar and water-soluble metabolites, facilitating drug excretion from the body through the kidney or bile, though there are some exceptions. For example, acetylation reactions generally reduce the water solubility of drugs. Most drugs will be inactivated following the formation of a phase II conjugate. However, there are some important exceptions to this, such as the morphine glucuronidation product, morphine-6-glucuronide, which is significantly more potent than its parent compound morphine.

Table 1.5: Phase II metabolism – conjugation reactions

Conjugation reaction(s)	Conjugating substrate	Enzyme(s)
Glucuronidation	UDP-glucuronic acid	UDP-glucuronyl transferase
Sulphation/Sulfonation	3'-phosphoadenosine-5'-phosphosulfate	Sulfotransferases
Methylation	S-adenosyl methionine	Methyltransferase
Acetylation	Acetyl CO-enzyme A	N-acetyltransferases
Glycine conjugation	Glycine	N-acyltransferase
Glutathione conjugation	Glutathione	Glutathione S-transferases

Factors affecting drug metabolism

Apart from individual variations, physiological conditions (such as age, gender, hereditary and racial differences) all influence drug metabolism. In general, drugs are metabolised more slowly in foetal, neonatal and elderly people than in adults. Pathological conditions, such as liver disease, may also affect drug metabolism processes.

The most important factors affecting drug metabolism are induction and inhibition of the enzymes involved in drug metabolism. Certain drugs, environmental chemicals and food ingredients can increase the synthesis of one or more CYP isozymes. For example, phenobarbital induces CYP2B1 and 2B2; and rifampicin induces CYP3A4, 1A2, 2C9 and 2C19. This is referred to as enzyme induction.

Increasing levels and activities of CYP isozymes result in increased biotransformation of drugs and can lead to significant decreases in plasma concentration of the drugs metabolised by these CYP isozymes, with subsequent loss or attenuation of pharmacological activity. For example, smoking induces CYP1A2 and this significantly increases the clearance of theophylline and reduces its half-life in smokers. The onset of enzyme induction is gradual, as more enzyme needs to be synthesised. The effects of induction also persist beyond removal of the inducing agent, as enzyme levels are gradually reduced.

In contrast, drug metabolising enzymes (in particular the CYP isozymes) may also be inhibited by certain drugs, environmental chemicals and food ingredients, as in inhibition of CYP3A4 by clarithromycin. The most common type of inhibition is competitive and reversible. The inhibitors are usually also a substrate of the inhibited isozymes (i.e. they are normally metabolised themselves by the same isoenzyme) but some inhibitors are capable of inhibiting isozymes to which they are not substrates. Some other factors affecting drug metabolism are summarised in Table 1.6 (below).

Table 1.6: Other factors affecting drug metabolism

Factor	Effect(s)	Example(s)
Age	Neonates are deficient in phase II conjugating system.	Chloramphenicol accumulation in infant due to insufficient activity of UDP-glucuronyl transferase, causing 'grey baby syndrome'.
	Elderly people have a marked depression of hepatic oxidative metabolism.	The total hepatic clearance of theophylline is reduced in older people.
Sex	Higher clearance is found in men than in women, due to increased glucuronide and sulphate conjugations.	Due to more active phase II metabolism, some medicines are metabolically cleared faster. Examples include paracetamol, caffeine and digoxin.
Nutritional status	A low intake of protein will cause a decrease in drug clearance by reducing oxidative metabolism.	Theophylline
Liver disease	Hepatitis A impairs the function of human hepatic CYP, resulting in decreased drug clearance.	Metabolic clearance of coumarin by CYP2A6 is reduced.
	Fatty liver disease affects the phase II conjugation reactions.	Clearance of paracetamol through sulfonation is decreased in steatohepatitis.
Intestinal flora	Microbial strains in intestinal flora can be involved in drug metabolism. Changes in the environment of intestinal flora will affect drug metabolism.	Digoxin is inactivated by gastrointestinal bacteria. Concurrent administration of antibiotics such as clarithromycin can therefore increase digoxin bioavailability.
Pharmaco-genetic variation	Polymorphisms have been identified for isozyme CYP2C, 2D6 and acetyltransferase, showing different metabolising capacities in different populations.	Reduced conversion of codeine to morphine, due to genotypes associated with lower CYP2D6 activity.

Case study: Statin toxicity

A 64-year-old African-American man has been receiving simvastatin for approximately six months. About three weeks ago, he started suffering from sinusitis and was prescribed the macrolide antibiotic clarithromycin to control the infection. However, he was admitted to hospital later with diffuse muscle pain and severe muscle weakness. Dark-coloured urine was noted. His creatinine kinase was found to be elevated and over the next few days the serum creatinine increased to 156 micromol/l (usual baseline for this patient was 90 micromol/l). A diagnosis of rhabdomyolysis was made. It was suspected that this was related to statin toxicity.

Activity 1.3 (Case study)
1. What is the most likely reason for statin toxicity in this case?
2. What is the major enzyme involved in the metabolism of simvastatin?
3. What is the potential interaction between macrolide antibiotics and statins?

Drug excretion

There are a number of ways by which drugs are excreted from the body. As shown in Figure 1.2 (below), the most important excretion routes are through the kidney and liver. Other routes include respiration through the lungs, sweating, or milk in nursing mothers. The forms of the excreted drug include the unchanged parent drug, phase I metabolites and phase II conjugates. Generally, the greater the polarity of a drug (the more hydrophilic it is), the more likely it is to be excreted through the kidney. Hydrophobic drugs, on the other hand, are more likely to be excreted through bile.

Renal excretion

Drugs and their metabolites are excreted via the kidneys into urine. Glomerular filtration is the main process in renal excretion of drugs. The normal kidney glomerular rate is 125 ml/min, which is about 20% of the normal renal blood flow rate. In addition, active secretion plays an important role in drug excretion via the kidney. For example, methotrexate is excreted through active secretion. The secretion primarily occurs in the proximal tubular area of the kidney.

Intestinal and biliary excretion

Due to incomplete absorption of enterally administered drugs, the unabsorbed drug will be excreted directly from the intestinal tract. The absorbed drug and its metabolites can be secreted into the bile in the liver, then secreted into the intestine and eventually excreted out of the body through defecation.

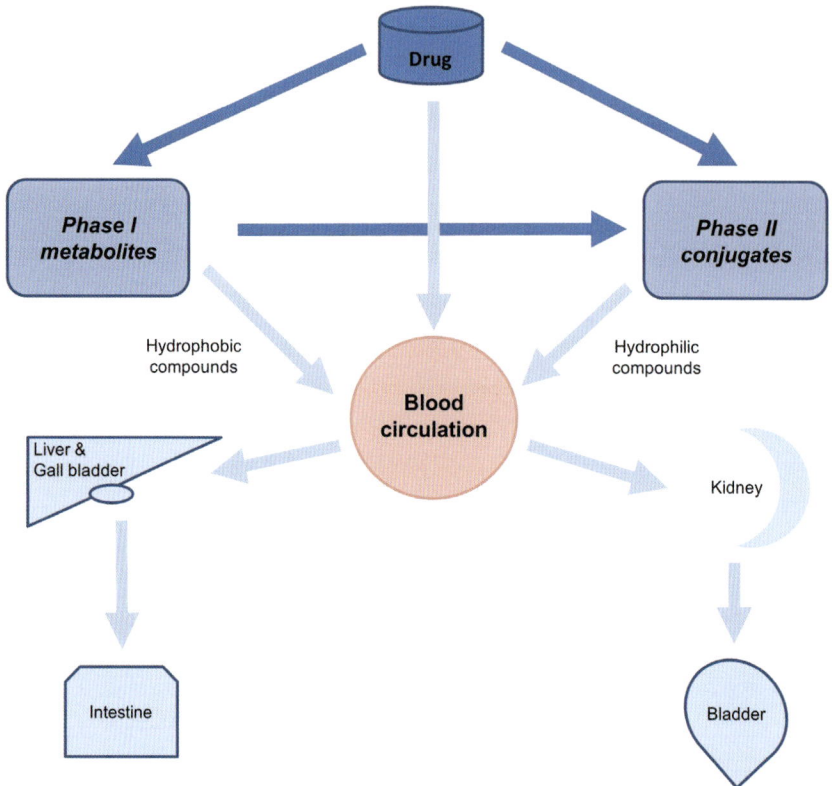

Figure 1.2: The major routes of drug excretion – kidney and biliary excretion. Phase 1 and Phase 2 metabolism occur in the liver

Factors affecting drug excretion

Drug excretion is affected by various factors. Reabsorption is an important process that may significantly affect the excretion of a drug. This is also a process during which drug interactions are likely to occur.

In kidney proximal tubular reabsorption, the drug (including its metabolites excreted from the kidney) can be reabsorbed back into the systemic circulation. The reabsorption process occurs in the distal tubular area of the kidney. Active transportation is also involved in the drug reabsorption.

In enterohepatic circulation, the drug (and its metabolites secreted from the bile) can be reabsorbed in the intestine and re-enter the systemic circulation. Conjugated metabolites can also be reabsorbed, following hydrolysis of the conjugates in the intestine, a process that often involves the gut flora. This reabsorption process from the gut is known as enterohepatic circulation or recycling.

Apart from reabsorption, there are many other factors that affect drug excretion. Table 1.7 (below) details some of these.

Table 1.7: Factors affecting drug excretion

Factor	Effect(s)	Example(s)
Blood flow to the liver and kidney	• Both hepatic and renal excretion of the drug are dependent on blood flow to these organs. Reduced blood flow, as in cardiogenic shock, heart failure or haemorrhage, may reduce excretion by these routes.	• Clearance of diltiazem, nifedipine and verapamil are dependent on liver blood flow.
Renal and liver diseases	• Dysfunction of liver and kidney will affect drug excretion.	• Accumulation of colchicine may be caused by reduced biliary excretion in patients with advanced liver disease and cholestasis. • Digoxin dose needs to be reduced, due to decreased excretion in patients with impaired kidney function.
Age	• Kidney tubular secretion is not completely developed in infants and neonates. • Renal clearance is reduced in older people.	• Around 90% of a benzylpenicillin dose is excreted through kidney tubular secretion. It is administered 12-hourly in neonates, but 4- to 6-hourly in adults. • Piptazobactam is administered three times a day, but reduced to twice a day if creatinine clearance is lower than 20ml/min.
Drug interaction	• Competitive inhibition of renal tubular secretion.	• Non-steroidal anti-inflammatory drugs (e.g. aspirin) and probenecid compete with methotrexate and penicillin respectively for the tubular secretion. Concurrent use of aspirin with methotrexate therefore potentially results in methotrexate toxicity. Conversely, probenecid is sometimes administered with penicillins to prolong their effects, e.g. in the treatment of syphilis.

pH	• Influences the degree of ionisation of weakly acidic and weakly basic drugs. Changes in urinary pH can result in 'ion-trapping', reducing reabsorption in the distal tubule.	• Forced alkaline diuresis for treatment of salicylate overdose – administration of IV sodium bicarbonate promotes renal elimination. Un-ionised aspirin, filtered by kidney, becomes ionised in alkalinised urinary filtrate, which reduces its reabsorption.

Activity 1.4

1. What are the most important pathways for drug elimination?
2. Where can excreted drugs be reabsorbed back into the systemic circulation?

Drug monitoring and pharmacokinetics

Half-life of a drug ($t_{1/2}$)

As mentioned at the beginning of this chapter, a drug's journey through the body can be monitored by measuring the blood concentration of that drug. Once a drug is delivered into the body, it will start to be absorbed and distributed. At the same time, the drug elimination process also begins. The changes in blood concentration of a drug reflect its kinetic course in the body.

A key parameter used to describe changes in blood drug concentration is the plasma half-life $t_{1/2}$, which is the time needed for 50% of the drug in the plasma to be eliminated, or the blood concentration of a drug to decrease by 50%. Most drugs exhibit first-order elimination kinetics. This means that the proportion of drug eliminated from the body per unit of time is constant, which in turn means that the half-life is independent of both the dose and blood concentration of a drug. As shown in Figure 1.3 (below), more than 95% of an administered drug is eliminated from the body after a period equivalent to four or five half-lives, following a single intravenous dose.

Changes in any of the relevant pharmacokinetic processes described above will change the half-life of any drug. Generally, the $t_{1/2}$ of a drug will be reduced by decreased distribution, such as lowered protein binding or enzyme induction, and increased by factors such as enzyme inhibition or impaired liver and kidney function. It is important for prescribers to be aware of such factors, as it may be necessary to adjust the dose in such circumstances to either maintain therapeutic efficacy or reduce the risk of toxicity.

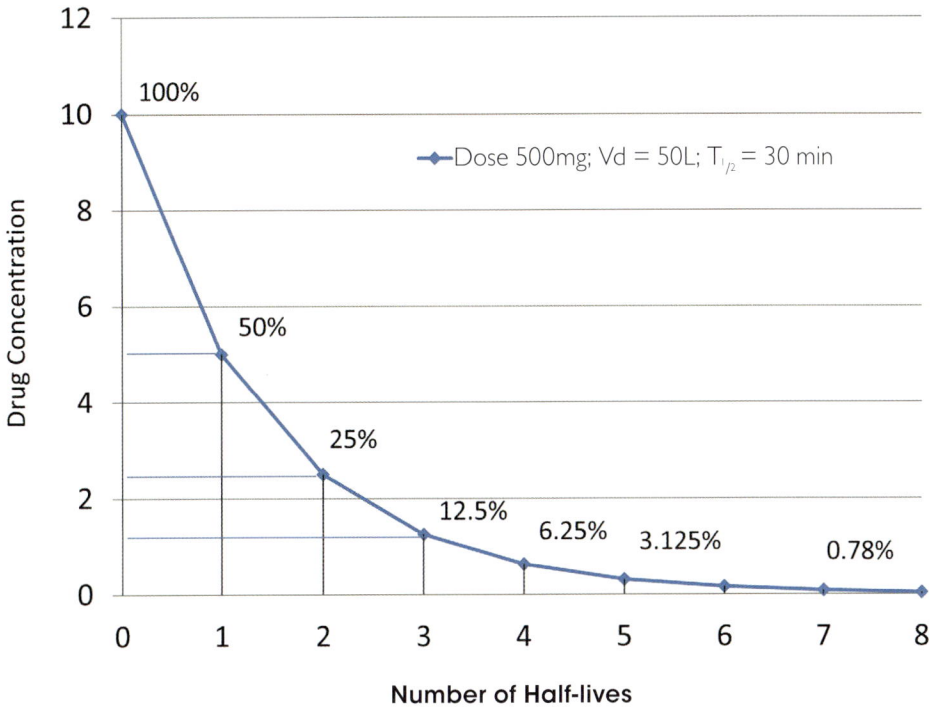

Figure 1.3: The time course of a single drug dose administered intravenously

Multiple doses and plateau levels of plasma drug concentrations

In clinical practice, it is more common to administer drugs with multiple doses at regular intervals. When a drug is given repeatedly at a fixed dose, and at regular intervals, the amount of the drug will accumulate in the body. The blood drug concentration will increase until equilibrium is achieved between the administration (or absorption) rate and the elimination rate. This is referred to as steady state equilibrium, at which point accumulation of the drug stops and the plasma concentration remains at a stable level.

In case of first-order kinetics, as the elimination rate of a drug is constant, steady state of a drug will always be achieved after 4–5 half-lives, regardless of the dose and frequency of administration. The actual steady state concentration achieved is, however, influenced by factors such as the size of the dose and the administration rate.

Effects of dose on the steady state concentration

If the administration frequency is fixed, the dose of a drug given per unit of time determines the steady state plasma concentration, as shown in Figure 1.4 (below). Higher doses of a drug will produce a higher steady state plasma concentration.

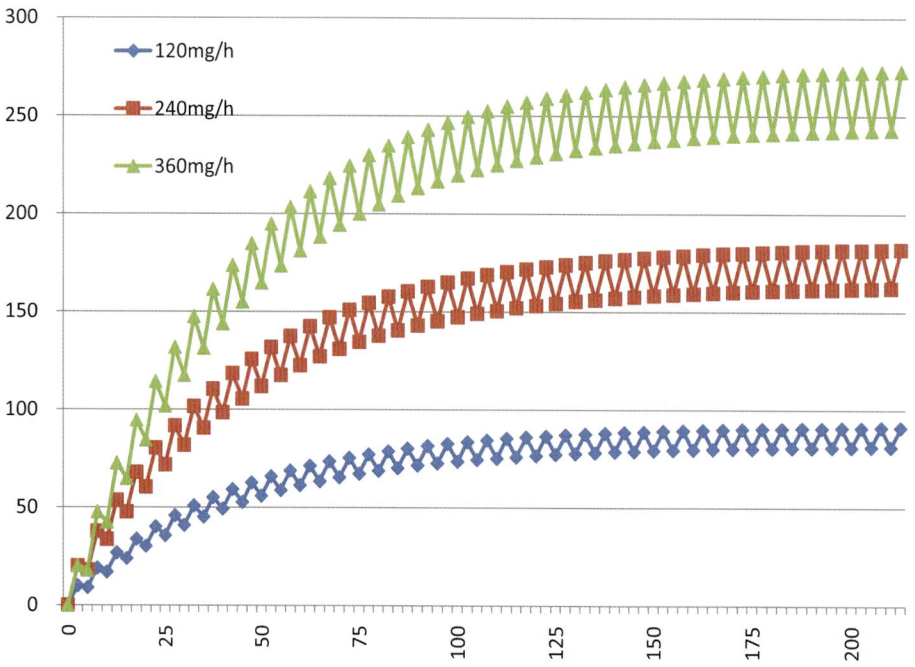

Figure 1.4: Steady state level of a drug at different doses given per unit of time

Effects of administration frequency on the steady state concentration

During the time period between the administration of repeated doses of a drug, all the pharmacokinetic processes described above (ADME) occur concurrently. Initially, absorption of the drug predominates and the plasma drug level increases until it eventually reaches a maximum or peak concentration (C_{max}). As absorption is completed, the effects of drug elimination (metabolism and excretion) become prominent, and the plasma drug level begins to fall. When the next dose of drug is administered, the plasma level begins to rise once again. When plasma drug concentration reaches steady state level, the highest and lowest plasma levels reached during the dosing interval are known as 'the steady state maximum' and 'minimum plasma concentration', or peak and trough levels respectively.

The steady state level of a drug is determined by both the dose and the frequency of administration. Figure 1.5 (page 21) illustrates this, with a fixed dose of a drug given at different dosing intervals.

In Figure 1.5a, a dose regimen has been chosen that produces peak and trough concentrations within the therapeutic range at steady state. This means that, at steady state, the drug would be exerting its desired effect(s) without significant toxicity – although no drug is free of adverse effects, which may occur even when plasma levels are within the therapeutic window.

In Figure 1.5b, the same dose of drug is administered at twice the frequency. In this example, at steady state the peak plasma concentration exceeds the MTC (minimum toxic level), at which point an unacceptable level of toxicity is likely to be seen.

Figure 1.5c shows the same dose of drug being given at half the frequency of that shown in Figure 1.5a. In this case, the plasma reaches a level within the therapeutic window. However, for a significant part of the dosing interval, the level is below the MEL (minimum effective level), during which time there would be no significant beneficial effect from the drug.

Figures 1.5a, 1.5b and 1.5c also show that the administration frequency affects the fluctuation of plasma drug concentration – in other words, the difference between the peak and trough levels. The longer the administration interval, the bigger the fluctuation in plasma drug concentration. The relevance of this is that smoother plasma drug concentration profiles are achieved when the dosing interval is reduced. As patients are likely to experience more adverse effects at peak plasma concentrations, the use of modified-release preparations in these circumstances may be helpful, as the same median plasma level of drug is achieved and peak concentrations are reduced. (Note: Although modified-release preparations are administered less frequently, they can be considered to be approximately equivalent to continuous release; so in terms of drug release, dosing can be said to be more frequent.)

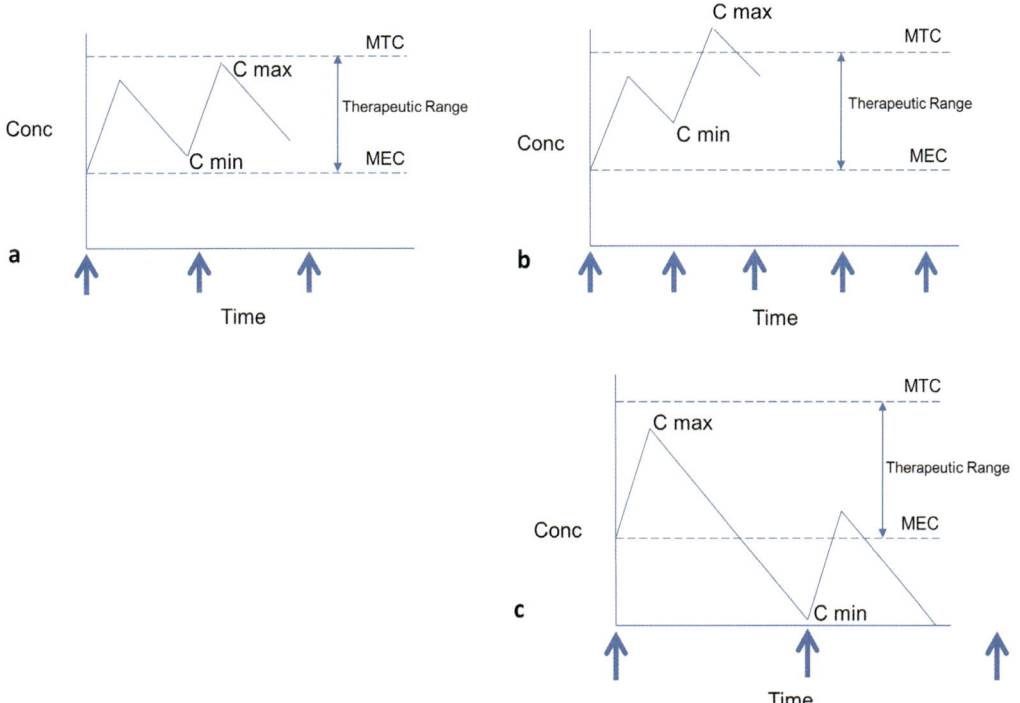

Figure 1.5: Steady state levels of a drug administered with a fixed dose but at different intervals

Loading dose

The range of plasma concentration of a drug, at which the pharmacological effectiveness is achieved but no toxicity appears, is called the therapeutic range of the drug. Dosage regimens are designed to achieve a steady state plasma concentration that is within the therapeutic range of a drug. A near steady state concentration is achieved after a period of time equivalent to 4–5 half-lives of the drug. In many clinical situations, the time taken to achieve steady state may be clinically unacceptable. In such cases, a larger loading dose of the drug is administered in order to rapidly achieve a therapeutic level of the drug. The loading dose is then followed by administration of a series of maintenance doses that help to achieve and maintain the therapeutic level as a steady state, as illustrated in Figure 1.6 (below).

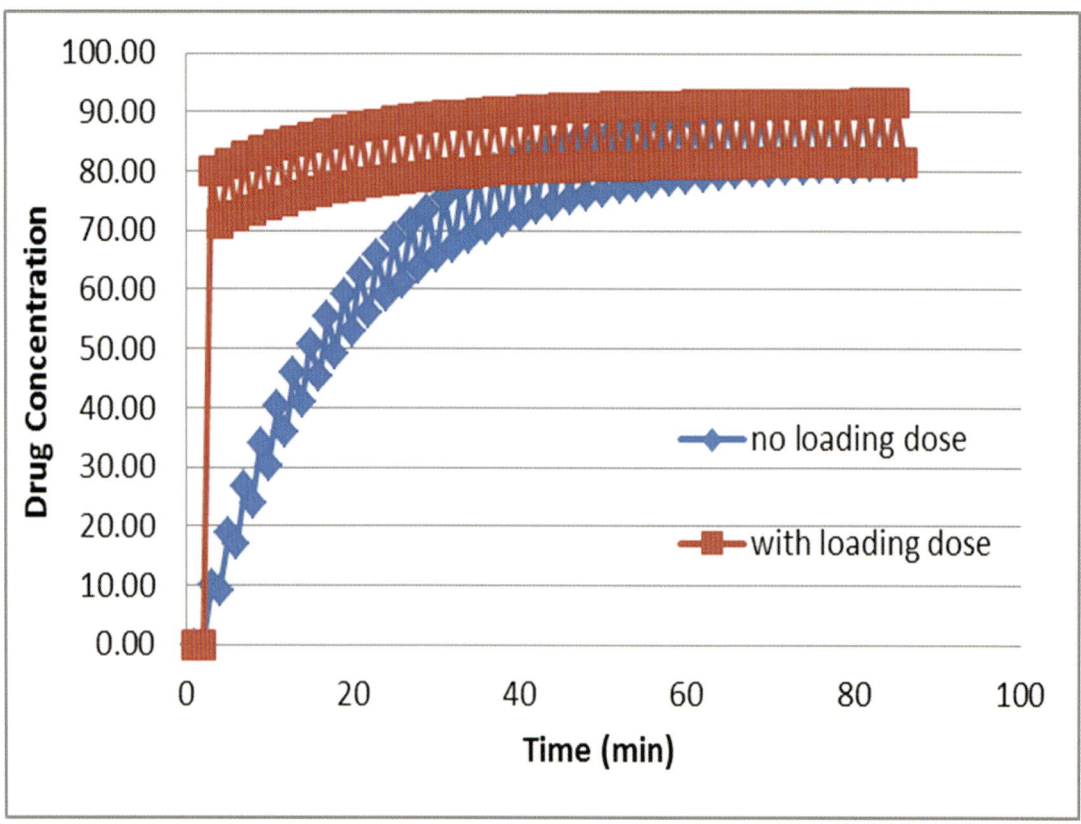

Figure 1.6: With a loading dose, an effective plasma concentration is achieved more quickly

Activity 1.5

1. What does the 'half-life of a drug' mean?
2. Define the term 'steady state level of a drug' and state how long it takes for this level to be reached, following the start of drug administration.
3. Name two drugs with long half-lives that often require a loading dose to achieve a therapeutic plasma concentration rapidly.

Summary

This chapter has discussed the processes of drug absorption, distribution and elimination (including metabolism and excretion). These processes determine the pharmacokinetic profile of a drug. It is essential to understand the factors that can affect the pharmacokinetics of a drug when designing appropriate drug administration regimens, selecting appropriate dosage forms and helping prescribers avoid side effects or toxicities.

Answers to activities

Activity 1.1

1. List the main factors that can affect drug absorption.

Drug absorption can be affected by drug-related factors such as molecular size, lipid solubility, degree of ionisation, concentration at the absorptive site, and route of administration. It can also be affected by human body-related factors such as blood flow, absorbing surface area and individual variations. (For further details, see Table 1.3, p. 6.)

2. Explain the term 'first-pass effect' and give examples of two drugs that undergo significant first-pass effect.

First-pass effect is the metabolic process that occurs before an orally administered drug reaches the circulatory system. A drug showing a high first-pass effect, such as glyceryl trinitrate, will have significantly reduced bioavailability and may be clinically ineffective if given by a route that has a first-pass effect. Propranolol is another drug with a high first-pass effect. This means that the IV dose used for arrhythmia and thyrotoxicosis is typically 1mg, which is significantly less than the oral doses of 10–40mg used for these indications.

3. Identify at least three routes of drug administration that avoid 'first-pass' hepatic effects.

The following administration routes can avoid 'first-pass' metabolism: sublingual, transdermal, rectal and inhalation.

Activity 1.2

1. Briefly explain what is meant by the term 'drug distribution'.

Once a drug enters the main circulation system through an absorption process, it is distributed into the body fluids, various tissues and organs via the blood. Drug distribution is normally very fast, and a moving equilibrium is quickly achieved whereby a drug can reversibly move between the bloodstream and the interstitial tissues or extracellular fluid and/or the organ cells. The distribution of a drug through the body is not uniform, and its concentration in some tissues may be high, whilst in others it may be low. Distribution is influenced by a number of factors, as summarised in Table 1.4 (see p. 9).

2. If a drug's distribution volume is significantly larger than normal human body volume, what does that mean?

A large volume of distribution suggests that a drug is widely distributed in the body. Conversely, a drug with a low volume of distribution may penetrate tissues poorly, and in some cases may be largely restricted to the circulatory system – for example, if the drug is highly bound to plasma proteins.

Activity 1.3 (Case study)

1. What is the most likely reason for statin toxicity in this case?

The most likely reason for statin toxicity is an interaction between the clarithromycin and simvastatin. This interaction may cause a significant increase in plasma statin concentration, inducing rhabdomyolysis (Lee & Maddix 2001).

2. What is the major enzyme involved in the metabolism of simvastatin?

Several statin drugs, including simvastatin, lovastatin and atorvastatin, are mainly metabolised by enzyme CYP3A4. If the activity of this enzyme is affected by other drugs, the pharmacokinetic deposition of the statins will change. For example, if the enzyme CYP3A4 is inhibited, the plasma levels of the statins will increase, due to reduced hepatic metabolism.

3. What is the potential interaction between macrolide antibiotics and statins?

Macrolide antibiotics, including clarithromycin, azithromycin and erythromycin, are inhibitors of CYP3A4. Inhibition of this enzyme affects the metabolism of statins, which are substrates for this particular isozyme. In the presented clinical case, simvastatin toxicity occurred as a result of the reduced clearance of simvastatin, owing to concurrent use with clarithromycin. This could have been avoided by withholding simvastatin for the duration of the clarithromycin therapy.

Activity 1.4

1. What are the most important pathways for drug elimination?

The most important ways for drugs to be eliminated from the body include liver metabolism transformation and intestinal and renal excretion.

2. Where can excreted drugs be reabsorbed back into the systemic circulation?

Drugs excreted through the kidney and liver can be reabsorbed back into the systemic circulation through the renal proximal tubule and through enterohepatic circulation respectively.

Activity 1.5

1. What does the 'half-life of a drug' mean?

Half-life refers to the time needed for 50% of a drug to be eliminated from the body, or the blood concentration of a drug to decrease by 50%.

2. Define the term 'steady state level of a drug' and state how long it takes for this level to be reached, following the start of drug administration.

The steady state level of a drug refers to the level achieved when the drug administration rate (absorption) and elimination rate reach an equilibrium. To achieve the steady state level of a drug normally requires a time equivalent to 4–5 half-lives. The plasma concentration at steady state is determined by both the dose size and the administration frequency.

3. Name two drugs with long half-lives that often require a loading dose to achieve a therapeutic plasma concentration rapidly.

Both digoxin and warfarin have long half-lives. Digoxin's half-life is approximately 36 hours and warfarin's is 40 hours. In practice, to get to steady state levels rapidly, an initial loading dose is administered and then a smaller maintenance dose.

References and further reading

Aronow, W.S., Frishman, W.H. & Cheng-Lai, A. (2007). Cardiovascular drug therapy in the elderly. *Cardiology Review*. **15** (4), 195–215.

Lee, A.J. & Maddix, D.S. (2001). Rhabdomyolysis secondary to a drug interaction between simvastatin and clarithromycin. *Annals of Pharmacotherapy*. **35** (1), 26–31.

Privitera, M. (2011). Current challenges in the management of epilepsy. *American Journal of Managed Care*. **17** (7), S195–203.

Rang, H.P., Dale, M.M., Ritter, J.M., Flower, R.J. & Henderson, G. (2011). *Rang & Dale's Pharmacology*. 7th edn. Edinburgh: Elsevier Churchill Livingstone.

Schmidt, L.E. & Dalhoff, K. (2002). Food-drug interactions. *Drugs*. **62** (10), 1481–502.

Springhouse Publishing (2012). *Clinical Pharmacology Made Incredibly Easy*. 3rd edn. Philadelphia, PA: Lippincott Williams & Wilkins.

Walker, R. & Whittlesea, C. (2007). *Clinical Pharmacy and Therapeutics*. 4th edn. London: Churchill Livingstone Elsevier.

2
How drugs affect the body

Donna Scholefield
MSc, BSc (Hons), RN, PGDip HE
Senior Lecturer, Health and Education, Middlesex University, London

This chapter:
- Provides an overview of how drugs produce their effects
- Explains key terms such as receptor, agonist, antagonist and partial agonist, efficacy, potency and the importance of the log10 dose response curve
- Discusses how drugs produce their effects after receptor binding.

Introduction

Chapter 1 looked at the pharmacokinetics of drug actions or 'What the body does to the drug'. It covered some of the processes – absorption, distribution, metabolism and excretion (ADME) – involved in getting a drug into the body and to the site of action.

This chapter will provide an overview of some of the key principles of pharmacodynamics or 'What the drug does to the body'. Pharmacodynamics refers to how drugs alter body function at the cellular level. It addresses the therapeutic as well as the adverse effects of drugs.

Drugs and disease

Disease can be defined as an alteration in normal physiological processes. An important use of drugs is to treat disease by modifying or reversing changes in physiological processes and returning the body to its normal homeostatic balance.

For example, diabetes mellitus is a metabolic condition in which blood glucose remains chronically high. It is due to a lack, or relative lack, of endogenous (internal origin, produced by the pancreas) insulin that is needed to convey glucose into body cells. Exogenous (external origin, manufactured) insulin is given to replace depleted or absent insulin so that blood glucose levels are brought back within normal ranges. Similarly, high blood pressure is treated using a number of anti-hypertensive agents to return blood pressure (BP) back within normal ranges.

How drugs produce their effects

Drugs produce their effects in many ways. Classification may vary from one text to another. Table 2.1 (below) outlines some of these mechanisms: receptor interaction, enzyme inhibition, interference with transport processes across the cell membrane, by drugs acting as substrates, and non-specific drug action.

Table 2.1: Mechanisms of drug action

Mechanism	Description
Binding to specific receptors	• Most drugs produce their effects this way, acting as either agonists or antagonists. Examples of beta-agonists include salbutamol and atenolol.
Inhibition (blocking) of enzymes	• Non-steroidal anti-inflammatory drugs (NSAIDs) inhibit cyclo-oxygenase, resulting in the inhibition of prostaglandin synthesis. Examples of these drugs include aspirin and ibuprofen. • Angiotensin converting enzyme (ACE) inhibitors prevent conversion of angiotensin I to angiotensin II. Examples include captopril, lisinopril and enalapril.
Interfering with transport processes across the cell membrane	• Digoxin inhibits Na/K ATPase pump in cell membrane, altering distribution of ions across the cell membrane, resulting in an increased calcium ion influx and an enhancement of myocardial cell contractility. • Calcium antagonists block the entry of calcium into muscle cells, resulting in dilatation of arteries. Examples include nifedipine, diltiazem and amlodipine. • Tricyclic antidepressants block the re-uptake of noradrenaline and other neurotransmitters (serotonin) into the central nerve terminal, thus increasing their actions. Examples include amitriptyline and lofepramine.
Drugs acting as substrates	• These drugs, such as amphetamines, replace the endogenous (natural) substance. The drug enters the cell and stimulates the release of norepinephrine, dopamine or serotonin. Examples include cocaine and tyramine.
Non-specific drug action	• These drugs produce their effects by their physicochemical (both physical and chemical) properties. An example is mannitol, which raises plasma osmotic pressure and acts as an osmotic diuretic.

Drug–receptor interaction

Drugs can produce their effects by means of a number of different mechanisms (see Table 2.1 above). However, by far the most important mechanism is drug–receptor interactions. Receptors are protein molecules located on the cell membrane, cytoplasm or nucleus (see Figure 2.1 below) and they play a key role in the way drugs act on the body.

One of the first, and possibly best studied, is the nicotinic acetylcholine receptor. These were originally obtained from the electric organs of the Torpedo ray, which has an abundant supply of these receptors (Rang et al. 2011).

Another important term is 'ligand'. This is a molecule or chemical that binds specifically (and usually reversibly) to another molecule or chemical, forming a larger complex. In a pharmacological context, a ligand can be defined as a molecule or chemical, such as a hormone, neurotransmitter or drug, that binds to a receptor.

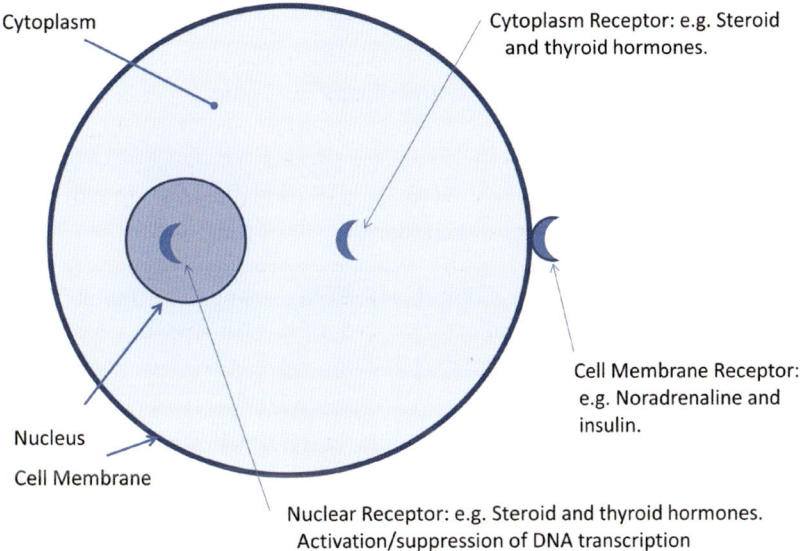

Figure 2.1: Receptor locations within a cell

Receptors

Over the last 35 years, our understanding of receptors has developed from that of theoretical concepts to real entities, with the use of receptor-labelling techniques, which later enabled the isolation, purification and now cloning of receptors.

Currently four main types of receptors have been identified (see Figures 2.2a, 2.2b, 2.2c and 2.2d). Although it is outside the scope of this book to examine these in any depth, the following section will provide a useful overview of their existence, as they are frequently referred to in both the pharmacological literature and the British National Formulary (BNF).

Ligand-gated ion channel receptors

These consist of subunits of proteins and an example is the GABA (Gamma amino butyric acid) receptor. Benzodiazepines, such as diazepam, bind to GABA-linked receptors in the brain, increasing the action of the endogenous neurotransmitter GABA, producing sedation and reducing anxiety as a result. Another example is nicotinic receptors in skeletal muscles. Normally, acetylcholine binds to these receptors, resulting in an opening of sodium channels, which results in muscle contraction. Muscle relaxants used in anaesthesia prevent acetylcholine from producing this effect, resulting in paralysis.

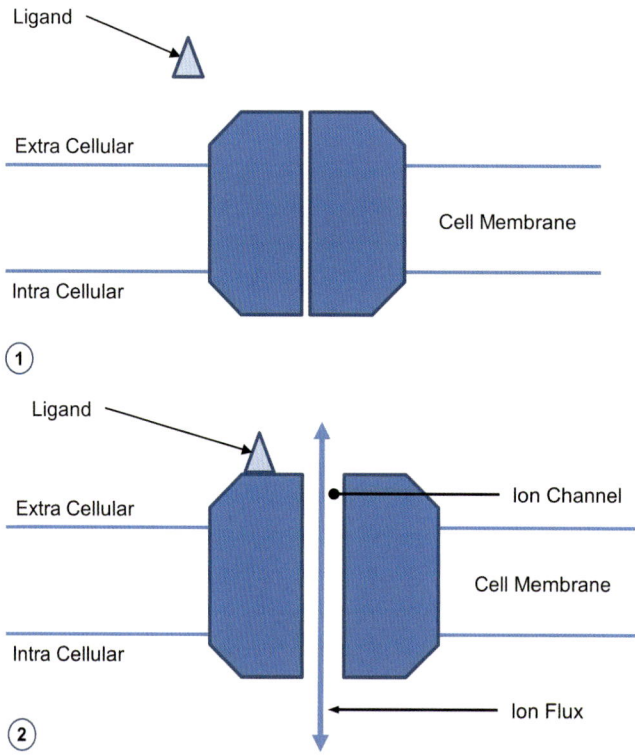

Figure 2.2a: Example of a ligand gated ion channel receptor – a multi-subunit protein receptor located in the cell membrane:
(1) Binding of a ligand (such as acetylcholine); (2) Binding results in the ion channel opening

G-protein coupled receptors (GPCRs)

This is a large and diverse family of transmembrane receptors that are a common target for therapeutic drugs. When the ligand binds to the receptor, G-protein is activated, which controls the action of the second messenger (the signalling molecules that produce physiological changes within the cell as described in Figure 2.2.b below). Examples of drugs that exert their effect in this way are salbutamol, atropine and noradrenaline.

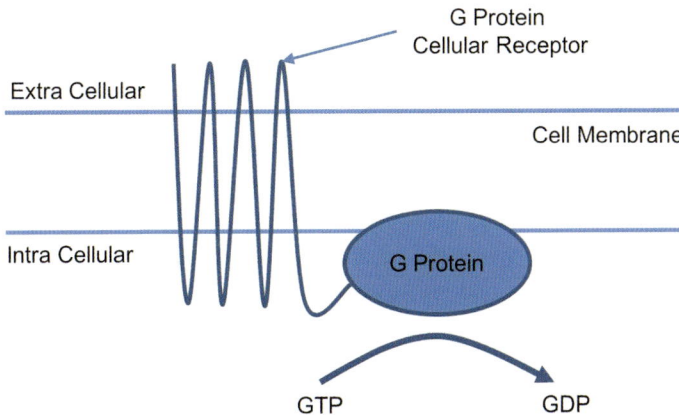

Figure 2.2b: With G-protein coupled receptors, the drug (e.g. salbutamol) combines and activates the G-protein receptor (guanosine triphosphate - GTP) and guanosine diphosphate (GDP) molecules bind to the receptor. Activation of G-protein stimulates the production of a second messenger such as cyclic adenosine monophosphate (cAMP), which brings about a change in the cell

Kinase-linked receptors

Examples of kinase-linked receptors include receptors for insulin, growth factors and peptide hormones.

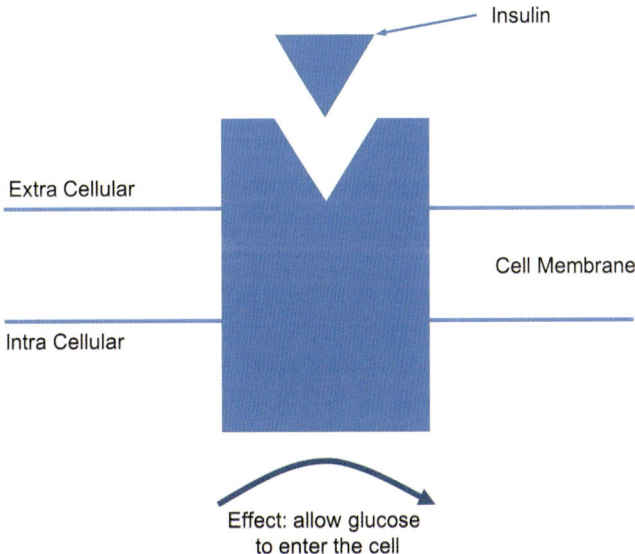

Figure 2.2c: This diagram shows a schematic example of a kinase-linked receptor. On binding, insulin induces a change in the structure of the tyrosine kinase receptor, causing a cascade of other changes that will eventually lead to glucose entering the cell

Nuclear receptors

Nuclear receptors are extremely important for drug targets and account for about 10% of the biological effects of prescription drugs. Examples include vitamin D, thyroid and steroid hormones. These substances are lipid-soluble so they pass through the cell membrane and bind to receptors within the cell. For example, a steroid hormone binds to the receptor, the receptor–hormone complex alters gene expression and turns the genes on or off. The activated receptor complex will direct the formation of a new protein, which will in turn alter the cell's activity.

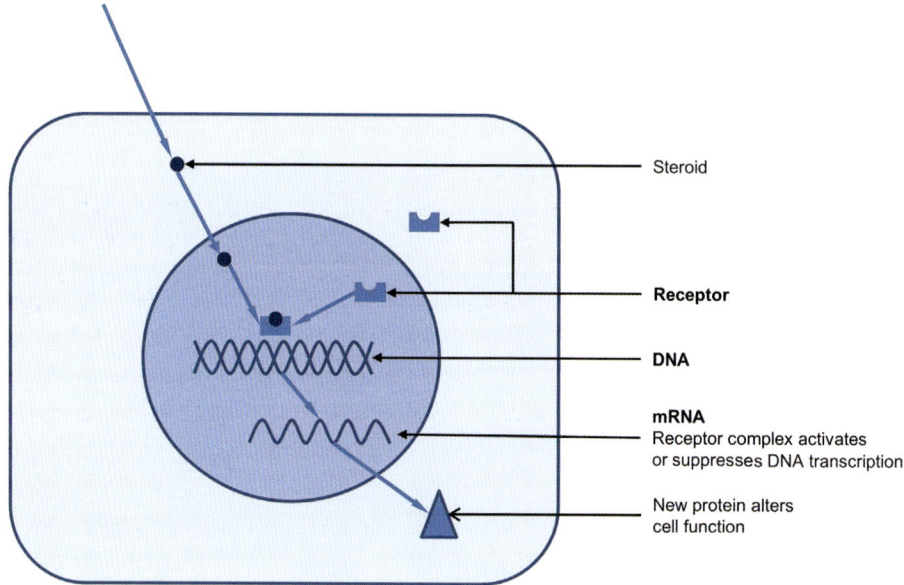

Figure 2.2d: This diagram shows a nuclear receptor, demonstrating the mechanism of action of a lipid-soluble hormone such as a steroid hormone (e.g. cortisol, oestrogen)

Having identified some common types of receptors that drugs bind to, the following section will briefly review different types of drugs and their interactions with receptors when they bind to them.

Agonists, antagonists and partial agonists

Many processes in the body are controlled by chemicals such as hormones and neurotransmitters. When these endogenous chemicals are bound to a receptor, they direct a change to occur in the cell, which alters the physiological and metabolic activity of that cell. For example, noradrenaline is an endogenous neurotransmitter that is released from one neurone, crosses the synapse and binds to several different types of receptors (see Figure 2.3 below) on the postsynaptic membrane of another neurone or muscle cell, producing a response. Many drugs (exogenous substances) have a similar structure to these endogenous chemicals, thus allowing them to bind to these receptors.

How drugs affect the body

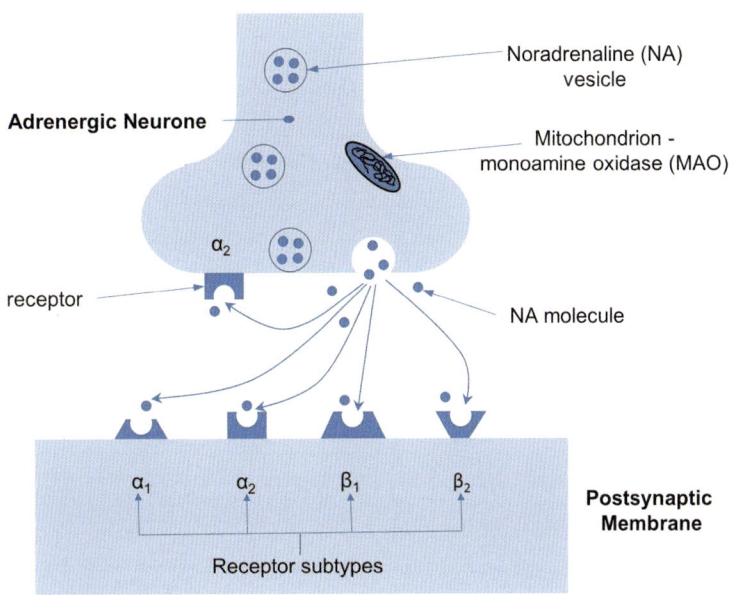

Figure 2.3: This diagram shows noradrenaline binding to two types of receptors – alpha (α) and beta (β). Subtypes for α and β receptors are also shown

When a drug binds to a receptor, it acts as an agonist, antagonist or partial agonist (see Table 2.2a).

Table 2.2a:
Drug activities: Agonists, antagonists and partial agonists

Classification	Definition
Agonist	A drug that binds and activates the receptor to produce a physiological response. For example, salbutamol (a beta-2 agonist) binds to and activates beta-2 receptors in the bronchiolar smooth muscles, producing bronchodilation.
Antagonist (blocker)	A drug that binds to a receptor but does not activate it. In other words, it blocks the receptor site, preventing the endogenous substance from gaining access to the receptor site. For example, a selective beta-blocker blocks beta-1 receptors in the heart, reducing the heart rate; and ranitidine blocks H-2 (histamine) receptors in the gastrointestinal tract, reducing gastric acid and promoting healing of duodenal and gastric ulcers.
Partial agonist	This is a drug that can either activate or block the receptor site. Partial agonists produce a submaximal response, unlike an agonist that produces a full response. Examples include buprenorphine and buspirone

Activity 2.1

Complete Table 2.2b (below) by writing each of the following drug classifications in one of the left-hand boxes, beside its corresponding description.

Drug classifications: agonists, partial agonists, antagonists.

Table 2.2b: Definition of agonists, antagonists and partial agonists

Classification	Description
a)	Binds tightly to receptor site, producing near maximal activity possible at that site. An example is morphine.
b)	Binds to receptor site less tightly than a pure agonist, producing a submaximal effect. An example is buprenorphine.
c)	Binds tightly to receptor site, stopping or blocking activity at that site. An example is naloxone.

Partial agonists

As indicated earlier, a drug's ability to activate a receptor is not an 'all or nothing' response - in other words, an agonist stimulates and an antagonist blocks receptors. In fact, stimulation of the receptor often results in a graded response. This means that if chemically related agonists are tested on the same biological system, the maximal response rate will be variable. This means that if chemically related agonists are tested on the same biological system, the maximal response rate will be variable. Some will produce a maximal response and therefore demonstrate the characteristics of a full agonist, while others will only produce a submaximal response. A partial response demonstrates the characteristic of a partial agonist or antagonist. The key point is that the difference between a full agonist and a partial agonist is determined by how many of the receptors are occupied by the drug, and the degree to which the drug activates the receptor and leads to a cellular response.

Antagonists

As mentioned previously, antagonists bind to receptors and block the effects of natural agonists. For example, atropine binds to muscarinic receptors in muscles and stops acetylcholine (a natural agonist) accessing the receptors. Most antagonists are competitive, which means the drug binds reversibly with the receptor. If the concentration of the agonist is increased, the effect of atropine (antagonist) can therefore be overcome. Irreversible antagonists, such as phenoxybenzamine, will bind irreversibly to smooth muscle alpha-adrenoreceptors. In this case, even if the agonist concentration is increased, the effects of the antagonist cannot be overcome.

Binding of the drug to the receptor site – affinity, specificity and efficacy

For a drug to bind to a receptor, the drug must be attracted to the receptor and have a suitable shape so that it can fit into the receptor site. Receptors in turn are specifically designed to recognise specific chemical forms (an endogenous substance or a drug) and bind to them selectively. In short drugs or endogenous substances have the ability to combine selectively with one particular type of receptor. This important property of receptors is known as specificity. For example, alpha- and beta-adrenergic receptors recognise and bind to adrenaline and noradrenaline molecules but will not bind to, for example, oestrogen or dopamine. These receptors will also recognise and bind exogenous adrenaline-like chemicals such as salbutamol. Salbutamol is a beta-2 agonist which binds to beta-2 receptors on smooth muscles producing bronchial dilatation and is used in the treatment of asthma. That said, readers should be aware pharmaceutical companies do design some drugs specifically to bind to several molecular targets so that they can be used in the treatment of a range of conditions. For example, bromocriptine binds to a number of receptors (e.g. serotonin, dopamine, alpha- and beta-adrenergic) and is used in the pharmacological management of conditions such as Parkinson's, diabetes and acromegaly.

Another important property of receptors is affinity, which refers to how tightly the drug binds to its receptors. This is largely determined by the type of bond that forms between the drug and the receptor. For example, morphine is an agonist that binds tightly and reversibly to opiate receptors, activates the receptor and produces an effect. Morphine is therefore said to have affinity and efficacy because it binds to the receptor site and produces a response. On the other hand, an antagonist, such as atenolol, will bind to beta receptor sites so have affinity but as it will not activate the receptor it has no efficacy.

Receptor subtypes

Cloning techniques have revealed many different types and subtypes of receptors in the body. It is important to identify these subtypes because the type of response that is produced by the drug or natural chemical depends on the subtype of receptor that it binds to. For example, noradrenaline (a natural substance) binds to many subtypes of receptors in the body, producing a range of different responses (see Figure 2.3, p. 33). Meanwhile a drug like propranolol, used to treat conditions such as anxiety and hypertension, selectively blocks just beta-1 and beta-2 receptors, and not alpha-1 and alpha-2 receptors. Indeed, the discovery of the existence of the many receptor subtypes explains why some drugs such as selective serotonin reuptake inhibitors (SSRIs) produce so many side effects like nausea, vomiting, diarrhoea and constipation.

Receptor subtypes are also differently distributed in certain tissues. For example, beta-1 receptors are mainly found in the heart and intestinal smooth muscle, while beta-2 receptors are largely in the bronchial, uterine and vascular smooth muscles.

Our understanding of receptor subtypes is continually advancing, and drugs are being developed that are selective for particular subtypes. For example, there are now beta-blockers, such as bisoprolol, that are more selective for beta-1 receptors, to reduce the side effects mediated by beta-2 blockade in the management of hypertension. In summary, it is important to recognise that the response produced is determined by the receptor subtype that the ligand (whether endogenous or exogenous) binds to.

Common drugs used to block or stimulate receptor subtypes

Clinically, it is important to be familiar with the location and function of different receptor subtypes, as many drugs are prescribed that either block or stimulate them. Some common subtypes are identified in Table 2.3 (see page 36).

Table 2.3: Examples of receptor subtypes

Receptor subtypes	Examples of drugs used to stimulate or block receptors

• Adrenergic receptors:
  alpha-1, alpha-2
  beta-1, beta-2
	• Propranolol blocks beta-1 and beta-2 receptors in the myocardium, reducing heart rate and contractility. Used in hypertension and angina.
	• Doxazosin blocks alpha-1 receptors in blood vessels, producing vasodilation. Used in treatment of hypertension.
	• Salbutamol stimulates beta-2 receptors on smooth muscles in bronchi, producing bronchodilation. Used in asthma.
	• Clonidine stimulates alpha-2 receptors in the brain stem, thus reducing the sympathetic nervous system outflow. Used in hypertension.

• Cholinergic receptors – bind acetylcholine
• Muscarinic receptors:
  M1 (neural, glandular), M2 (cardiac), M3 (glandular), M4 and M5 (neural)
• Nicotinic receptors:
  N1, N2
	• Atropine is a muscarinic antagonist that blocks the effect of acetylcholine. It is used to block the parasympathetic nerve. Resulting effects include: increased heart rate (M2) when used in the management of bradycardia; reduced bronchial and gastrointestinal secretions (M1) when used as a pre-med in surgery; dilation of the pupils (M3) as an adverse effect.
	• Galantamine is used in the treatment of dementia to increase levels of acetylcholine in the brain. It achieves this by inhibiting the action of acetylcholinesterase. Galantamine also acts on nicotinic receptors in the brain to increase the release of acetylcholine.

How drugs affect the body

• Serotonin receptors • 5-hydroxytryptamine • Subtypes: 5-HT$_{1, 2, 3}$ and $_5$	• 5-HT antagonists, such as ondansetron (5HT$_3$) and granisetron (5HT$_3$), are used to treat nausea by blocking the effect of serotonin in the gastrointestinal system and the vomiting centre in the medulla. These drugs are strong anti-emetics, which is useful in patients receiving cytotoxic drugs such as cisplatin, which releases 5-HT.
• Histamine receptors • Subtypes: H$_1$, H$_2$ and H$_3$	• H$_2$ (gastric) antagonists, such as cimetidine and ranitidine, reduce gastric acid production by blocking the effect of histamine on the parietal cell. Used in the treatment of peptic ulcer. • H$_1$ antagonists, such as cyclizine, are used to treat extreme nausea. H$_1$ receptors are mainly located in the bronchioles and gastrointestinal smooth muscles. Other examples of drugs that target these receptors are antihistamines such as bilastine and cetirizine.
• Dopamine receptors There are five subtypes of dopamine receptors (D1, D2, D3, D4 and D5). D1 is the most abundant in the CNS then D2 followed by D3, D4 and D5. These can be further subdivided into: • D1-like receptors (D1, D5) • D2-like receptors (D2, D3, D4)	• Neuroleptics, such as fluphenazine, are antagonists at D$_2$ receptors. • Neuroleptic drugs also block other receptor types such as muscarinic, alpha-adrenoreceptors and 5-HT; hence the many side effects associated with these drugs. See Chapter 17 for detailed pharmacology of these drugs.

Dose-response curve – potency and efficacy

Using experiments that observe the effect of increasing concentrations of a drug on a tissue, the response of the tissue can be plotted against the concentration of the drug. In pharmacology, the response is usually plotted against the dose using a log10 (logarithmic) scale and most drugs typically show a sigmoid dose-response curve (see Figure 2.4 below).

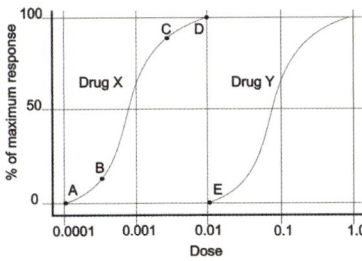

Figure 2.4: This graph shows the drug–dose-response curve for different strengths of a strong antagonist (Drug X) and a weak antagonist (Drug Y)
The response to the drug is related to the dose; an increased dose leads to a greater response

Figure 2.4 shows the following characteristics:

- The maximum (20–80%) response is on the steepest part of the curve (the straightest section).
- At a low concentration of a drug, a small response is elicited, e.g. points A–B.
- At a higher concentration of a drug, an increase in dosage produces a much greater response, e.g. points B–C. At points C–D, saturation is approached.
- The graph shows that both drugs produce the same maximum response – in other words, the same efficacy.
- The graph also illustrates that drug X is more potent than drug Y because it produces the same response as drug Y, but at a lower dose. For example, compare point A to point E.

In summary, the dose-response curve is a very important tool that gives information about the potency and efficacy of agonists and antagonists.

Activity 2.2

Complete Table 2.4 (below) by writing each of the following terms in one of the left-hand boxes, beside its corresponding definition.

Terms: *specificity, affinity, efficacy, potency.*

Table 2.4

Term used to describe drug's action at a receptor site	Definition
a)	A term for the strength of a drug, where the greater the strength, the smaller the amount of the drug that has to be present to produce the desired effect.
b)	The ability of a drug to produce a response when it binds to a receptor.
c)	The ability of a drug to combine with one particular type of receptor. Examples of receptors: acetylcholine, histamine and adrenoreceptors.
d)	The strength of attraction between a drug and a receptor.

Activity 2.3

Answer the following questions:

a) An agonist has affinity and efficacy at a receptor. TRUE/FALSE

b) An antagonist has affinity but no efficacy. TRUE/FALSE

Activity 2.4

Study Figure 2.5 and answer the following questions.

1. Look at the binding between the receptor and drug in the diagram. If the drug is to achieve an effect, what essential criteria must it have in common with an endogenous substance?
2. Name a drug that is an agonist and outline its therapeutic response.
3. Name a drug that is an antagonist and outline its therapeutic response.
4. How could the therapeutic response in question 3 be restored to normal?
5. Antagonists are termed 'reversible' or 'irreversible'. What is meant by these terms?

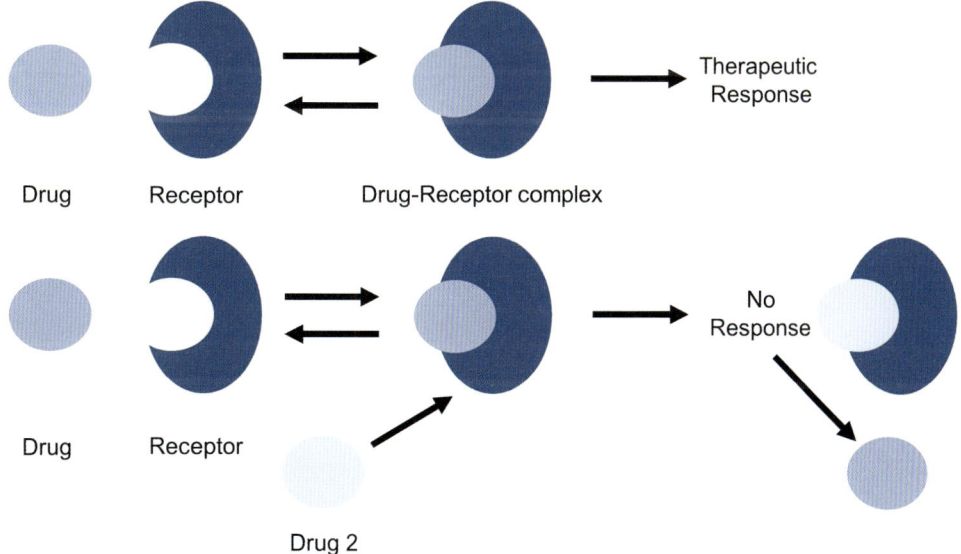

Figure 2.5: Drug–receptor interaction

How drugs achieve their effects on the cell after they bind to receptors

Second messenger systems

When drugs bind to receptors, they cause alterations in the conformation (three-dimensional shape) of the receptor, to produce changes in the cell. This is, in short, a drug response. Second messenger systems are chemicals that strengthen the signals from the receptor on the cell surface and then stimulate changes in the cell's activity. The best-known and most studied second messenger system is the cyclic adenosine monophosphate (cAMP) system. Others include inositol-1,4,5-trisphosphate (InsP3), calcium and diacylglycerol (DG) system.

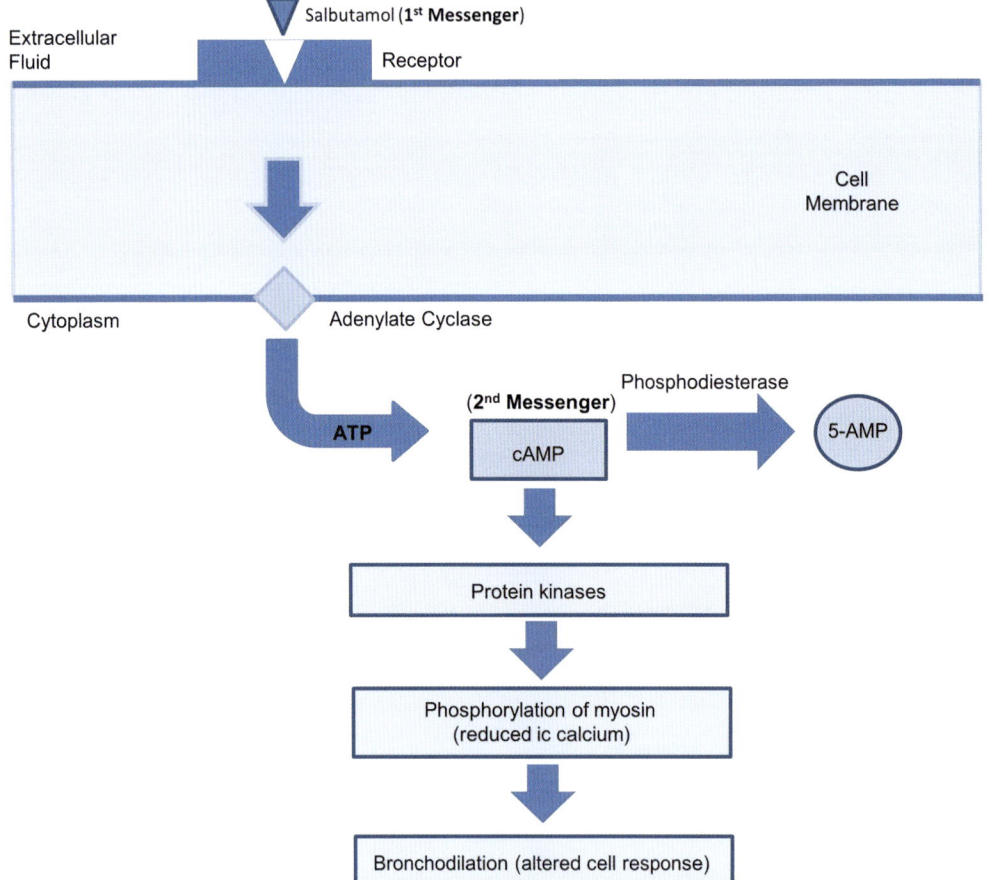

Figure 2.6: This diagram shows a second messenger system: cAMP increases the activity of protein kinases, which causes the phosphorylation of myosin (muscle protein), reducing intracellular calcium and leading to bronchodilation

How does it work?

The drug acts as a 'first messenger' and activates the enzyme adenylate cyclase, which stimulates the production of a 'second messenger' (cAMP). Cyclic adenosine monophosphate alters the activity of appropriate cellular enzyme systems to produce cell responses, such as a change in protein synthesis. For example, salbutamol is a beta-2 agonist used in the treatment of asthma. Salbutamol (first messenger) binds to the receptor (beta-2 receptor), activates it and increases levels of adenylate, which in turn enhances the production of cAMP (second messenger). The cAMP then activates more enzyme systems to produce a cellular response – in this case bronchodilation. The enzyme phosphodiesterase will then terminate the effects of cAMP (see Figure 2.6).

Receptor up and down regulation

Many drugs are used for their short-term effects. An advantageous property of such drugs is that they can rapidly come off the receptors after they have achieved their effect and then be eliminated from the body as quickly as possible. This reduces their capacity to cause toxicity. Examples are diamorphine, which is used to relieve the pain of coronary heart disease, and the inhaler salbutamol for treating severe acute asthma.

Receptor down regulation

Some drugs are given for their long-term effects. Examples are the use of L-dopa in Parkinson's disease and opioids in the management of chronic pain. When tissues are continually exposed to agonist drugs, the number of receptors decreases. This is known as receptor down regulation. In this case, the receptors are internalised by endocytosis, which has the effect of making the tissue less responsive to the drug.

> ### Activity 2.5
> If an asthmatic patient uses a bronchodilator such as salbutamol excessively, what is the likely outcome with regard to efficacy and side effects?

Receptor up regulation

When tissues are continually exposed to antagonist drugs, new receptors are formed. This is called receptor up regulation (the reverse of receptor down regulation). The effect is to increase the sensitivity of the target cells, and increase the number of cell receptors for binding agonists. For example, if beta-blockers continually block beta-receptors, these receptors will increase their sensitivity to the endogenous agonists (i.e. adrenaline and noradrenaline), due to the formation of new receptors. The clinical implication is that the patient is likely to experience rebound hypertension on sudden discontinuation of a beta-blocker.

Summary

- Pharmacodynamics refers to the effects the drug has on the body – both therapeutic and adverse effects.
- Drugs can produce their effects in many ways but most drugs act by binding to specific receptors.
- There are many types and subtypes of receptors. The type of response that is produced by the drug or natural chemical depends on the type of receptor that it binds to.
- Agonists activate receptors and produce a cellular response.
- Antagonists combine with receptors but do not activate them and therefore block the effect of endogenous agonists.
- Partial agonists bind to receptor sites less tightly than pure agonists, producing a submaximal effect.
- Most drugs bind reversibly to receptors.
- A drug must have an affinity for the receptor to achieve a therapeutic effect. A drug's affinity means how strongly it binds to the receptor.
- Efficacy is a drug's ability to produce an effect at a receptor.
- Many drugs produce a change in the cell by stimulating the production of second messengers such as cAMP and IP3.
- The dose response curve is a very important tool. It gives information about the action, potency and efficacy of drugs such as agonists and antagonists.

Answers to activities

Activity 2.1

Complete Table 2.2b (below) by writing each of the following drug classifications in one of the left-hand boxes, beside its corresponding description.

Drug classifications: agonists, partial agonists, antagonists.

Table 2.2b: Definition of agonists, antagonists and partial agonists

Classification	Description
a) Agonist	Binds tightly to receptor site, producing near maximal activity possible at that site. An example is morphine.
b) Partial agonist	Binds to receptor site less tightly than a pure agonist, producing a submaximal effect. An example is buprenorphine.
c) Antagonist	Binds tightly to receptor site, stopping or blocking activity at that site. An example is naloxone.

Activity 2.2

Complete Table 2.4 (below) by writing each of the following terms in one of the left-hand boxes, beside its corresponding definition.

Terms: specificity, affinity, efficacy, potency.

Table 2.4

Term used to describe drug's action at a receptor site	Definition
a) Potency	The amount of drug that has to be present to produce the desired effect. The greater the potency, the smaller the amount of the drug that has to be administered.
b) Efficacy	The ability of a drug to produce a response when it binds to a receptor.
c) Specificity	The ability of a drug to combine with one particular type of receptor. Examples of receptors: acetylcholine, histamine and adrenoreceptors.
d) Affinity	The strength of attraction between a drug and a receptor.

Activity 2.3

Identify the correct answer to the following questions:

a) An agonist has affinity and efficacy at a receptor. TRUE

b) An antagonist has affinity but no efficacy. TRUE

Activity 2.4

1. Look at the binding between the receptor and drug in the diagram. If the drug is to achieve an effect, what essential criteria must it have in common with an endogenous substance?

It must have a similar structure and it must have affinity.

2. Name a drug that is an agonist and outline its therapeutic response.

Morphine attaches to a mu receptor (drug receptor complex), abolishing or reducing pain. Other examples, such as benzodiazepines (e.g. diazepam), bind to GABA receptors in the brain, reducing anxiety.

3. Name a drug that is an antagonist and outline its therapeutic response.

Atenolol (beta-blocker) binds to beta-1 receptors in the heart, reducing heart rate and contractility.

4. How could the therapeutic response in question 3 be restored to normal?

By increasing the concentration of the agonist.

5. Antagonists are termed 'reversible' or 'irreversible'. What is meant by these terms?
A reversible drug binds briefly and transiently to the receptor (weak bond). The effect can be reversed by increasing the amount of the natural agonist. Most competitive antagonists are reversible. An irreversible drug binds tightly to the receptor (strong bond, e.g. covalent). Its effect cannot be reversed. Wait for elimination of the drug from the system.

Activity 2.5

If an asthmatic patient uses a bronchodilator such as salbutamol excessively, what is the likely outcome with regard to efficacy and side effects?
Reduced efficacy secondary to receptor down regulation with prolonged use. Possible side effects include fine tremor, tachycardia, headaches and nervous tension. These adverse effects are generally not seen at the dosage used to stimulate bronchodilation.

References and further reading

Alexander, S.P.H., Mathie, A. & Peters, J.A. (2009). Guide to Receptors and Channels (GRAC). 4th edn. *British Journal of Pharmacology.* **158** (1), S1–S254.

Greenstein, B. (2009). *Trounce's Clinical Pharmacology for Nurses.* 18th edn. Edinburgh: Elsevier Churchill Livingstone.

Halliwell, R.F. (2007). A short history of the rise of the molecular pharmacology of ionotropic drug receptors. *Trends in Pharmacological Sciences* **28**, 214–19.

Neal, M.J. (2012). *Medical Pharmacology at a Glance.* 7th edn. Chichester: Wiley-Blackwell.

Rang, H.P., Dale, M.M., Ritter, J.M., Flower, R.J. & Henderson, G. (2011). *Rang & Dale's Pharmacology.* 7th edn. Edinburgh: Elsevier Churchill Livingstone.

3

Types of adverse drug reactions and interactions

Alan Sebti
BPharm, DipPharmPrac, Pharmacy Manager, Chase Farm Hospital,
Royal Free London NHS Foundation Trust

Dr Kaicun Zhao
PhD, MSc, MB, Clinical Pharmacology; Senior Lecturer Traditional Chinese Medicine, Mental Health, Social Work and Interprofessional Learning, Middlesex University, London

This chapter:
- Discusses the concept of adverse drug reactions and drug side effects
- Explains the classification of adverse drug reactions
- Outlines drug interactions and their potential risk of causing adverse drug reaction
- Explains the procedures used to prevent adverse drug reactions
- Discusses the concepts behind adverse drug reaction reporting mechanisms.

Introduction

Drug therapy is an important treatment modality used for various clinical conditions. The pharmacological activities of drugs are beneficial in treating different pathological disorders to relieve clinical symptoms. However, drugs not only have beneficial therapeutic effects; they may also produce side effects or cause adverse reactions. Adverse drug reactions (ADRs) or side effects are common. A UK-based prospective observational study has shown that 6.5% of hospital admissions are related to adverse drug reactions (Pirmohamed *et al.* 2004).

However, many of these incidents are avoidable. Prescribers have to consider the risk benefit ratio before prescribing a particular drug, and be aware that any patient taking regular medication may develop an adverse reaction. Healthcare professionals should know how to monitor, recognise and manage adverse drug reactions or side effects, and this may involve stopping or changing the drug before harm is done to patients.

Adverse drug reactions and side effects

The terms 'adverse drug reactions' (ADRs) and 'side effects' (SEs) are commonly used to describe unintended effects following administration of a drug. Although ADRs and SEs are frequently used interchangeably, there are differences in definition between the two terms.

According to the World Health Organisation (WHO) and the Medicines and Healthcare Products Regulatory Agency (MHRA), the UK medicine regulation authority, ADRs can be defined as 'unwanted and harmful reactions occurring after the administration of a drug or combination of drugs under normal conditions of use and at normal doses, which are suspected or known to be related to the drug or combination of drugs'.

The European legislation, EU Directive 2010/84, extends the definition of the term 'adverse drug reaction' to cover noxious and unintended effects resulting from medication errors and uses outside the terms of the marketing authorisation, including the misuse and abuse of medicinal products.

Side effect generally means 'those unintended effects of a drug administered under normal conditions of use and at normal doses, which are related to the pharmacological properties of the drug'. A side effect is usually an extension of the drug's pharmacological actions, but the effects are secondary to the one intended for the drug to work in the body. When discussing side effects, it is important to consider the range of a drug's pharmacological actions. For example, atropine, as an anti-muscarinic agent, exerts a wide range of pharmacological actions. When used to treat bradycardia, atropine may cause a dry mouth. Atropine has also been used therapeutically to treat hypersalivation, and patients receiving atropine for hypersalivation may experience tachycardia as an unintended effect of this treatment. An observed pharmacological effect may therefore be the desired 'therapeutic effect' in one context and a 'side effect' in another, depending on what a drug is being used for.

Classification of adverse drug reactions

There are many different ways to classify various adverse drug reactions. The most commonly accepted categorisation method classifies ADRs into type A (augmented) or type B (bizarre). This was first proposed in the 1980s (Rawlins & Thomson 1985). The key difference between the two types of ADRs is that type A reactions are augmented effects of the drug's pharmacological activities, while type B reactions are idiosyncratic effects that are not directly related to the drug's pharmacological activities.

Type A ADRs are therefore dose-dependent and predictable; type B ADRs are neither predictable nor dose-dependent. Type A ADRs are side effects that are normally associated with high morbidity and low mortality. In contrast, type B ADRs are often severe or bizarre reactions and are associated with low rates of morbidity but potentially high rates of mortality. The immune system is commonly involved in type B ADRs. Type A adverse reactions are more common than type B reactions and account for 80–90% of all reactions (Pirmohamed et al. 1998, Einarson 1993).

Later, more types of ADRs were proposed, based on the features and characteristics of the reactions. As shown in Table 3.1, some ADRs are also categorised as type C, D and E, which each have some specific features or characteristics. More recently, it has been suggested that dose-related, time-related and susceptibility factors (DoTS) should be taken into account for classification of ADRs (Aronson & Ferner 2003).

Table 3.1: Classification of adverse drug reactions

Type	ADRs	Definition	Examples
A	Augmented pharmacological effects	• Exaggerated normal pharmacological activities at usual therapeutic dose • Dose-dependent • Commonly seen • High morbidity and low mortality	• Opioid-induced respiratory depression • Warfarin-associated bleeding • Anti-diabetic-related hypoglycaemia • Beta-blocker-associated bradycardia
B	Bizarre effects	• Novel and unexpected reaction • Not related to drug's normal pharmacological activities • Uncommon • Not dose-related • Low morbidity and potentially high mortality	• Penicillins causing anaphylaxis • Chloramphenicol-induced bone marrow suppression
C	Chronic continuing reactions	• Occurring after continuous and long-term therapy • Persist for a relatively long time	• Bisphosphonate-related osteonecrosis of the jaw • Neuroleptic-induced tardive dyskinesia
D	Delayed effects	• Occurring some time or even a long period after the use of a medicine	• Lomustine causing leucopenia • Diethylstilbestrol-associated cervical and vaginal adenocarcinoma in female offspring exposed in-utero • Isotretinoin-associated teratogenesis – craniofacial malformations in infants
E	End-of-use reactions	• Occurring on discontinuation of therapy	• Insomnia, anxiety and perceptual disturbances following the withdrawal of benzodiazepines • Adrenocortical insufficiency after long-term and/or repeated steroid therapy • Seizures following withdrawal of long-term anticonvulsant treatment

Pharmacology case studies for nurse prescribers

Activity 3.1

Adverse drug reactions are mainly classified into reactions related to the main pharmacological action of the drug (type A) and reactions that are unpredictable and are not dose-related (type B).

Complete the table below, using the key words and phrases provided in the box.

	Type A adverse drug reactions	Type B adverse drug reactions
Predictable or unpredictable		
Dose-dependent		
Augmented or Bizarre		
Morbidity		
Mortality		
Incidence		
Example		

Keywords and phrases

High mortality; Low mortality; Unpredictable; Yes; Uncommon; Common; No; Predictable; Insulin – causing hypoglycaemia; Bizarre; Associated with inherited abnormalities; Augmented; Warfarin – producing bleeding; Often involves hypersensitivity reactions, e.g. penicillin – anaphylaxis; Chloramphenicol – produces bone marrow suppression; Beta-blocker – causing bradycardia; High morbidity; Low morbidity; Opioids – respiratory depression

Therapeutic index and ADRs

Drugs that have a low therapeutic index (which means there is little difference between the therapeutic dose and the toxic dose) are often associated with dose-related adverse drug reactions. These include some of the most commonly prescribed drugs, such as anticoagulants (e.g. warfarin), hypoglycaemic drugs (e.g. insulin), antiarrhythmics (e.g. digoxin), aminoglycosides (e.g. gentamicin), cytotoxic drugs (e.g. methotrexate) and xanthines (e.g. theophylline).

Hypersensitivity reactions

In many instances, the reasons and mechanisms for type B ADRs are not clear. However, these ADRs are often related to allergic and genetic factors. The most common problems involve hypersensitivity reactions. These reactions occur in a minority of patients who receive the drug, and the seriousness of the reaction is sometimes unrelated to the dose. It is most likely to occur in patients with a history of atopic disease such as hay fever, asthma and eczema.

Hypersensitivity reactions imply previous exposure to a drug that triggers an immune response, which is usually the production of specific antibodies. When the individual is exposed to the same drug a second time, an immunological reaction may occur – in the form of a skin rash, joint pain or anaphylactic reaction – due to the binding of the drug and the specific antibodies. Anaphylaxis is one of the most serious allergic reactions caused by drugs and can be potentially fatal if not treated promptly.

In the light of all this, simply asking a patient whether they are allergic to the drug you are about to prescribe or administer is a very important part of the nurse's role. Hypersensitivity reactions are normally classified into four different types as shown in Table 3.2 (below).

Table 3.2: Types of hypersensitivity reactions

Reaction type	Hypersensitivity reactions	Examples
Type I Immediate	<ul><li>On first exposure to drug, antibody becomes attached to surface of mast cells.</li><li>On second exposure, the drug interacts with antibodies (IgE) that are fixed onto mast cells, triggering the release of histamine, inducing anaphylaxis.</li></ul>	<ul><li>Penicillin</li><li>Iodine-based contrast media</li></ul>
Type II Cytotoxic	<ul><li>On first exposure, antibody attached to surface of red cells.</li><li>On second exposure, antibody and drug combination on surface of red blood cell activates complement, resulting in destruction/lysis of red cells. White cells may also be destroyed. Outcome depends on blood cells involved in reaction.</li></ul>	<ul><li>Methyldopa</li><li>Clozapine-induced agranulocytosis</li></ul>
Type III Serum sickness	<ul><li>Antibody and antigen combine in the circulation forming an immune complex. This complex stays in the circulation or in the tissue, activating complement which then stimulates inflammation. The inflammatory response damages the walls of blood vessels or tissue complex becomes lodged in tissues such as the joints and kidneys.</li><li>Resulting symptoms include: rash, fever arthritis, swollen lymph nodes.</li></ul>	<ul><li>Gold or penicillamine therapy used in rheumatoid arthritis</li></ul>

(table continued overleaf)

Table 3.2 continued

Reaction type	Hypersensitivity reactions	Examples
Type IV Rashes	• T-lymphocytes react with the drug to stimulate an inflammatory response. This type of reaction may be delayed for at least 12 hours and usually causes rashes, contact dermatitis and eczema. • Most are non-life threatening but toxic epidermal necrolysis (an inflammatory skin condition resulting in breakdown of the skin) can occur very rarely. This is associated with a 35% mortality rate.	• Gold therapy (serious rashes) • Ampicillin (mild rashes)

How to identify adverse drug reactions

As discussed earlier, different types of ADRs may show some specific symptoms that are helpful for identification. Patients may also tell you about undesirable symptoms they have experienced after taking a particular medicine. Healthcare professionals should be alert to the possible occurrence of ADRs. ADRs due to current or previously prescribed drug treatment (including herbal products and over-the-counter drugs) should be considered and excluded as possible causes of the patient's presenting signs or symptoms.

To help identify potential ADRs, healthcare professionals should be alert to the following:

- Unexpected or suspicious symptoms, such as asthma, skin rash, headache, dizziness, nausea, vomiting or diarrhoea
- Changes in clinical observations, including temperature, heart rate, blood pressure, blood glucose level and body weight
- Patients' complaints regarding their drug(s) therapy
- Abnormalities in biochemical or haematological tests, including blood profile, liver function profile and kidney function profile.

Reporting adverse drug reactions — The Yellow Card Scheme

The Yellow Card Scheme is an important ADRs reporting procedure, which is managed by the MHRA in the UK. Healthcare professionals and patients can report any potential ADRs, even if causality has not been fully established. In other words, only a reasonable level of suspicion is required.

A Yellow Card report should be completed for:

- Any reaction, minor or major, suspected to be associated with use of a drug or vaccine highlighted by an inverted black triangle symbol (▼), i.e. drugs that are new to the market.

- Serious reactions suspected to be due to any established drug or vaccine (including over-the-counter and herbal medicines). Serious reactions are those that:

  Are fatal

  Are life-threatening

  Are disabling

  Are incapacitating

  Can result in, or prolong, hospital admission

  Are medically significant

  Can lead to congenital abnormalities.

- Reactions associated with areas of special interest that include:

  ADRs in children

  ADRs in the elderly

  Biologicals and vaccines

  Delayed drug effects

  Congenital anomalies

  Herbal products.

For further details, see: https://yellowcard.mhra.gov.uk/the-yellow-card-scheme/ (last accessed 22 September 2020).

The following essential pieces of information need to be included in the Yellow Card report:

- The suspect drug(s) – including details of dose, route, date(s) of administration
- Suspect reaction(s) – including a diagnosis if appropriate, details of onset, severity, treatment given and outcome
- Patient details – sex, age, weight if known, local identifier such as hospital or practice reference number
- Reporter's name and full address to contact for further information if necessary.

ADRs should be reported whether they occur under conditions of 'normal' use or as a result of error, misuse/abuse, or off-label use. The MHRA collates the information from Yellow Card reports and carries out further assessment on the suspected ADRs to identify any emerging patterns to evaluate the potential risk. Whenever necessary, action will be taken to ensure that medicines are used in a way that minimises risk while maximising patient benefit.

Drug interactions

Drug interactions occur when the pharmacological effect(s) of a drug are altered by other drug(s) or other substances, such as food, co-administered with the drug. This modification is not necessarily harmful, and may be exploited therapeutically.

For instance, antihypertensive medicines are often combined in the treatment of high blood pressure. Combined use in this manner results in a better balance between the desired therapeutic effect and side-effects than the use of a single agent at a higher dose. However, drug interactions also contribute to the increasing number of adverse drug reactions and can be harmful. Furthermore, as the number of drugs administered together increases, so does the potential incidence of harmful interactions (Pirmohamed et al. 2004, Duerden, Avery & Payne 2013). ADRs are frequently caused by drug interactions, particularly in the following conditions:

- Older patients – likely to be taking a number of different drugs (polypharmacy) due to multiple health-related problems. The elderly may be more sensitive to small changes in the blood concentration of certain drugs due to either natural or pathological deterioration in their ability to detoxify foreign drugs (see Chapter 19).
- Drugs with a narrow therapeutic index, such as warfarin, digoxin, lithium and gentamicin
- Individuals with kidney and/or liver disease, as these are the main organs involved in the metabolism and excretion of drugs.

Mechanisms of drug–drug interaction

Drug interactions can be classified as pharmacodynamic or pharmacokinetic. Pharmacodynamic interactions are associated with the biomedical mechanisms of actions of drugs. Pharmacokinetic interactions are related to the changes of drug behaviour in the body. Some examples of pharmacodynamic interactions are described in Table 3.3, and examples of pharmacokinetic interactions are described in Table 3.4.

Table 3.3: Examples of pharmacodynamic drug interactions

Key drug	Additional drug	Likely therapeutic/adverse outcome
Benzodiazepines, e.g. diazepam	Alcohol	Enhanced sedation or severe central nervous system depression resulting from additive effects, as both drugs have similar actions.
Beta-blocker	Salbutamol	In asthmatic patients, beta-blockers may cause bronchoconstriction and precipitate an asthma attack.
Loop diuretics, e.g. furosemide	NSAIDs	NSAIDS result in sodium and water retention opposing the effects of loop diuretics.
Potassium supplements	ACE-inhibitors	Combination results in hyperkalaemia.

Table 3.4: Pharmacokinetic drug interactions

Pharmacokinetic phase	Drug combination	Rationale	Likely outcome
Absorption	Antacids and tetracyclines	• Antacids chelate with tetracyclines, reducing their absorption.	• Antibiotic treatment failure
	Oestrogen and antibiotics	• Entero-hepatic recycling of oestrogen in oral contraceptives may be decreased by antibiotics. Antibiotics kill the bacteria that cleave the oestrogen-conjugate complex which normally allows reabsorption of some oestrogen.	• Potential reduction in effectiveness of the oral contraceptive – potential for pregnancy
Distribution	Aspirin and warfarin	• Aspirin displaces warfarin from plasma proteins, enhancing its effects.	• Increase in international normalisation ratio (INR) and bleeding complications of warfarin
Metabolism	Phenobarbital and warfarin	• One drug can reduce or increase the metabolism (breakdown) of another. Phenobarbital increases the activity of the liver enzymes involved with the breakdown of warfarin.	• Increased clearance of warfarin and decrease in INR
		• Ciprofloxacin inhibits theophylline metabolism.	• Decreased clearance of theophylline and potential toxicity
Excretion	Thiazide diuretics and lithium	• Thiazide diuretics cause a reduction in sodium reabsorption, leading to retention of lithium.	• Lithium toxicity

Activity 3.2

As described above, drug interactions can take place at different sites in the body. The table below lists the sites where drug interaction may occur. Give at least one example for each site.

Site	Examples
In the intestine	
In the blood	
At site of action of drug	
At site of metabolism	
At site of elimination, e.g. kidney, liver	

Drug-food interactions

Food and drink can also interact with drugs, increasing or decreasing their effectiveness. Conversely, particular drugs can alter the effects of substances in food. For example, monoamine oxidase inhibitors (MAOIs) reduce the breakdown of neurotransmitters such as adrenaline and noradrenaline. MAOIs also break down dietary tyramine – a precursor for adrenaline and noradrenaline. If individuals taking MAOIs eat foods such as cheese (which are rich in tyramine) they could experience a hypertensive crisis, both as a direct result of the increased effects of tyramine – a potent vasopressor – and due to potentiation of the effects of adrenaline and noradrenaline. However, because people have varying intakes of many foods these interactions tend to be less predictable than drug–drug interactions

Table 3.5: Potential drug-food interactions and their likely outcomes

	Rationale	Likely outcome
Pharmacokinetic	• Large meals and foods with high fat content can decrease stomach emptying.	• Reduced absorption rate
	• Certain medicines are best taken with food to increase their absorption (e.g. griseofulvin).	• Increased systemic availability of the drug
	• Dairy products are high in calcium and iron content.	• Decreased absorption

	Rationale	Likely outcome
	• Grapefruit juice contains flavonoids – substances that can inhibit one of the P450 metabolic enzymes involved in the metabolism of many drugs as they pass through the gut wall.	• Increased bioavailability of the drug, due to reduced metabolism, e.g. statins and calcium channel blockers
	• The uptake of levodopa into the central nervous system (CNS) can be affected by high-protein diets due to competition between amino acids and levodopa at the blood–brain barrier.	• Reduced uptake of levodopa into the CNS
	• Foods (e.g. barbecued meals, cabbage, broccoli) that contain enzymes which speed up the reaction of enzymes involved in breaking down drugs can affect how effectively the drug is cleared from the body.	• Increased drug clearance
Pharmacodynamic	• Foods containing a high level of Vitamin K (e.g. liver, broccoli, Brussels sprouts and green leafy vegetables) antagonise the effects of warfarin by increasing production of vitamin K-dependent clotting factors.	• Reduced efficacy of warfarin

Drug-herb interactions

As a major part of complementary medicine, herbs are being used more widely across the world. Whilst herbal medicine is often beneficial in treating various clinical conditions, it also produces a number of safety problems due to drug–herb interactions. Table 3.6 (below) lists different kinds of drug–herb interactions, some of which may be clinically significant.

Table 3.6: Common drug-herb interactions

Drugs	Herbs	Interactions
Amitriptyline, ciclosporin, digoxin, indinavir, irinotecan, warfarin, alprazolam, dextrometorphan, simvastatin and oral contraceptives	St John's Wort (Hypericum perforatum L)	Decreased plasma concentrations of the drug

(table continued overleaf)

Table 3.6 continued

Drugs	Herbs	Interactions
Ciclosporin, tacrolimus	Citrus grandis peel, grapefruit juice	Increased plasma level of the drug
Digoxin	Eleutherococcus Senticosus (Siberian Ginseng)	Increased digoxin levels
	Yellow Foxglove, Thevetia peruviana	Synergism, as the herbs contain digoxin-like substances
	Hawthorn Berry	Potentiate digoxin action synergistically
Diuretics, thiazides	Hibiscus sabdariffa L. (Family Malvaceae)	Decreased plasma clearance and decreased elimination rate constant of hydrochlorothiazide
Hypoglycaemic agents, e.g. sulfonylureas, metformin, and insulin	Butcher's Broom, Buchu, Dandelion, Juniper	Diuretics, which may compromise hypoglycaemic effects
	Allium sativum, prickly pear cactus, Chromium, Vanadium, Gymnema Sylvestri, Karela	Improved glucose tolerance and enhanced hypoglycaemic effects
	Cassia auriculata	Significantly reduced absorption of metformin
Lorazepam	Valeriana officinalis L., Passiflora incarnata L.	Increased inhibitory activity of benzodiazepines binding to the GABA receptors, causing severe secondary effects including hand tremor, dizziness, throbbing and muscular fatigue
Midazolam	Green tea, grape seeds	Green tea increases elimination of intravenously administered midazolam due to induction of CYP3A in the liver, but grape seeds increase absorption of orally administered midazolam
Phenytoin	Rheum palmatum	Markedly decreased oral bioavailability of phenytoin via activation of P-gp
Warfarin	Cayenne, Feverfew, Garlic, White Willow Bark, St John's Wort, Ginkgo Biloba	Decreased platelet aggregation, causing haemorrhage
	Danshen, Devil's claw, Dong quai, Papaya (papain)	Enhanced anticoagulant effect
Anti-hypertensives, losartan	Curcumin	Significantly increased plasma concentrations of losartan and its metabolite

Case study: Warfarin–amiodarone interaction

A 75-year-old man suffering from heart disease has a permanent pacemaker implanted. He has been taking warfarin and sotalol for chronic atrial fibrillation and atorvastatin for hyperlipidaemia for several years. Since last year, his atrial fibrillation has been getting worse. Due to persistent episodes of atrial fibrillation, his doctor decided to prescribe the anti-arrhythmic amiodarone to replace sotalol. Approximately two weeks later, the INR (a measure of how fast the blood clots, used for monitoring and determining the dose of warfarin) had increased to 4.8 (normal range is 2–3), indicating over-anticoagulation.

Activity 3.3 (Case study)

Answer the following questions:

1. Why did the INR increase above the normal range?
2. What were the potential adverse effects?
3. What is the major mechanism underlying the warfarin–amiodarone interaction?

What actions should the healthcare professional take in this situation?

Summary

Adverse drug reactions and interactions are responsible for significant numbers of morbidities and mortalities in many countries. In the UK they are an important cause of hospital admissions, resulting in significant costs to the NHS. Many of the consequences of ADR could be avoided or minimised by improving prescribing. In order to do this, prescribers need to be more informed and vigilant in recognising and addressing the factors that increase the occurrence of adverse drug reactions and interactions.

Answers to activities

Activity 3.1

Adverse drug reactions are mainly classified into reactions related to the main pharmacological action of the drug (type A) and reactions that are unpredictable and not dose-related (type B). Complete the table below, using the key words and phrases provided.

Adverse drug reactions	Type A	Type B
Predictable or unpredictable	Predictable	Unpredictable
Dose-dependent	Yes	No
Augmented or Bizarre	Augmented	Bizarre
Morbidity	High	Low
Mortality	Low	High (potentially)
Incidence	Common	Uncommon
Examples	• Opioids – respiratory depression • Warfarin – producing bleeding • Insulin – causing hypoglycaemia • Beta-blocker – causing bradycardia	• Associated with inherited abnormalities • Often involves hypersensitivity reactions, e.g. penicillin – anaphylaxis • Chloramphenicol – produces bone marrow suppression

Activity 3.2

As described above, drug interactions can take place at different sites in the body. The table below lists the sites where drug interactions may occur. Give at least one example for each site.

Site	Examples
In the intestine	• Opioids slow intestinal motility so they may increase drug absorption. • Purgatives increase intestinal motility so they may decrease enteral drug absorption. • Absorption of tetracycline is reduced if it is given with iron. • Antacids reduce the absorption of many commonly used drugs, e.g. angiotensin-converting enzyme inhibitors (ACEIs), angiotensin II antagonists, digoxin, oral iron and lansoprazole.
In the blood	• There is competition for plasma proteins if two drugs that are highly bound are taken concurrently. Drug X may be displaced from the carrier site by drug Y. The plasma level of drug X then increases, leading to toxicity. For example, the effect of warfarin could be enhanced when given with aspirin. • Phenytoin, with 88% plasma protein binding, may interact with sodium valproate, which shows 95% plasma protein binding.
At site of action of drug	• Quinidine affects the binding of digoxin in the tissues of various organs including the heart.

| At site of metabolism | - Many drugs are metabolised in the liver.
- Enzyme induction: One drug can increase the enzyme activity of another, causing a reduction in concentration. For instance, rifampicin, if given with warfarin, can reduce warfarin's anticoagulant effect.
- Phenytoin accelerates the metabolism of oestrogens through induction of CYP450, reducing the contraceptive effect of oestrogens.
- Enzyme inhibition: One drug can inhibit the enzymes that metabolise another, thus increasing plasma concentration and potential toxicity. A number of drugs potentiate (enhance) the effects of warfarin. These include cimetidine and diltiazem.
- Cimetidine inhibits CYP450, affecting the metabolism of propranolol, theophylline, warfarin and phenytoin. |
|---|---|
| At site of elimination, e.g. kidney or liver | - Aspirin excretion is increased by sodium bicarbonate, which causes pH change in the renal tubules.
- Penicillin and probenecid interact by competitive binding to the active transferring protein in the renal tubules. This results in reduced excretion of penicillin.
- Salicylates can reduce the active renal excretion of methotrexate, leading to methotrexate toxicity. |

Activity 3.3 (Case study)

1. Why did the INR increase above the normal range?

The patient had been using warfarin for several years without significant side effects being reported. The increase in the INR occurred after the initiation of the antiarrhythmic medication amiodarone. This temporal relationship provides good reasons to suspect that the INR increase was the result of an interaction between warfarin and amiodarone.

2. What were the potential adverse effects?

The high INR indicated over-anticoagulation with warfarin, which significantly increases the risk of bleeding.

3. What is the major mechanism underlying the warfarin–amiodarone interaction?

Warfarin is metabolised primarily by CYP2C9. Inhibition of CYP2C9 by amiodarone, and its major metabolite, potentiates the anticoagulant effects of warfarin.

4. What actions should the healthcare professional consider taking in this situation?

The healthcare professional should immediately reduce or stop the dose of warfarin, depending on whether any bleeding has occurred and its severity. Vitamin K may also need to be administered. The BNF provides appropriate guidance on how to manage a raised INR in these circumstances – http://www.bnf.org. The INR should then be monitored more regularly to re-establish an appropriate warfarin dosage level for the patient. Note that amiodarone has an extremely long half-life (in the order of 35 days) so this particular interaction may take several weeks to stabilise.

References and further reading

Aronson, J.K. & Ferner, R.E. (2003). Joining the DoTS: a new approach to classifying adverse drug reactions. *British Medical Journal.* **327**, 1222–25.

Atkin, P.A. & Shenfield, G.M. (1995). Medication-related adverse reactions and the elderly: a literature review. *Adverse Drug Reactions and Toxicological Reviews.* **14**, 175–91.

Borrelli, F. & Izzo, A.A. (2009). Herb–drug interactions with St John's Wort (Hypericum perforatum): an update on clinical observations. *The American Association of Pharmaceutical Scientists Journal.* **11**, 710–27.

Duerden, M., Avery, T. & Payne, R. (2013). *Polypharmacy and Medicines Optimisation: Making it safe and sound.* London: King's Fund. Available at: https://www.kingsfund.org.uk/sites/default/files/field/field_publication_file/polypharmacy-and-medicines-optimisation-kingsfund-nov13.pdf (Accessed: 11 February 2021).

Einarson, T.R. (1993). Drug-related hospital admissions. *Annals of Pharmacotherapy.* **27**, 832–40.

Griffiths, R. (2006). Adverse drug reactions and non-compliance with prescribed drugs. *Nurse Prescribing.* **4**, 121–23.

Harada, T., Ohtaki, E., Misu, K., Sumiyoshi, T. & Hosoda, S. (2002). Congestive heart failure caused by digitalis toxicity in an elderly man taking a licorice-containing Chinese herbal laxative. *Cardiology.* **98** (4), 218.

Hughes, S.G. (1998). Prescribing for the elderly patient: Why do we need to exercise caution? *British Journal of Clinical Pharmacology.* **46**, 531–33.

Jordan, S. (2007). Adverse drug reactions: Reducing the burden of treatment. *Nursing Standard.* **21** (34), 35–41.

Mallett, L., Spinewine, A. & Hauang, A. (2007). The challenge of managing drug interactions in elderly people. *Lancet.* **370**, 185–91.

Masnoon, N., Shakib, S., Kalisch-Ellett, L. & Caughey, G.E. (2017). What is polypharmacy? A systematic review of definitions. *BMC Geriatrics.* **17** (230), 2–10. DOI 10.1186/s12877-017-0621-2

McGavock, H. (2009). *Pitfalls in Prescribing and How to Avoid Them.* Oxford: Radcliffe Publishing.

Meyer, U.A. (2000). Pharmacogenetics and adverse drug reactions. *Lancet.* **356**, 1667–71.

Mills, E., Montori, V.M., Wu, P., Gallicano, K., Clarke, M., & Guyatt, G. (2004). Interaction of St John's Wort with conventional drugs: systematic review of clinical trials. *British Medical Journal.* **329**, 27–30.

National Institute for Health and Clinical Excellence (NICE) (2017). [KTT 18] *Multi-morbidity and Polypharmacy.* London: NICE.

Ogu, C., Pharm, D., Jan, L. & Maxa, R.P.H. (2001). Drug interactions due to cytochrome P450. *Baylor University Medical Center Proceedings.* **13**, 421–23.

Pirmohamed, M., Breckenridge, A.M., Kitteringham, N.R. & Park, K.B. (1998). Adverse drug reactions. *British Medical Journal.* **316**, 1295–98.

Pirmohamed, M., James, S., Meakin, S., Green, C., Scott, A.K., Walley, T.J, Farrar, K., Park, B.K. & Breckenridge, A.M. (2004). Adverse drug reactions as a cause of admission to hospital: prospective analysis of 18820 patients. *British Medical Journal.* **329**, 15–19.

Rawlins, M.D. & Thomson, J.W. (1985). 'Mechanisms of adverse drug reactions' in Davies, D.M. (ed) *Textbook of Adverse Drug Reactions.* 3rd edn. Oxford: Oxford University Press.

Vidushi, S.N.-B. (2013). Underestimating the toxicological challenges associated with the use of herbal medicinal products in developing countries. *BioMed Research International.* **2013**, Article ID 804086, http://dx.doi.org/10.1155/2013/804086.

4

Understanding and using the British National Formulary

Iram Husain
BPharm, MScAPP, MFRPSII, UKMi member,
Regional Medicines Information Manager (Governance & Training), Specialist Pharmacy Services

This chapter:

- Explains the scope and purpose of the BNF and how to access it
- Covers the useful information that can be found in the BNFs and the limitations of the BNFs
- Provides 'test yourself questions' within activities to assist you in using the electronic BNFs effectively.

The BNF 78 and BNF for Children (2019–2020) form the main basis of this chapter.

Medicines Information Services and the BNFs

Every year, over half a million questions about medicines are handled by Medicines Information Services – and these are just questions from healthcare professionals working in medical and patient care fields across the NHS. Many other healthcare professionals are based in secondary and tertiary NHS services and they also have questions.

Medicines Information Services have a proven positive impact on patient care and medicines safety. These services are run by clinical problem-solving experts, trained at a national level, to ensure that service users get good-quality, relevant, safe responses. The BNFs are just one of the core resources that these experts use in their day-to-day practice. A list of all the current UKMi approved resources, and some of their common limitations, can be found on the open-access Specialist Pharmacy Services website: https://www.sps.nhs.uk

Introduction to the BNFs

British National Formularies (BNFs) were originally created after the Second World War and have been published and maintained jointly by the British Medical Association (BMA) and the Royal Pharmaceutical Society (RPS) since then. In 2005 the BNF for Children (BNFc) was published, due to the lack of national consensus in paediatric prescribing. It is a unique resource and should be used to aid medicines management in children up to the age of 18. Both BNFs are used widely in the UK as a 'gold standard' resource for prescribing and dispensing information. They are also available in a number of other languages and used internationally.

The BNFs are written for all healthcare professionals involved in the prescribing, dispensing and/or administration of medications in the UK. The information in the BNFs originates from a variety of resources, such as the Summary of Product Characteristics (SmPC) produced by drug manufacturers, guidelines produced by the National Institute for Health and Care Excellence (NICE), alerts from the Medicines and Healthcare Products Regulatory Agency (MHRA), and expert practice groups such as the Royal Colleges.

The Joint Formulary Committee is responsible for the content of the BNF; and the Paediatric Formulary Committee, which includes the Neonatal and Paediatric Pharmacists Group (NPPG), the Royal College of General Practitioners (RCGP), the MHRA, and the Department of Health (DH), is responsible for the content of the BNFc.

The BNFs should always be used alongside professional judgement and clinical knowledge and may not always be the sole source of medicines information in clinical practice. By using an evidence-based, nationally recognised formulary, healthcare professionals reduce the risk of medication errors when prescribing for their patients.

Accessing the content of the BNF

The platforms for accessing the BNF content have evolved extensively over the years. Each platform has advantages and disadvantages, a few of which are listed in Table 4.1.

Table 4.1: Comparison of the current BNF platforms

BNF platform	Notable remarks
Books	**Advantages** • Some organisations provide a free copy for prescribers (check with your employer) • Updated every 6 months. **Disadvantages** • Lag time between content creation and actual publication can render paper-based publications out of date at point of purchase • Difficult to update in the light of frequent changes in medical practice so user will still need a means of accessing current updates • Requires user to be familiar with how to use each chapter, e.g. general statements prior to each drug class
Medicines Complete (RPS)	**Advantages** • BNF updates are available to both registered and non-registered users • Registered users can request BNF updates to be emailed • The website is easy to use via a simple search box or browsing the contents page • Hyperlinks within the text allow for easy retrieval of relevant information from particular chapters of the BNFs • Hyperlinks to external pages (such as NICE guidance) are included • Each page has a date when it was last updated • The website is updated monthly. **Disadvantages** • Part of a purchased suite of information resources • NHS employees based in the UK need to register for a Medicines Complete account to prove they are entitled to free access to the BNF resources (BNF and BNFc); a 1-year single-user access to the online BNFs is provided after registration.
NICE	**Advantages** • Offers free UK access to BNFs without registration • Easy to locate via the NICE home page • Can browse by Dental Practitioners' Formulary • Can browse by Nurse Prescribers' Formulary • The website is easy to use via a simple search box or browsing the contents page • Hyperlinks within text allow for easy retrieval of relevant information from particular chapters of the BNFs • Includes hyperlinks to external pages such as NICE guidance • Each page has a date of last update • Website is updated monthly. **Disadvantages** • Need to switch between BNF and BNFc (these are not integrated when searching or browsing).

(table continued overleaf)

Table 4.1 continued

BNF platform	Notable remarks
Personal Digital Assistant (PDA)	**Advantages** • The Pharmaceutical Press (RPS publishers of the BNFs) offer a PDA version • Updated monthly. **Disadvantages** • Can become out of date if user does not update version on device.
Local Formulary integration	**Advantages** • Some organisations have integrated their local formulary into the online BNF; check your local formulary to see if you already have access to the BNFs • Your local formulary website lists the products and strengths it has in stock and may advise on restricted prescribing and include hyperlinks to organisation guidelines. **Disadvantages** • The local formulary requires maintenance and updating of the BNF links, which could cause a time lag in ensuring the accuracy of the information.

Based on Table 4.1 and the author's experience, readers are advised to use the online versions of the BNFs whenever possible, in preference to the printed versions. The online versions provide monthly updates which include changes, corrections and clarifications.

Regardless of platform, all BNF users should read the 'how to use' section of the BNF and/or BNFc. In the print versions, this section appears as Chapter xii.

Medicines optimisation and the BNFs

NICE guidance (2015 NG5) states that in 2003 it was estimated that between 30% and 50% of medicines prescribed for long-term conditions were not taken as intended. As medicines are the most common healthcare intervention, and we have a growing and ageing population, optimising a patient's medication is clearly key to successful patient care and treatment. Medicines optimisation is defined as 'a person-centred approach to safe and effective medicines use, to ensure people obtain the best possible outcomes from their medicines'.

Shared decision-making is an essential part of evidence-based medicine. The RPS Framework asserts that the prescribing of medicines is based on shared decision-making between the clinician and the service user and is respectful of the individual's preferences, diversity and expectation of treatment.

The safety of medicines, and the avoidance of adverse effects, are important considerations when optimising medicines. The BNFs provide evidence-based choices of medicines and give guidance on the safe use of these medicines. Healthcare professionals will therefore find the BNFs a useful resource when discussing the best medication options with their patients, since they include consideration of issues such as comorbidities, concurrent drug therapies and formulation options for each medicine. The BNF alone will not optimise a patient's medication use but it should be one of the first sources consulted when reviewing medicines used by a patient.

The 'test yourself' questions in the activities in this chapter demonstrate how the BNFs can be used to reduce the risk of harm from medicines and ensure their safe and appropriate use.

Types of medicines information provided by the BNFs

The online BNFs (via https://bnf.nice.org.uk/ – NICE platform) will be used to explain how to navigate the information provided by the BNF and BNFc. Readers are advised to access the online BNFs when reviewing this chapter. The following subheadings relate to the home page for the online BNFs and refer to the printed BNFs where relevant.

What's changed?
The BNF and the BNFc have their own sections for cumulative changes made since the last print versions so make sure that the correct publication is selected when viewing changes. The 'significant changes', 'dose changes' and 'new preparations' are listed alphabetically. The print versions list these in Chapter xix. The BNFs do not provide information on drug shortages and so, even if a product is listed in the BNF, users must ensure they have the latest information on current drug shortages and advice through other routes.

Treatment summaries
These are alphabetical lists of the general statements that appear at the beginning of each chapter in the BNFs. They are different for the BNF and the BNFc. This section can be searched or browsed, depending on the user's familiarity with the BNFs' contents. It is useful to review the relevant treatment summary before considering the drug options if you are unfamiliar with, or unclear about, current treatment options. The summaries provide hyperlinks to relevant drug monographs and may contain external links to current UK guidance.

> ### Activity 4.1
> 1. Using the BNF online (via the NICE platform), what initial treatment is recommended for type 2 diabetes?
> 2. Using the BNFc online (via the NICE platform), what advice is given regarding the administration of ear drops in children?

Interactions
This section provides useful background information on drug interactions, explaining pharmacodynamic and pharmacokinetic interactions in a bit more detail. The section also explains

the way in which the BNF publishers have graded drug interactions, using the severity of interaction and the strength of the evidence base. The interactions can be browsed online by clicking on a drug monograph and then 'interactions'. The interactions will always be between two drugs and it is not possible to search multiple drugs simultaneously. Appendix I of the print version provides a table of drug–drug interactions in a similar fashion. Interactions relating to a drug class are not listed online but can be found in Appendix I of the printed BNFs.

In addition, Appendix I of the printed BNFs contains tabulated lists of the drugs most commonly associated with specific adverse drug reactions (ADRs). Concurrent use of two or more drugs from the same table may therefore increase the risk of an adverse event due to synergistic interactions. The printed tables are not exhaustive but cover drugs that commonly cause:

- Hepatotoxicity
- Nephrotoxicity
- Anticoagulant effects
- Antiplatelet effects
- Thromboembolism
- Bradycardia
- First dose hypotension
- Hypotension
- Prolongation of QT interval
- Antimuscarinic effects
- Central nervous system (CNS) depressant effects
- Peripheral neuropathy
- Serotonin syndrome
- Antidiabetic effects
- Myelosuppression
- Hyperkalaemia
- Hypokalaemia
- Hyponatraemia
- Ototoxicity
- Neuromuscular blocking effects

The drugs listed in the BNF and BNFc differ so make sure you use the correct publication when reviewing drug interactions for a patient. The BNFs do not provide clinical advice on what action to take regarding a drug interaction since this decision must be taken on a case-by-case basis. Other drug interaction resources are available, which can provide advice on what adjustments to make to drug therapy in the light of a drug–drug interaction.

Activity 4.2

1. What information does the online BNF (via NICE) give about the interaction between erythromycin and diltiazem?
2. How strong is the evidence for the interaction between erythromycin and warfarin?

Drugs

These sections allow the user to browse the drug monographs in the BNFs alphabetically. This is, in essence, the index page of the print BNFs by drug name.

Activity 4.3

1. Using the 'drugs' feature on the online BNF (via NICE) home page, locate the entry for omeprazole. What monitoring should be considered for patients on proton pump inhibitors and when?
2. Staying on the omeprazole entry, how would you change to the BNFc entry for omeprazole?

Searching the BNF

Both BNFs can be searched by typing a text word or phrase into the online search box. It is also possible to search for pairs of drugs here, to review drug interaction entries. The print BNFs are generally searchable by contents page or index listing.

Activity 4.4

1. In the search bar at the top of the online BNF (via NICE) screen, type in 'simvastatin side effects'. What do you notice?
2. Using the online BNFc (via NICE), search the database for the dose of fluconazole. What is the dose for children with tinea capitis and is this a licensed use?

Other useful information to browse

The 'useful information to browse' differs between the BNF and BNFc home pages. This information also appears as appendices in the print BNFs.

The BNF wound management section reviews the stages of wound healing and provides a useful table of suggested dressings based on the stage of healing. This is Appendix 4 in the printed BNF but does not appear in the BNFc print version.

The BNF and BNFc medical devices sections provide basic information on products, such as device indication, but do not provide advice on choice or suitability. This information is searchable in the printed BNFs by product name only.

The BNF and BNFc borderline substances sections provide guidance on conditions in which some foods (and skin treatments) have the characteristics of a drug. The Advisory Committee on Borderline Substances (ACBS 2020) advises on when these products can be included on an NHS prescription. Prescriptions issued in accordance with the Committee's advice and endorsed 'ACBS' will normally not be investigated. Appendix 2 of the printed BNFs provides this information.

The BNF and BNFc Dental Practitioners' and Nurse Prescribers' Formularies list the approved preparations and appliances that can be prescribed by these practitioners. These formularies are listed separately in the printed BNFs.

The BNF medicines guidance section is useful to all healthcare professionals. Table 4.2 summarises the main topics covered.

Table 4.2: Main topics covered within each medicines guidance section

Section	Content
Guidance on prescribing	Covers considerations involving never events, multimorbidity, deprescribing, taking medicines to best effect, advanced pharmacy services, medicines use review, biological medicines, biosimilar medicines, complementary and alternative medicine, abbreviation of titles, prescribing unlicensed medicines, oral syringes, excipients, extemporaneous preparation, drugs and driving, patents, safety in the home, labelling of prescribed medicines, security and validity of prescriptions, and patient group directions.
Prescription writing	Prescription writing requirements are explained and an example prescription provided.
Emergency supply of medicines	The legal requirements are explained for an emergency supply of medication when requested by a prescriber or a member of the public.
Controlled drugs and drug dependence	The classifications and schedules for controlled substances and their prescription requirements are explained. Also covers instalments and repeatable prescriptions, private prescriptions, drugs commonly involved in dependence and misuse, supervised consumption, who to notify when patients are receiving structured drug treatment for substance dependence, and the prescribing of diamorphine (heroin), dipipanone, and cocaine for addicts.
Adverse reactions to drugs (ADRs)	Explains the Yellow Card Scheme: what it is and how to report adverse drug/device reactions and where to find monthly drug safety updates. The ADRs listed in the BNFs for each drug are not exhaustive and users should consult the manufacturer's literature (Summary of Product Characteristics or SmPC) for a full list with incident data. The BNF ADRs are generally listed alphabetically, in order of frequency. Guidance is given on how to reduce the risk of ADRs in practice. Some serious ADRs are discussed, where they are attributed to a specific drug or drug class. Different types of drug hypersensitivity are also explained, to aid recognition.

Guidance on intravenous infusions	Advice to multidisciplinary teams (MDTs) on giving intravenous drugs via: • Continuous infusion • Intermittent infusion • Addition via drip tubing. Includes information on common additives and gives best practice guidance.
Prescribing in children	Detailed advice on medicines used in children can be found in the BNFc. General advice is provided here, including routes to avoid, use of drugs outside their UK licence (off-label), particular ADRs in children, prescription writing requirements, drug dosing and drug calculations.
Prescribing in hepatic impairment	Liver disease may alter the body's response to drugs in several ways and so drug dosing needs to be individualised. No resource provides a comprehensive list of drug dosing in liver disease. The BNF provides brief information on some liver disease complications and it is not a comprehensive resource for drug dosing in liver disease. The manufacturer's information (SmPC) is preferable, or the practitioner should seek advice from a liver specialist.
Prescribing in renal impairment	Discusses the issues encountered in renal impairment and provides general guidance. The information on dosage adjustment in the BNF is usually stated as estimated glomerular filtration rate (eGFR). However, some drug doses are calculated using creatinine clearance (CrCl). The calculations for kidney function are provided in this section with an interpretation of GFR and albumin:creatinine ratio (ACR) to diagnose the severity of chronic kidney disease. The manufacturer's prescribing information (SmPC) provides renal dosing advice in greater detail.
Prescribing in pregnancy	The BNF and BNFc identify drugs which: • May have harmful effects in pregnancy (and will indicate the trimester of risk) • Are not known to be harmful in pregnancy. Drug dose adjustments due to changes in maternal physiology are beyond the scope of the BNFs. Other resources, such as the UK Teratology Information Service (UKTIS), provide more in-depth advice on drugs in pregnancy for healthcare professionals and members of the public.
Prescribing in breast-feeding	An overview of breast-feeding is provided. The BNF identifies drugs: • That should be used with caution or are contra-indicated in breast-feeding • That can be given to the mother during breast-feeding because they are present in milk in amounts which are too small to be harmful to the infant • That might be present in milk in significant amounts but are not known to be harmful. A more comprehensive resource for drugs in breast feeding is the UK Drugs in Lactation Advisory Service (UKDILAS) database, accessible via the Specialist Pharmacy Services (SPS) website – www.sps.nhs.uk

(table continued overleaf)

Table 4.2 continued

Section	Content
Prescribing in the elderly	Appropriateness in prescribing is discussed, including formulations and drugs requiring caution, such as hypnotics, diuretics and non-steroidal anti-inflammatory drugs (NSAIDs).
Prescribing in dental practice	Advice on the drug management of dental and oral conditions is included in the appropriate sections of the BNFs. This section provides particular advice on dealing with dental patients who have medical conditions such as heart conditions, indwelling catheters, anticoagulant therapy, prosthetic joints, and thromboembolic disease.
Drugs and sport	Includes signposts to information about the prohibited status of specific medications, based on the current World Anti-Doping Agency Prohibited List.
Index of manufacturers	An alphabetical list of manufacturers and their contact details as referenced in the BNF. Note that this is not an exhaustive list of manufacturers.
Special order manufacturers	List of manufacturers, by region, that provide special orders.
Life support algorithm	Summarises the current adult life support steps.
Non-medical prescribing	Defines the range of non-medical healthcare professionals and explains the terms 'independent' and 'supplementary' prescriber.

The Medicines Guidance presented in the BNFc varies slightly and should be consulted for all paediatric drug prescribing, dispensing and administration. Additional topics include managing medicines in school, use of medicines off-label, oral syringes, issues with excipients, and estimating body surface area based on body weight alone.

The printed BNFs provide this information in the introductory chapters and the post-appendix chapters (as listed in the contents page).

Activity 4.5

1. By either using the search box or browsing the medicines guidance section in the online BNF (via NICE), decide if a footballer could take a cannabidiol out of competition. You will need to use an external link signposted by the BNF.
2. Using the online BNF (via NICE), what do you need to consider when deciding whether to prescribe a drug for a pregnant woman?

Tabulated information

The BNFs contain a number of tables to assist healthcare professionals. The online BNF tables are not so easy to find and so some commonly used ones are listed in Table 4.3. The BNF tables can be located by typing the 'table name' (or similar) into the search box of the relevant BNF or by browsing the relevant section. They are also accessible via hyperlinks from relevant pages in the online BNFs. The printed BNFs do not provide a dedicated list of useful tables and the table names do not appear in the contents or index pages.

Table 4.3: Other useful tables listed in the BNF

Table name	Section
Approximate Conversions and Units	About – Approximate Conversions and Units
Equivalent anti-inflammatory doses of corticosteroids	Treatment summary – Glucocorticoid therapy
Ingredient nomenclature in sunscreen preparations	Treatment summary – Sunscreen
Suitable quantities of dermatological preparations to be prescribed for specific areas of the body	Treatment summary – Skin conditions, management
Suitable quantities of corticosteroid preparations to be prescribed for specific areas of the body	Treatment summary – Topical corticosteroids
Topical corticosteroid preparation potencies	Treatment summary – Topical corticosteroids
Electrolyte concentrations – intravenous fluids	Treatment summary – Fluids and electrolytes
HRT risks – endometrial cancer, ovarian cancer, venous thromboembolism, stroke, coronary heart disease	Treatment summary – Sex hormones
Acetylcysteine dose and administration for paracetamol overdose	Treatment summary – Poisoning, emergency treatment
Drugs unsafe for use in acute porphyrias	Treatment summary – Acute porphyrias
Drugs with definite and possible risk of haemolysis in most G6PD-deficient individuals	Treatment summary – Anaemias
Recommended regimens for helicobacter pylori eradication	Treatment summary – Peptic ulceration
Blood infections, antibacterial therapy	Treatment summary – Blood infections, antibacterial therapy
Hormonal contraceptive preparation choice	Treatment summary – Contraceptives, hormonal
Routine immunisation schedule – children and adults	Treatment summary – Immunisation schedule
Medical emergencies in a community: acute asthma, unstable angina, myocardial infarction, croup, anaphylaxis, meningitis, hypoglycaemia, and convulsions (including febrile)	Treatment summary – Medical emergencies in the community

(table continued overleaf)

Table 4.3 continued

Table name	Section
Latin abbreviations commonly used on prescriptions. Also listed inside the back cover of the printed BNFs.	About – Abbreviations and Symbols
Common E numbers and their associated ingredients. Also listed inside the back cover of the printed BNFs.	About – Abbreviations and Symbols

> ### Activity 4.6
> 1. Using the treatment summary for topical steroids, how much corticosteroid preparation should be prescribed to an adult for treatment of both arms for 4 weeks?
> 2. Which 7-day helicobacter pylori eradication regimens would be suitable for an adult patient with a true penicillin allergy?

Drug monographs

The BNF does not cover herbal or homeopathic medicines although it includes a few in the drug interactions section, such as St John's Wort (hypericum). European law requires the use of the Recommended International Non-proprietary Name (rINN) for medicinal substances. In most cases, the British Approved Name (BAN) and the rINN are identical. Where these are different in the BNFs, the BAN has been amended to conform to the rINN. The only exceptions to this are adrenaline and noradrenaline.

The BNF data presented in the drug monographs comes mainly from the manufacturers' prescribing information (SmPC). However, the BNF and BNFc data may not always agree with the SmPC due to internal editorial guidelines. Where there is a difference in dosing, the BNF drug monograph will note that doses may be different from those in the SmPC for the same indication, e.g. methadone for opioid dependence, or chloroquine for malaria chemoprophylaxis.

The BNFs may occasionally give information on the use of unlicensed medicines, or the use of licensed medicines in an unlicensed (off-label) manner, e.g. clopidogrel 600 mg loading dose prior to percutaneous coronary intervention, rectal diazepam in children under 1 year, or fluconazole for tinea infections in children. The BNFc includes information on drugs when there is sufficient evidence for the drug to be considered relatively safe and effective in children. In most cases, the drug will be unlicensed or off-label.

The drug monographs in all BNF platforms are structured in the same way. The online BNFs allow searching by drug or product name, or by browsing the alphabetical drug name. The printed BNFs require the user to consult the index.

Using the printed BNFs, it is easy to see how the drug monographs are divided into 15 chapters, since each chapter represents a body system (e.g. gastrointestinal, respiratory, infections, eye and skin). These chapter headings are not seen when using the online versions. Instead the drug monograph can be located directly, and links are provided to relevant areas of the BNFs based on topic. For example, the drug monograph for sertraline links to treatment summaries such as antidepressant drugs, cholestasis and premature ejaculation. The monograph also lists and hyperlinks to other drugs in the same class, i.e. serotonin re-uptake inhibitors (SSRIs).

The drug monographs are subdivided further, as described in Table 4.4. The subsection headings are very similar to those found in SmPC, which contain more in-depth information than the BNF drug monographs.

Table 4.4: Drug monograph subsections

Subsection	Content
Drug action	A brief summary of the pharmacological action.
Indications and doses	For each indication, the route of administration and dose is given. Specific dosing for the elderly, or other relevant patient populations, may be provided where relevant. Dosing data for children is best located in the BNFc rather than the BNF.
	Doses are either expressed in terms of a definite frequency or as a total daily dose. In the total daily dose format, the dose should be divided into individual doses.
	The dose section also contains, where known, considerations that may affect the choice of dose, and dose equivalence information, which may aid the selection of dose when switching between drugs or preparations.
	The BNF includes unlicensed uses of medicines when a clinical need cannot be met by a licensed medicine.
Contraindications	Administration of the drug should be avoided in the circumstances listed. If the contraindication applies to the drug class, this will be stated.
Cautions	Outlines the precautions to be taken for patients with the comorbidities listed and gives details of monitoring to be undertaken, if applicable. If the caution applies to the drug class or specific formulation, this will be stated. Important safety advice provided by regulatory authorities or guideline producers will also be found here.
Interactions	This subsection usually hyperlinks to the interaction table for the specific drug, listing all known interactions. The online monograph does not link to drug class interactions, whereas the printed version does. For example, the online sertraline monograph hyperlinks to drug–drug interactions with sertraline but the printed Appendix 1 entry for sertraline refers the user to the entry for SSRIs.

(table continued overleaf)

Table 4.4 continued

Subsection	Content
Side effects	These are listed as: • Common/very common • Uncommon • Rare/very rare • Frequency not known. Data is usually provided for the drug class and the individual drug, and may also include overdose symptoms if relevant. Any products under intense monitoring by the MHRA must have all ADRs (no matter how minor) reported. In the case of children, all ADRs should be reported (even if not under intense MHRA monitoring).
Pregnancy	Provides manufacturer's advice in most cases. Also includes prescribing considerations for females of childbearing potential or men who might father a child.
Breast-feeding	Provides manufacturer's advice in most cases.
Hepatic impairment	Provides manufacturer's advice in most cases.
Renal impairment	Provides manufacturer's advice in most cases.
Additional information	Regimens to deprescribe, advice on monitoring, and information on effects on laboratory tests, interchangeability of drug brands, and NHS funding status is provided where relevant.
Patient and carer advice	Warnings are given here, e.g. where medication may impair the performance of skilled tasks. The advice in this section does not replace that provided in manufacturers' patient information leaflets (PILs). The NHS website (www.nhs.uk) provides more comprehensive patient-friendly information leaflets and should be used to supplement medication PILs and information about health.
Medical forms	Hyperlinks to the various formulations available in the UK are listed here, including references to any unlicensed and special formulations. The hyperlinks provide formulation, strength, pack size and NHS price (see 'BNF pricing', p. 76). Excipients are sometimes included but are not listed exhaustively. The SmPCs and PILs provide a full list of excipients for a particular product and should be consulted in the first instance. The BNFs also denote legal status here: prescription only medicine (POM), controlled drug (CD), pharmacy medicine (P), and general sales listed (GSL). The BNF does not provide information on drug shortages or guidance on alternative measures. Any products under intense monitoring by the MHRA will have a black triangle symbol by their brand name: ▼

Understanding and using the British National Formulary

> **Activity 4.7**
> 1. What important safety information is given about sodium valproate?
> 2. When prescribing diltiazem, should the brand name be used to identify the product?

Common abbreviations and symbols

A few abbreviations have already been mentioned and Table 4.5 provides a collective list of common (non-medical) BNF abbreviations that healthcare professionals may find useful. A full list is provided in the inside cover of the print BNFs and on the 'Abbreviations and Symbols' page (in the 'About' section) of the online versions.

Table 4.4: Drug monograph subsections

Abbreviation/symbol	Definition
ACBS	Advisory Committee on Borderline Substances
BAN	British approved name
CD1	Preparation in schedule 1 of the Misuse of Drugs Regulations
CD2	Preparation in schedule 2 of the Misuse of Drugs Regulations
CD3	Preparation in schedule 3 of the Misuse of Drugs Regulations
CD4-1	Preparation in schedule 4 (part 1) of the Misuse of Drugs Regulations
CD4-2	Preparation in schedule 4 (part 2) of the Misuse of Drugs Regulations
CD5	Preparation in schedule 5 of the Misuse of Drugs Regulations
DT	Drug tariff price
e/c	Enteric coated or gastro-resistant formulation
f/c	Film-coated formulation
GSL	General Sales List
m/r	Modified release
NCL	No cautionary labels (endorsement by prescriber)
P	Pharmacy medicine only
PGD	Patient group direction
POM	Prescription only medicine
rINN	Recommended international non-proprietary name
s/c	Sugar-coated
SLS	Selected list scheme
▼	Newly licensed medicine under intensive monitoring by the MHRA

BNF pricing

Basic NHS net prices are given in the BNF to provide an indication of relative cost. Where there is a choice of suitable preparations for a particular disease or condition, it may be useful to know the relative cost when selecting. Cost-effective prescribing should be considered, such as dose frequency, treatment duration, and reduction of time spent in hospital. BNF prices are not suitable for quoting to patients seeking private prescriptions or asking if products are cheaper to purchase over the counter, since VAT, professional fees, and other overheads are not accounted for. Patients enquiring about the private cost of medications should be referred to local pharmacies to obtain quotes.

Summary

The BNFs are an essential resource for all healthcare professionals involved in medication provision. The content is tailored to the UK user and provides a condensed version of the SmPCs, national guidance, and specialist information in easy-to-use formats.

NHS-based healthcare professionals can seek further assistance with questions about medicines by contacting the Regional and District Medicines Information Services, as listed in the 'About' section of the online BNFs (About – medicines information services) or on the inside front cover of the printed BNFs.

Answers to activities

Activity 4.1

1. Using the BNF online (via the NICE platform), what initial treatment is recommended for type 2 diabetes?

Metformin hydrochloride is recommended as the first choice for initial treatment for all patients, due to its positive effect on weight loss, reduced risk of hypoglycaemic events and the additional long-term cardiovascular benefits associated with its use.

2. Using the BNFc online (via the NICE platform), what advice is given regarding the administration of ear drops in children?

To administer ear drops, lay the child down with the head turned to one side; for an infant pull the earlobe back and down, for an older child pull the earlobe back and up.

Activity 4.2

1. What information does the online BNF (via NICE) give about the interaction between erythromycin and diltiazem?

Erythromycin is predicted to increase the exposure to diltiazem. The manufacturer makes no recommendation.

2. How strong is the evidence for the interaction between erythromycin and warfarin?
The online BNF (via NICE) notes that the evidence for the interaction is based on anecdotal data, though the interaction is rated as severe.

Activity 4.3

1. Using the 'drugs' feature on the online BNF (via NICE) home page, locate the entry for omeprazole. What monitoring should be considered for patients on proton pump inhibitors and when?
Measurement of serum-magnesium concentrations should be considered before and during prolonged treatment with a proton pump inhibitor, especially when used with other drugs that cause hypomagnesaemia or with digoxin.

2. Staying on the omeprazole entry, how would you change to the BNFc entry for omeprazole?
The online BNF (via NICE) states that the BNF is currently being viewed at the top of the screen. A hyperlink is provided to view the BNFc. Click on the hyperlink to go to the home page and then browse for the drug omeprazole to view the drug monograph.

Activity 4.4

1. In the search bar at the top of the online BNF (via NICE) screen, type in 'simvastatin side effects'. What do you notice?
The database initially tries to map the entered terms to one in its indexing but it is possible to bypass this and enter the phrase. The search takes the user directly to the side effects section in the drug monograph.

2. Using the online BNFc (via NICE), search the database for the dose of fluconazole. What is the dose for children with tinea capitis and is this a licensed use?
Searching for 'dose of fluconazole' in the BNF produces numerous results, but the first one is the most relevant. The hyperlink for 'fluconazole (indications and dose) drug' links directly to the dosing section for fluconazole in the BNFc. The dose advised for tinea capitis in children is 6mg/kg daily (max. per dose 300mg) for 2–4 weeks. The 'unlicensed use' note further down indicates that fluconazole is not licensed in children for tinea infections.

Activity 4.5

1. By either using the search box or browsing the medicines guidance section in the online BNF (via NICE), decide if a footballer could take a cannabidiol out of competition. You will need to use an external link signposted by the BNF.
The medicines guidance for drugs and sport provides links to two resources: The UK Anti-Doping (UKAD) website and the Global Drug Reference Online (GDRO) website. The UKAD provides a number of PDFs and the GDRO provides a searchable database. In either case, the information regarding cannabidiol is that it is not prohibited in sports.

2. Using the online BNF (via NICE), what do you need to consider when deciding whether to prescribe a drug to a pregnant woman?

Review the medicines guidance for 'drugs in pregnancy'. Here the advice is to prescribe in pregnancy:
- If the expected benefit to the mother is thought to be greater than the risk to the foetus.
- Taking care to avoid the first trimester where possible.
- Using a drug which has been extensively used in pregnancy and appears to be safe.
- Using the smallest effective dose.

Activity 4.6

1. Using the treatment summary for topical steroids, how much corticosteroid preparation should be prescribed to an adult for treatment of both arms for 4 weeks?

The online BNF (via NICE) treatment summary for topical corticosteroids suggests 30–60g would be suitable for a once-daily application for an adult for 2 weeks. Therefore, 60–120g would be a suitable amount to prescribe.

2. Which 7-day helicobacter pylori eradication regimens would be suitable for an adult patient with a true penicillin allergy?

The online BNF (via NICE) treatment summary for peptic ulceration provides advice on helicobacter pylori eradication regimens. It does not specifically list a regimen for penicillin-allergic patients and relies on the user to check the appropriate drug monograph. Searching 'penicillin allergy' separately will provide a list of hyperlinks to drugs which carry a caution or contraindication.

The BNF suggests options such as:
- Esomeprazole with clarithromycin + metronidazole
- Lansoprazole with clarithromycin + metronidazole
- Omeprazole with clarithromycin + metronidazole
- Pantoprazole with clarithromycin + metronidazole
- Rabeprazole sodium with clarithromycin + metronidazole.

Clarithromycin is a macrolide and unlikely to have cross sensitivity in a penicillin-allergic patient.

Activity 4.7

1. What important safety information is given about sodium valproate?

The drug monograph for sodium valproate highlights the MHRA alert issued in 2018. Valproate must not be used in women and girls of childbearing potential unless the conditions of the Pregnancy Prevention Programme are met, due to its teratogenicity and the risk of neurodevelopmental disorders and congenital malformations.

2. When prescribing diltiazem, should the brand name be used to identify the product?

Using the drug monograph for diltiazem, review the information regarding 'prescribing and dispensing information'. The standard formulations containing 60mg diltiazem hydrochloride are licensed as generics and there is no requirement for brand name dispensing. However, different versions of modified-release preparations containing more than 60mg diltiazem hydrochloride may not have the same clinical effect. To avoid confusion between these different formulations of diltiazem, prescribers should specify the brand to be dispensed.

References and further reading

Advisory Committee on Borderline Substances (ACBS). (2020). https://www.gov.uk/government/groups/advisory-committee-on-borderline-substances (Last accessed 13 August 2020).

Innes, A.J., Bramley, D.M. & Wills, S. (2014). The impact of UK Medicines Information services on patient care, clinical outcomes and medicines safety: an evaluation of healthcare professionals' opinions. *European Journal of Hospital Pharmacy*. Published Online First: 9 June 2014.

Joint Formulary Committee (2020). *British National Formulary* (online), London: BMJ Group and Pharmaceutical Press. https://bnf.nice.org.uk (Last accessed 13 August 2020).

Medicines and Healthcare Products Regulatory Agency (MHRA) (2020). https://www.gov.uk/government/news/welcome-to-our-new-mhra-website (Last accessed 13 August 2020).

National Health Service (NHS) (2020). https://www.nhs.uk/ (Last accessed 13 August 2020).

National Institute for Health and Care Excellence (NICE) (2015). Medicines optimisation: the safe and effective use of medicines to enable the best possible outcomes (NICE guideline NG5) Available at: https://www.nice.org.uk/guidance/NG5/chapter/introduction (Last accessed 13 August 2020).

Paediatric Formulary Committee. *BNF for Children* (online), London: BMJ Group, Pharmaceutical Press, and RCPCH Publications. https://bnfc.nice.org.uk (Last accessed 13 August 2020).

Royal Pharmaceutical Society (RPS) (2020). Medicines Complete. https://www.rpharms.com/publications/medicinescomplete (Last accessed 9 August 2020).

Royal Pharmaceutical Society (RPS) (2020). Quick reference guides: How to use your BNF. https://www.rpharms.com/resources/quick-reference-guides/how-to-use-your-bnf (RPS members only access); https://bnfc.nice.org.uk

Specialist Pharmacy Services (SPS) (2016). UKMi Recommended Resource Lists and Tools. Updated May 2020. https://www.sps.nhs.uk/articles/ukmi-recommended-resource-lists-and-tools/ (Last accessed 13 August 2020).

Specialist Pharmacy Service (2020). https://www.sps.nhs.uk/ (Last accessed 12 August 2020).

5

Adherence

Suzanne Everett

MSc, BSc (Hons) PG Cert HE
Senior Nurse Practitioner and Independent Prescriber.
Senior Lecturer and Senior Teaching Fellow, Middlesex University, London

This chapter has been revised and updated by Suzanne Everett, based on work originally produced by **Elizabeth Haidar**, MSc, BSc (Hons), RN Cert T/L Advanced Nurse Prescriber, Extended Independent and Supplementary Prescriber

This chapter:

- Explores how certain behaviour and personal traits can reduce or support adherence to medicine regimens
- Looks at the impact of poor adherence on clinical outcome and costs of care
- Shows how an understanding of an individual's patterns of adherence to taking prescribed drugs can be used to facilitate a richer consultation, which may prevent non-adherence to a medicines regimen
- Considers techniques that a healthcare provider may adopt when encouraging adherence to a medicine regimen.

Terms used when discussing medication-taking behaviour

'Adherence' is the term used for medication-taking behaviour and refers to whether someone takes the prescribed medication and whether they continue to take it. Whilst some individuals do take their prescribed medication (adherence), others may fluctuate in their adherence or stop taking their medication over time (showing 'lack of medication persistence'). There are further differentiations to be made between 'intentional' non-adherence (where patients do not take the medication because they do not accept the diagnosis) and 'non-intentional' non-adherence (where patients forget a dose or do not follow the regimen correctly through lack of knowledge).

'Compliance' and 'non-compliance' are useful terms but can have negative connotations, implying that the patient or client is passive and/or incompetent to follow instructions. Another term that is sometimes employed is 'concordance', which relates to the interaction between the patient and the individual healthcare practitioner and not the patient's medication-taking behaviour.

Medicines optimisation

However, adherence is not just about patients' failure to take their medication; it is a collaboration between healthcare professionals and patients to achieve medicine optimisation. Medicine optimisation involves prescribing the right medicine for the right patient, with the patients' involvement being central to the decision (NICE 2009). The aim of medicine optimisation is to improve patients' health by ensuring that they take their medication correctly. This process will avoid unnecessary polypharmacy and will reduce the wastage of medicines and improve medicine safety (RPS 2013, Duerden, Avery & Payne 2013). *Medicines Optimisation* (Royal Pharmaceutical Society 2013) addresses the four guiding principles for medicine:

1. Aiming to understand the patient's experience
2. Choosing evidence-based medicine
3. Ensuring medicine safety
4. Making medicine optimisation part of routine practice.

Principle 1, aiming to understand the patient's experience, is about having a dialogue with the patient about their personal journey in medication, to discover how it impacts upon their activities of daily living. This is to ensure that patients have a greater understanding of the choice of medication, there is shared decision-making, they can use their medication as agreed and that they are confident about discussing its impact on their daily life.

Principle 2, choosing evidence-based medicine, ensures that the best available and most appropriate and cost-effective medication is selected for the patient. This entails following NICE and local formulary guidelines, **reviewing treatment that is no longer required** and being transparent about access to medication.

Principle 3, ensuring medicine safety, helps avoid incidents, reduces hospital admissions/readmissions, and gives patients the confidence to ask about their treatment, to find out about issues such as side effects and safe disposal of unused medicines.

Principle 4, making medicine optimisation part of routine practice, encourages regular discussions between patients, carers and health professionals about medicine optimisation. This promotes consistency of care along with the realisation that activities of daily living alter and these changes may need to be reflected in the medication prescribed.

These principles are central to the Royal Pharmaceutical Society *Competency Framework for All Prescribers* (RPS 2016, NICE 2009). All prescribers should use this framework within their prescribing to ensure that they are prescribing safely and involving patients.

Characteristics that support adherence

Patients are more likely to adhere to prescribed medication if they are involved in their own plan of care and if they believe that the medication will work for them. A discussion of likely adverse and unpleasant side effects, and how they can be reduced, is also likely to improve adherence. Patients need to know how long to continue the regimen and how to get repeat prescriptions.

Knowledge, attitudes and beliefs

Adherence is usually better when healthcare professionals take care to address the patient's knowledge, attitudes and beliefs when discussing their medication. Incorporating coaching and counselling techniques and patient-focused cognitive work may be effective in challenging non-adherent behaviour when combined with other interventions (NICE 2009).

Interventions to support adherence in long-term conditions

The most effective interventions to support adherence in the long term include reinforcement, self-reporting questionnaires, clinical nurse specialist-led intervention, electronic monitoring and education behaviour. Clinical nurse specialist-led interventions do tend to result in higher levels of patient satisfaction, with fewer medication errors. The evidence suggests that a combination approach is most helpful in gaining adherence to a medication regimen (NICE 2009).

Activity 5.1

1. Can you suggest other strategies to support adherence?
2. Reflect on your own experience or that of your peers and outline one or two case studies that support the efficacy of the strategies that you suggested.

When identifying the statistical significance of an intervention, reinforcement, reminding and self-reporting questionnaires have been shown to be effective. Medication event monitoring systems (MEMS) are electronic devices that are attached to a pill bottle.

The device downloads data to a computer system each time the bottle is opened, recording medication adherence. This is seen as an effective method in comparison to alternative methods of measuring adherence (such as self-reporting pill counting). However, there has been criticism of the methods used to analyse research on these methods (El Alili *et al.* 2016). With self-reporting, research shows that there is a risk of patients potentially over-estimating their pill-taking and adherence (El Alili *et al.* 2016).

The healthcare agency Spoonful of Sugar (SoS) aims to provide evidence-based adherence solutions to healthcare providers and the pharmaceutical industry. They do this by means of behavioural mapping and engineering to diagnose intentional and unintentional barriers to adherence. One example is the development of smartphone apps for people with diabetes. NHS England is trialling an app library to help patients use safe and effective tools to support medication adherence (Oswald 2018). However, it is important to remember that technology is not suitable for everyone, and this highlights the need for healthcare practitioners to know their patients well and involve them in any interventions.

Non-adherent behaviour patterns

Predictors of non-adherence can also be seen as patterns in a patients' behaviour. Having a basic understanding of these may be helpful for prescribers during consultations.

Non-adherent patterns usually take the form of complete discontinuation, drug holidays and skipping doses due to forgetfulness or psychological resistance to adherence. Patients may stop medication because they are no longer experiencing symptoms, not realising that they need to continue in order to stay symptom-free.

It is important to consider how easy particular regimens will be for patients and involve them in the choice, as dosing regimens that do not fit in with patient's lives will be difficult for them to adhere to. Patients may lack confidence in the treatment or may find prescription charges too expensive. The patient's situation is also an important factor, as non-adherence most commonly occurs at particular times, such as during hospital transition of care or situations involving change like acute illness (Laven & Arnet 2018).

Case study: Choosing a combined pill

Jane has been treated for breast cancer twice and, as she was not menopausal, has taken Tamoxifen for five years. She stopped Tamoxifen after five years because of benign endometrial polyps and now feels happier and more like herself.

On visiting her oncology clinic for a routine follow-up appointment, she is advised that she should take Letrozole to reduce her risk of getting cancer again. Jane is now menopausal. However, Jane has a number of friends who have experienced joint problems with Letrozole so she is not keen to take it. Nevertheless, the doctor writes up the prescription and says 'I think this is a really good idea. Come and see me again in six months.'

Jane does not take the Letrozole but attends the appointment after six months. At this appointment she sees a different doctor, who listens to her concerns and explains that her risk of getting breast cancer a third time could be hugely reduced by taking Letrozole.

The doctor also explains that, whilst some people do get joint pain, most women do not get these side effects. If Jane experiences these symptoms, she can change to an alternative treatment or stop. The benefit of taking Letrozole was not adequately explained in the first consultation. The approach was autocratic and showed lack of consultation with the patient. The second consultation was a facilitative approach clearly explaining the reduction in risk, the risk of side effects and what could be done if Jane experienced them.

Following the second consultation, Jane took Letrozole and experienced no side effects. She was followed up regularly by the second doctor.

Having an understanding of a patient's lifestyle may be useful when identifying possible challenges to adherence. Individuals tend to adopt a particular behaviour when faced with practical obstacles in daily life, such as running out of medication or being unable to afford the prescription charge, or travelling through different time zones (which may interfere with their regimen).

It is therefore important to be aware of negative attitudes towards continuous medication-taking. These attitudes are as important as cultural beliefs and life experiences and ought to be explored fully before prescribing. In addition, prescribers should always reflect on their own practice and consider whether they hold biases or beliefs that affect the way they deal with certain patients. If so, they should work to reduce these biases.

How big a problem is non-adherence?

The scale of non-adherence to medication regimens is significant. In developed countries, approximately 50% of patients do not adhere to their medication regimen, and the figure is higher in developing countries.

The implications of non-adherence are evident in the outcomes for many diseases, including HIV, cardiovascular disease, type 2 diabetes and high cholesterol. When adherence is poor, targets may not be achieved, and disease-related complications and adverse outcomes may increase. There is a personal cost to the patient and to the NHS. For example, the implications of non-adherence to contraceptive methods may result in an unwanted pregnancy and result in an abortion. Hazell and Robson (2015) found that the estimated overall cost of wasted medication in the NHS in England was 300 million pounds; and this figure does not take into account the cost of further hospital visits or investigations or even abortions.

Surprisingly, the extent of non-adherence has not altered in over three decades, despite the delivery of preventative services to patients. Yet the significance of adherence to regimen is fundamental, not only for a successful outcome but also to reduce the spread of resistance – as has been seen in antibiotic use. Adherence to short-term medication, such as antibiotics, is thought to be greater than when taking medication for a longer period.

Non-adherence may be compounded by drug form, dose and timing and by adverse side effects. Here, prescribers can promote adherence by ensuring that patients are started on the lowest therapeutic dose, and titrating it upwards slowly, using a regimen that is as simple as possible while also giving accurate information on side effects and tolerability.

Failure to complete treatment is a simplistic interpretation of non-adherence, as the term actually covers a wider spectrum of behaviour, including:

- Not starting the medication (non-acceptance)
- Not taking the right dose daily (dosing problem)
- Not maintaining the dose at the correct time (timing problem)
- Not continuing the medicine for the prescribed period (non-persistence).

Non-adherence is not confined to a distinct location or to a particular group of people; suboptimal adherence to medication can be seen across all settings and all groups. Nevertheless, there does appear to be evidence of some predictors that inhibit adherence but these need to be further explored.

Characteristics that inhibit adherence

Ethnicity, socioeconomic status and LGBT issues and sexual preferences

There is some evidence of a link between demographic regions, ethnicity, health and socioeconomic status for non-adherence in long-term condition medication. Reports suggest that younger age groups and people from Black, Asian and Minority Ethnic groups (BAME) groups are more likely not to adhere to long-term condition medication. Langley, Bush, et al. (2012) carried out research in the UK and found that patients from BAME groups, under the age of 60, Islamic, and speakers of Urdu or Bengali, were more likely to have a lower adherence to medication.

When this ethnicity-based research is reviewed (Basanez, Collazo, et al. 2013), lower rates of adherence have been found to be associated with certain beliefs and experiences of prescribed drugs and with the nature of the patient–prescriber relationship. For example, black patients have reported feeling discriminated against by their white physicians. Connolly (2010) compared treatment of mental illness in BAME groups and white patients and found significant differences in rates of admission, detention and seclusion.

There are many reasons for lower adherence, including cost and poor availability of certain medications. In addition, certain cultural beliefs and life experiences can inhibit adherence. Income, level of education and employment status have been found to be significantly associated with the level of adherence to medicine regimens and BAME patients have unequal access to these, in comparison to white patients. Van Houtven, Voils, et al. (2005) carried out an observational study in the USA which found that patients who perceived that they had received unfair treatment were more likely to delay investigation and treatment and this tendency was significantly higher in people who believed the unfair treatment was the result of racism.

Somerville (2015) found that 57% of health and social care staff did not consider sexuality to be important to patients' health needs. However, LGBT patients are less likely to trust healthcare professionals and share information, and this is particularly hard for BAME patients who are LGBT who may originate from countries where this is illegal.

All these studies highlight the need for prescribers to understand their patients in order to increase adherence. Prescribers need to reflect on prescribing practice and listen to patients, being open to changing the way they work, to reduce racism and discrimination.

Age

Older people are identified as being 'at risk' of non-adherence to a regimen because of a range of factors such as multimorbidity, physical and cognitive deterioration (NICE 2017b, Duerden, Avery & Payne 2013). So, for example, they are likely to get confused by taking a multitude of medications, as is seen in patients taking medication for multimorbidity and/or long-term conditions.

Polypharmacy also increases the risk of drug interactions (NICE 2017b). For example, diuretics will increase micturition, which may cause some elderly patients to worry about incontinence, resulting in them reducing their fluid intake and increasing their risk of urinary tract infections.

Activity 5.2

1. Search the literature and identify three sources that explore the difference in non-adherence between males and females.
2. Structure a short argument that supports your own conclusions as to what these statistics demonstrate.

Children and teenagers with long-term condition medication (such as the bronchodilators used to treat asthma or insulin-dependent diabetics) may also be at risk of non-adherence to their regimen, possibly rejecting and rebelling against their diagnosis and treatment. In this situation, counselling may be useful to address these issues.

Young people have been found to be the highest users of antibiotics, and also the highest misusers, in terms of sharing them with others. This group appear to hold misconceptions about antibiotics. They may have left home and/or may lack experience of looking after themselves. They may also need to be educated about antibiotics and how to keep their use to a minimum by following a healthy lifestyle and getting medical advice at an early stage (Hawking *et al.* 2017, NICE 2017a).

Gender

There has been conflicting data on the effect of gender on adherence, with some research showing women to be worse at adhering to medication (Eindhoven, Hilt, et al. 2018). Meanwhile, a study of 76 GP practices serving patients in Birmingham found no major differences in adherence rates between females and males (Langley, Bush, et al. 2012).

A review of the literature on adherence to prescribed medication in pregnancy found that between 39% and 59% of women reported non-compliance during pregnancy. Their reasons included doubts about the use and safety of the prescribed drug during pregnancy (Matsui 2012).

Long-term medication

When studying the conditions of non-adherent patients, researchers have found specific long-term condition medication to be a major factor in non-adherence. They list those with hypertension, beta-blocker usage after heart attacks, asthma and depression as being high on the list of non-adherence candidates, possibly due to the lengthy period of adherence that is required. With long-term conditions and non-adherence, it is prudent to consider depression as an underlying reason, and whether patients fully understand why they are taking the medications and the risks if they do not adhere to it.

Short-term/acute medication

Short-term medication and treatment for acute conditions often involve antibacterial medications. In order to reduce resistance to antibiotics, antibiotic stewardship encourages healthcare professionals to consider whether they are prescribing antibiotics appropriately. Ensuring that the right prescription is given for the right infection is vital to reduce increasing drug resistance to antibiotics (NICE 2017a). Antibiotic stewardship has identified the need to educate patients as a vital component. Patients need to understand how to take medication, and when to contact a healthcare practitioner if their symptoms are worsening. Patients also need to understand drug resistance so that they understand the importance of using antibiotics appropriately.

Case study: Barriers to adherence

Anne is a 48-year-old woman with type 2 diabetes and hypertension. She lives in London, is a single parent and has a child with special needs. Anne attends the community hypertensive clinic with sitting blood pressure of 184/97 and heart rate of 60bpm.

Her medications consist of: irbesartan 2 × 150mg; doxazosin 1 × 4mg; bendroflumethiazide 1 × 2.5mg; glimepiride 6 × 1mg; metformin 2 grams MR; atorvastatin 20mg; fexofenadine 120mg and colecalciferol 20,000u. Anne also produces two other medications (atenolol and perindopril) which she is no longer prescribed.

During the consultation Anne admits that she regularly misses taking her tablets several times during the week and that she feels her eyesight has deteriorated.

Activity 5.3 (Case study)

1. Can you outline your approach during the consultation?
2. What are some of the factors highlighted within the scenario that could be barriers to Anne adhering to her medication regime?
3. Can you list some of the strategies used by healthcare practitioners to encourage adherence?

Case study continued: Barriers to adherence

Despite the strategies put in place to support and encourage adherence to her medication after the first visit to the community hypertension clinic, Anne's BP remains high on subsequent appointments at the clinic. Her BP is 200/88 mmHg.

Furthermore, she does not always attend appointments and on one occasion she has mislaid the irbesartan and produced atorvastatin which had been discontinued. Anne also confirms that she does not like taking blister packs, as taking everything in it makes her dizzy so she has decided she won't use it.

With support and implementation of the strategies considered above, Anne's BP returns to acceptable limits as her adherence to medication and lifestyle changes improve. At her last clinical visit, BP readings were within the following range: 146/80–138/76.

She is now maintained on a regime of: irbesartan 300mg daily; amlodipine 10mg daily; glimepiride 6mg daily; sitagliptin 100mg daily and insulatard 22 units in a morning. She also appears more in control and comfortable with the agreed approach to managing her conditions, especially the reduction in the number of medications.

> ### Activity 5.3 (Case study continued)
>
> 4. What approaches could the hypertension specialist nurse use to monitor Anne's adherence to her medication? Can you give some examples?

The information in this case study is adapted from a real-life scenario and shows that Anne was finding it difficult to manage all the different tablets she had been prescribed. In addition, the scenario indicates that she had limited understanding (before seeing the hypertension nurse specialist) of the different types of medication and the impact of not taking them appropriately.

This example also demonstrates that managing adherence is not straightforward and there may be periods of relapse. It therefore takes time and patience to improve adherence, and patients and healthcare practitioners need to work in partnership.

Summary

Ensuring the patient's adherence to their medicine regimen is fundamental to effective treatment and the general consensus is that adherence support requires a systems approach. It is therefore important to understand and explore adherence and non-adherence with the patient before prescribing treatment. There are numerous factors that may influence a patient's decision-making when it comes to taking medication. For the healthcare professional, having a good understanding of these factors is paramount. The healthcare professional should also be aware of typical behaviour patterns and take these into consideration to help the patient gain the highest possible level of adherence and the most successful clinical outcome.

Answers to activities

Activity 5.1

1. Can you suggest other strategies to support adherence?
You could have included: Support for behaviour change, risk minimisation and skills acquisition, knowledge and clinical service use outcomes, self-management programmes (training, counselling, education), self-monitoring, simplified dosing regimens, liaising with pharmacists (follow-ups, care plans, medication reviews), delayed antibiotic use, reminders, cues, incentives, recall, home visits, free vaccination (Ryan *et al.* 2014).

2. Reflect on your own experience or that of your peers and outline one or two case studies that support the efficacy of the strategies that you suggested.
As this is a reflective account, there are no prescribed answers to this activity.

Activity 5.2

1. Search the literature and identify gender differences in factors associated with adherence.

Experts have suggested there are no definitive gender differences regarding non-adherence. However discrepancies in some papers have suggested that women are slightly more inclined to be non-adherent to regimen, and there is a need to collect data on whether there has been support for the individual, previous health literacy and other psychosocial variables in order to explain non-adherence barriers. Other variables suggested to explain greater female medication non-adherence relate to balance and risk factors, less personal control and enhanced illness coherence problems. Further possibilities have included increased alcohol use, along with other social factors, such as lack of long-term housing, not belonging to a support group, medication side effects and current drug use (Kardas, Devine, *et al.* 2005, Granger, Ekman, *et al.* 2009, Berg, Demas, *et al.* 2004).

2. Structure a short argument that supports your own conclusions as to what these statistics demonstrate.

This may include:
- Statistical significance
- Imbalance of females to males in a study
- Too few participants in a study
- Differences in culture and attitudes to females
- Data not available to identify whether females were given full information on their medication
- Background of authors.

Activity 5.3 (Case study)

1. Can you outline your approach during the consultation?

The following answers outline important aspects – they do not give a comprehensive account.

- Refer to information in chapter: RSP framework & NICE (2009)
- Carry out medication review: Anne is a candidate due to her polypharmacy, long-term conditions (hypertension, diabetes), evidence of non-adherence (subjective as confirmed by patient, and objective BP levels). Enough time should be allowed to obtain a comprehensive history and assessment.
- The medicine review should also focus on: addressing Anne's needs and preferences; considering how to involve Anne in her own treatment; exploring Anne's understanding of her condition and medication; exploring the reasons for Anne's non-adherence and the complexities of her family life; the adverse effects of her non-adherence; any interactions between her prescribed medication and over-the-counter drugs; the effectiveness and safety of her regimen in managing her condition; and whether any of the medication is unnecessary.

- Manage polypharmacy: reducing number of medications.
- Work with other members of the MDT, including the diabetic nurse specialist, the optometrist/ophthalmologist and the social worker.
- Consider what practical support can be provided: Anne may need financial and social support; reminder strategies that she is comfortable engaging with; written information regarding medication and list of medication.
- Provide individualised self-documented medication plan.

2. What are some of the factors highlighted within the scenario that could be barriers to Anne adhering to her medication regime?

Examples may include:.
- Her long-term condition (hypertension) tends to cause few clinical signs or symptoms
- She may be struggling with polypharmacy
- Her social situation – how she is coping with her home life
- Her possible lack of a support network
- Physical barrier – deterioration in her eyesight.

3. Can you list some of the strategies used by healthcare practitioners to encourage adherence?

Examples may include:.
- Medication review
- Patient involvement
- Effective communication
- Strategies that are tailored to the patient's needs
- Involvement of a specialist practitioner
- Involvement of several practitioners through the multidisciplinary team (e.g. diabetic nurse specialist and social service support)
- Offering support, including education, electronic reminders and social support.

4. What approaches could the hypertension specialist nurse use to monitor Anne's adherence to her medication?

Examples may include:.
- Clinical BP measurements
- Monitoring of blood glucose levels
- Self-reporting.

References and further reading

Basanez, T.B., Collazo, L., Berger, J.L. & Crano, W.D. (2013). Ethnic groups' perception of physicians' attentiveness: implications for health and obesity. *Psychological Health and Medicine*. **18** (1), 37–46.

Beena, J. & Jose, J. (2011). Patient Medication Adherence: Measures in Daily Practice. *Oman Medical Journal*. **26** (3), 155–59.

Berg, K.M., Demas, P.A., Howard, A.A., Schoenbaum, E.E., Gourevitch, M.N. & Arnsten, J.H. (2004). Gender differences in factors associated with adherence to antiretroviral therapy. *Journal of General Internal Medicine*. **19** (11): 1111-17. doi: 10.1111/j.1525-1497.2004.30445.x.

Chambers, S.A. (2008). An assessment of outcomes and adherence to medications in patients with systemic lupus erythematosus with reference to ethnicity. University College London Repository.

Connolly, A. (2010). Race and prescribing. *The Psychiatrist*. 34, 169–71. https://www.cambridge.org/core/journals/the-psychiatrist/article/race-and-prescribing/32C1474CF0A540888F9CB28C033BB8FA (Last accessed 1 September 2020).

Duerden, M., Avery, T. & Payne, R. (2013). *Polypharmacy and Medicines Optimisation: Making it safe and sound*. London: King's Fund.

Eindhoven, D.C., Hilt, A.D., Zwaan, T.C., Schalij, M.J. & Willem Borleffs, C. (2018). Age and gender differences in medical adherence after myocardial infarction: Women do not receive optimal treatment – The Netherlands claims database. *European Journal of Preventive Cardiology*. **25** (2), 181–89. https://journals.sagepub.com/doi/10.1177/2047487317744363 (Last accessed 1 September 2020).

El Alili, M., Vrijens, B., Demonceau, J., Evers, S.M. & Hiligsmann, M. (2016). A scoping review of studies comparing the medication event monitoring system (MEMS) with alternative methods for measuring medication adherence. *British Journal of Clinical Pharmacology*. **82**, 268–79. https://bpspubs.onlinelibrary.wiley.com/doi/full/10.1111/bcp.12942 (Last accessed 1 September 2020).

Granger, B.B., Ekman, I., Granger, C.B., Ostergren, J., Olofsson, B., Michelson, E., McMurray, J.J., Yusuf, S., Pfeffer, M.A. & Swedberg, K. (2009). Adherence to medication according to sex and age in the CHARM programme. *European Journal of Heart Failure*. **11** (11), 1092–98 doi:10.1093/eurjhf/hfp142. (Last accessed 1 September 2020).

Hawking, M.K., Lecky, D.M., Touboul Lundgren, P., Aldigs, E., Abdulmajed, H., Ioannidou, E., Paraskeva-Hadjichambi, D., Khouri, P., Gal, M., Hadjichambis, A.C., Mappouras, D. & McNulty, C.A. (2017). Attitudes and behaviours of adolescents towards antibiotics and self-care for respiratory tract infections: a qualitative study. *BMJ open*. **7** (5), e015308. https://bmjopen.bmj.com/content/7/5/e015308 (Last accessed 1 September 2020).

Hazell, B. & Robson, R. (2015). Pharmaceutical waste reduction in the NHS. 18 June 2015. https://www.england.nhs.uk/wp-content/uploads/2015/06/pharmaceutical-waste-reduction.pdf (Last accessed 1 September 2020).

Kardas, P., Devine, S., Golembesky, A. & Roberts, C. (2005). A systematic review and meta-analysis of misuse of antibiotic therapies in the community. *International Journal of Antimicrobial Agents*. **26**, 106–13.

Langley, C.A., Bush, J., Harvey, J.E. & Patel, A. (2012). The Aston Medication Adherence Study (AMAS). Establishing the extent of patient nonadherence to prescribed medication in the Heart of Birmingham teaching Primary Care Trust (HoBtPCT).

Laven, A. & Arnet, I. (2018). How pharmacists can encourage patient adherence to medicines. *The Pharmaceutical Journal*. https://www.pharmaceutical-journal.com/cpd-and-learning/learning-article/how-pharmacists-can-encourage-patient-adherence-to-medicines/20205153.article (Last accessed 1 September 2020).

Matsui, D. (2012). Adherence with drug therapy during pregnancy. *Obstetrics and Gynecology International*. On-line Dec 26, 2011. https://core.ac.uk/download/pdf/193417669.pdf (Last accessed 1 September 2020).

National Institute for Health and Clinical Excellence (NICE) (2009). CG 76. Updated 2019). Medicines adherence: involving patients in decisions about prescribed medicines and supporting adherence. https://www.cntw.nhs.uk/resource-library/medicines-adherence-nice-clinical-guideline-76/ (Last accessed 1 September 2020).

National Institute for Health and Clinical Excellence (NICE) (2017a). Antimicrobial stewardship: changing risk related behaviours in the general population. https://www.nice.org.uk/guidance/ng63 (Last accessed 1 September 2020).

National Institute for Health and Clinical Excellence (NICE) (2017b). [KTT 18] Multi-morbidity and polypharmacy. London: NICE. https://www.nice.org.uk/advice/ktt18/resources/multimorbidity-and-polypharmacy-pdf-58757959453381 (Last accessed 1 September 2020).

Oswald, K. (2018). Non-adherence: medicine's weakest link. The *Pharmaceutical Journal.* https://www.pharmaceutical-journal.com/news-and-analysis/features/non-adherence-medicines-weakest-link/20204378.article (Last accessed 1 September 2020).

Royal Pharmaceutical Society (2013). Medicines Optimisation: Helping patients to make the most of medicines. https://www.rpharms.com/Portals/0/RPS%20document%20library/Open%20access/Policy/helping-patients-make-the-most-of-their-medicines.pdf (Last accessed 1 September 2020).

Royal Pharmaceutical Society (RPS) (2016) Competency Framework for all Prescribers. Available at: https://www.rpharms.com/Portals/0/RPS%20document%20library/Open%20access/Professional%20standards/Prescribing%20competency%20framework/prescribing-competency-framework.pdf (Accessed: 10 July 2019)

Ryan, R., Santesso, N., Lowe, D., Hill S., Grimshaw, J., Prictor, M., Kaufman, C., Cowie, G. & Taylor, M. (2014). Interventions to improve safe and effective medicines use by consumers: an overview of systematic reviews. The Cochrane Library. http://onlinelibrary.wiley.com/doi/10.1002/14651858.CD007768.pub3/abstract (Last accessed 1 September 2020).

Somerville, C. (2015). *Unhealthy Attitudes. The treatment of LGBT people within health and social care services.* London: Stonewall.

Van Houtven, C.H., Voils, C.I., Oddone, E.Z., Weinfurt, K.P., Friedman, J.Y., Schulman, K.A. and Bosworth, H.B. (2005). Perceived discrimination and reported delay of pharmacy prescriptions and medical tests. *Journal of General Internal Medicine.* **20** (7). https://doi.org/10.1111/j.1525-1497.2005.0123.x

World Health Organization (2003). *Adherence to Long-term Therapies – evidence for action.* WHO edn. Geneva, Switzerland: WHO. http://whqlibdoc.who.int/publications/2003/9241545992.pdf (Last accessed 1 September 2020).

6

Pharmacological case studies: Pregnancy and breastfeeding

Maria Yousif
MRPharmS, MPharm, PGDipGPP, PgCert Leadership in Health.
Pharmacist Specialist, Medicines Optimisation Team, Care Quality Commission

This chapter:
- Provides best practice guidance for prescribing in pregnancy and breastfeeding
- Discusses how the mode of action and pharmacokinetics of medicines are altered due to physiological changes in pregnancy
- Discusses the effects that drug exposure in pregnancy and lactation can have on the foetus or the neonate
- Describes the management of common symptoms and medical conditions during pregnancy.

Introduction

The use of medicines in pregnancy is very common but the safety of many medicines in pregnancy is unknown. Some medicines can increase the chances of congenital malformation, stillbirth, miscarriage, learning difficulties or other developmental issues in the foetus which may only be noticed later in life. Prescribing in pregnancy is therefore complex and can be further complicated by the physiological changes that occur during pregnancy. The risks and the benefits to the mother and to the developing foetus should therefore be considered before prescribing a medicine.

Good practice principles

In accordance with the Nursing and Midwifery Council (2019), collaborative working is key when providing care to pregnant women. All pregnant women should have a named midwife throughout pregnancy, labour and the postnatal period. Care under a midwife should commence as soon as possible. Before making a prescribing decision, midwife prescribers should follow *The Prescribing Competency Framework* (2016) as set out by the Royal Pharmaceutical Society (RPS) and Trust prescribing policies. Nurse prescribers should exercise their professional judgement based on best practice guidance such as the National Institute for Health and Care Excellence (NICE) pathways. They must also be able to recognise if a situation falls outside their competence and seek advice or refer to specialists accordingly.

When offering care during pregnancy, healthcare professionals should enable a woman to make informed decisions, tailored to her needs, having discussed matters fully beforehand. Medicines should be prescribed only if the expected benefit to the mother outweighs the risk to the foetus. Where use of a medicine in pregnancy is unavoidable, medicines that have been extensively used in pregnancy and appear to be generally safe should be used in preference to those which are new or have not been tried before. All medicines prescribed in pregnancy should be prescribed at the lowest effective dose for the shortest possible duration.

Midwives, exemptions

Midwives may supply and administer, without a prescription or written direction from a doctor, any substances specified in medicines legislation under midwives' exemptions, as long as it is within their professional midwifery practice. If a medicine is not included in midwife exemptions, a prescription will be required. However, as Trust employees, the medicines that midwives may supply must be approved by the Trust due to vicarious liability.

Midwives have an exemption clause in the Prescription Only Medicines (Human Use) Order 1997, which links to the 1968 Medicines Act. 'Exemptions' are distinct from 'prescribing'. Midwives may only prescribe if they have completed a recognised prescribing course and have the qualifications recorded on the NMC's professional register. *Practising as a Midwife in the UK* (NMC 2020) provides an overview of midwives' exemptions, which includes up-to-date information and legislation.

Stages of foetal development

In order to assess the foetal risk of drug exposure, it is important to understand the different stages of foetal development. There are three main stages of antenatal development – pre-embryonic, embryonic and foetal.

Pre-embryonic stage (0–2 weeks post-conception)

This stage refers to the first 2 weeks post-conception when the fertilised ovum is implanted in the uterus. Exposure during the pre-embryonic stage to a teratogen is thought to prompt the 'all or nothing' response. This response will either cause death of the embryo (if most cells are affected), leading to a spontaneous miscarriage, or survival of the embryo (if only a few cells are affected) and progression of normal foetal development.

Embryonic stage (3–8 weeks post-conception)

During this stage, cell differentiation and major organ formation (organogenesis) occur. This is thought to be the most critical time for embryonic exposure to teratogens as the embryo is at its most vulnerable. If the differentiated cells are harmed, it could lead to permanent defects to organs as these cells will be irreplaceable. If possible, all drugs should therefore be avoided in the first trimester.

Foetal stage (9–38 weeks post-conception)

The foetus continues to grow, develop and mature during this stage. The foetus therefore remains vulnerable to teratogenic drug effects. Damage to the central nervous system and renal dysfunction, for instance, can occur with exposure to certain drugs as the cerebral cortex and renal glomeruli are still developing. The placenta is fully functioning at 12 weeks.

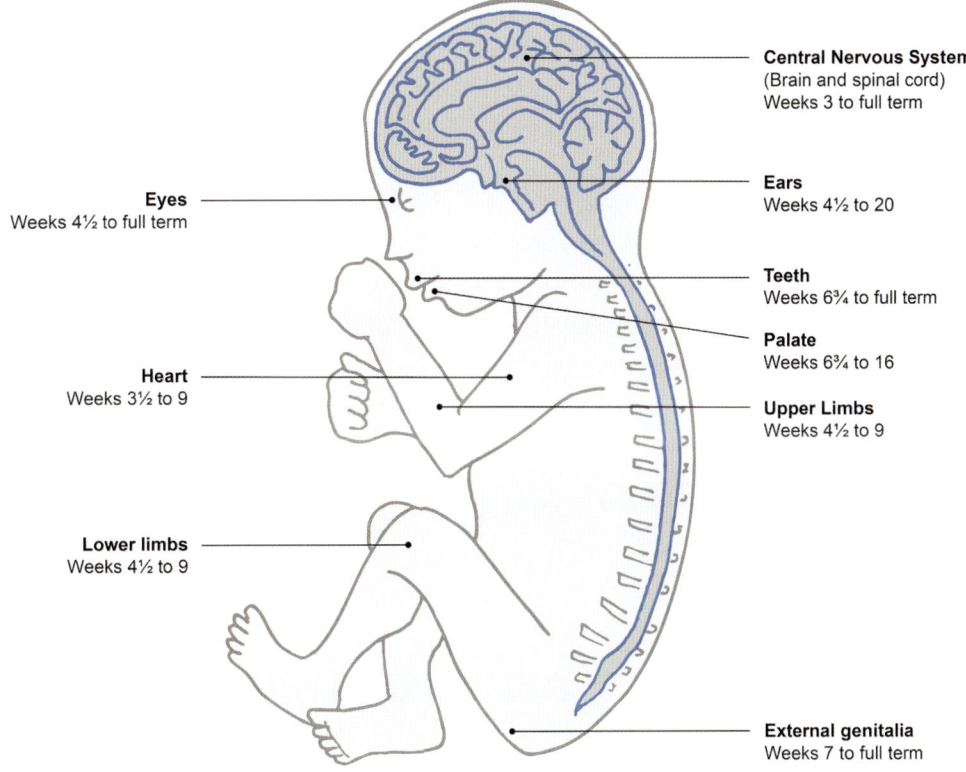

Figure 6.1: Stages of foetal development

Teratogenicity

Teratogenicity occurs when an agent or a factor can cross the placenta and cause congenital malformations. These factors/agents are known as teratogens. However, the definition of a teratogen extends to any agent that can directly or indirectly cause structural or functional abnormalities in the foetus and is therefore not only limited to agents that cross the placenta. The incidence of major congenital malformations is estimated to be between 2 and 3%. However, most of these defects (>75%) have an unknown cause. Only a small percentage (1–2%) are thought to be due to drugs and not all exposures will cause abnormalities.

One of the most famous potent teratogens is thalidomide. Thalidomide was first marketed in 1957 in Germany as a sedative. It was later found that the drug had anti-emetic properties and was also effective against morning sickness. As thalidomide was available to purchase over the counter, thousands of pregnant women in many countries took the drug to remedy their morning sickness symptoms.

Following its use, many babies were born with severe anatomical birth defects such as amelia and phocomelia. Amelia is the complete absence of one or more limbs and phocomelia is defined as the loss, or severe shortening, of the long bones of the limb (upper and/or lower). In the UK thalidomide was withdrawn from the market in 1961.

The thalidomide disaster prompted many countries to introduce more rigorous rules and regulations on the testing and licensing of medicines. Decades later, thalidomide was reintroduced and licensed for the treatment of myeloma. It is also used by dermatologists off-licence for several treatment-resistant skin conditions such as leprosy. If treatment is to be initiated, all women of childbearing potential should be counselled about the risk of severe birth defects and must be entered in a pregnancy prevention programme before starting thalidomide. Thalidomide must never be taken during pregnancy.

Principles of teratogenicity

When assessing the risk of reproductive or developmental toxicity associated with the use of a drug or other agent during pregnancy, it is important to consider four fundamental principles, which are discussed below.

Principle 1: Drug dose

The potential for teratogenicity to occur is usually dose dependent. Almost all drugs that are known to be toxic to the foetus or the embryo have a dose threshold below which the drug does not exert any teratogenic effects. It is therefore recommended to always use the lowest effective dose when prescribing medicines in pregnancy. Certain medicines also require more frequent blood monitoring to ensure that dosing is appropriate throughout pregnancy.

Principle 2: Susceptibility of the species

Some species are more susceptible to the teratogenic effects of a drug or other agent. A drug that produces birth defects in one species can have little or no effect in others. In some cases, although a drug can cause similar effects in multiple species, the defects may vary in the incidence of their occurrence. In other cases, one drug may cause various types of defects in different species. These variations are due to genetic differences (such as receptor sensitivity to a teratogen) and can also be affected by environmental factors.

Studies on rodents are usually used to evaluate the safety of medicines in pregnancy but rodents are physiologically, metabolically and developmentally very different from humans. If a drug causes toxicity to the foetus or embryo in various animal species, it may indicate that it has teratogenic potential in humans. However, if a drug does not exert teratogenic effects in animals, it cannot be assumed that it is safe to use in human pregnancies.

Principle 3: Timing of exposure

The timing of drug or chemical exposure during a pregnancy can determine the likelihood, severity and nature of the resulting foetal or embryonic toxicity. For instance, the period of greatest teratogenic risk with thalidomide exposure is between 20 and 36 days after conception. The risks therefore vary between different foetal developmental stages in different trimesters. This explains how exposure at an early stage of pregnancy can cause morphological issues for the foetus but at a later stage it can have adverse functional or development effects.

Principle 4: Mode of action of drug

It is vital to understand the actions of different drugs in order to understand how they can disturb the development of the foetus. When assessing the risk, it can be useful to identify which specific molecular components teratogens target during pregnancy.

Table 6.1: Examples of possible teratogenic effects caused by specific drugs or agents

Drug/agent	Possible teratogenic effect/s (non-exhaustive)
Isotretinoin	• Central nervous system abnormality (hydrocephalus, microcephaly), facial dysmorphia, cleft palate, external ear abnormalities, eye abnormalities, cardiovascular abnormalities
Tetracyclines	• Discoloration of teeth, bone growth adverse effects
Drug/agent	**Possible teratogenic effect/s (non-exhaustive)**

(table continued overleaf)

Table 6.1 continued

Carbamazepine	• Neural tube defects
Warfarin	• Foetal warfarin syndrome, characterised by nasal hypoplasia, short limbs and digits, stippled epiphysis
Methotrexate	• Craniofacial defects, malformations of the digits, defects of spine and ribs
Sodium valproate	• Neural tube defects (spina bifida in particular), orofacial clefts, cardiac effects
Alcohol	• Foetal Alcohol Spectrum Disorders (FASD); at the severe end of the spectrum, FASD effects may include growth retardation, characteristic facial features and central nervous system abnormalities leading to neuro-behavioural problems
Cocaine	• Spontaneous abortion, placental abruption, intra-uterine growth retardation, Sudden Infant Death Syndrome (SIDS)

The risk of birth defects increases with the number of drugs being taken at the same time. In women with epilepsy, it has been observed that the incidence of foetal malformations increases with the number of anti-epileptic medicines taken together.

Physiological and pharmacokinetic changes in pregnancy

During pregnancy several physiological and pharmacokinetic changes occur in the mother's body. Knowledge of these changes is important in order to understand how the body's handling of medicines is altered and what adjustments and monitoring may be needed. For example, blood flow to the skin and the lungs is increased, so there is greater absorption from these sites. Increased pulmonary perfusion can lead to increased absorption of pollutants, such as cigarette smoke, bronchodilators and other volatile agents.

Meanwhile, absorption from the gut slows down. Due to increased gastrointestinal emptying time and reduced gastrointestinal motility, absorption of medicines from the gut can be slower, leading to a delay before a particular medicine takes effect.

Total body water increases in pregnancy by approximately 8 litres; and a 30% increase in cardiac output results in an increased volume for medicines to be distributed in. When combined with an increase in renal perfusion (of up to 50%), this can lead to increased dosages being required

Pharmacological case studies: Pregnancy and breastfeeding

for certain medicines, unless this is counterbalanced by other factors.

Plasma proteins can also be affected during pregnancy. Albumin, which binds acidic drugs, is decreased so the concentration of the unbound drug may increase in the plasma. Monitoring is required to maintain the drug dose within therapeutic levels and avoid drug-related toxicity.

Changes in drug metabolism during pregnancy are more complex and more difficult to predict but can have a significant impact on drug dosing. For instance, knowledge of the effect of pregnancy on cytochrome P450 isoenzymes, and which isoenzymes are involved in the metabolism of specific drugs, can be useful to inform decisions about monitoring and dosing adjustments. In particular, an increase of approximately 50% in the glomerular filtration rate (GFR) leads to faster elimination of medicines, which are excreted unchanged by the kidneys.

In most cases there is no significant impact on the effectiveness of medicines but in some cases close monitoring may be required as treatment may be ineffective if drug concentrations drop below therapeutic levels.

Table 6.2: Summary of the key pharmacokinetic changes that occur in pregnancy

Parameter	Change in pregnancy	Possible consequences
Absorption	↓ Gastrointestinal motility	Delay in absorption, leading to a longer time to onset of action of some medicines.
Distribution	↑ Plasma volume	Higher doses of hydrophilic medicines may be required to achieve the same therapeutic effect.
	↑ Body water	
	↓ Plasma albumin	Increase in the unbound concentration of protein-bound medicines. More frequent monitoring may be required.
	↑ Fat deposition	Increased distribution of lipophilic medicines.

(table continued overleaf)

Table 6.2 continued

Parameter	Change in pregnancy	Possible consequences
Metabolism	↓↑ Hepatic activity	The metabolic activity of certain cytochrome P450 isoenzymes (such as CYP3A4, CYP2D6, CYP2A6 and CYP2C9) is increased in pregnancy, whereas it is decreased for CYP1A2 and CYP2C19. Depending on which cytochrome P450 isoenzyme metabolises, a drug dose adjustment may be needed.
Excretion	↑ Glomerular filtration ↑ Renal blood flow	Medicines which are excreted unchanged by the kidneys will be eliminated faster from the body and dosing frequency may therefore need adjusting.

Properties of drugs

It is estimated that most drugs cross the placenta by simple diffusion. The degree to which drugs will cross the placenta depends on several properties: molecular size, degree of ionisation, extent of protein binding and lipid solubility. The placenta is a lipid barrier between the maternal and foetal circulation. It therefore favours the transfer of fat-soluble over water-soluble drugs. Ionised hydrophilic dugs are less likely to cross the placenta than non-ionised lipid-soluble ones. Drugs with a high molecular weight, such as heparin, do not tend to cross the placenta.

Activity 6.1

Taking into consideration the properties of the drugs/agents below, describe whether or not each one is likely to cross the placenta:

1. Enoxaparin
2. Diazepam
3. Insulin
4. Alcohol

Pre-conception and planning a pregnancy

When prescribing medicines in women of childbearing potential, the choice of medicine should be carefully considered, as almost half of all pregnancies are unplanned. Women with pre-existing medical conditions, such as epilepsy, asthma and diabetes, should be advised to seek specialist assessment before trying to conceive and medicines should be reviewed and adjusted or changed to alternative safer options. In women with epilepsy, for instance, pharmacotherapy with one agent at the lowest effective dose is ideal.

When women with long-term conditions are planning a pregnancy, compliance with medicines is also a key factor for practitioners to consider. For many women, the fear of potential harm to the baby from medicines they are taking can lead to non-adherence. However, this non-adherence may result in inadequate control of their medical condition, which may be more detrimental to the health of both mother and foetus. Patient education should be provided to enable women to make decisions based on clear, up-to-date information.

Contraception and pregnancy testing

Women using medicines with known teratogenic potential should avoid getting pregnant during treatment and should be advised on the need to use contraception. In some cases, these patients are entered in a formal pregnancy prevention programme. The choice of the most effective contraceptive should take into account a woman's personal circumstances. The Medicines and Health Products Regulatory Agency (MHRA) continues to receive reports of inadvertent exposure to medicines with teratogenic potential, as women may sometimes be unaware that they are pregnant at the start of their treatment. Pregnancy testing is therefore advised as an additional measure to avoid inadvertent exposure to such medicines during early pregnancy. The MHRA have developed guidance for prescribers on the frequency of pregnancy testing needed, depending on the chosen contraceptive method, to avoid exposure to teratogens during pregnancy (MHRA 2019a, 2019b).

Sodium valproate, which is a medicine used for epilepsy, is highly teratogenic. It carries an approximately 30–40% risk of neurodevelopmental disorders and 10% risk of congenital malformations occurring if used in pregnancy. Sodium valproate must *not* be used in women and girls of childbearing potential unless the conditions of the Pregnancy Prevention Programme are met; and it must only be used if alternative treatments are not tolerated or a specialist does not think alternative treatments will be effective. Strict guidance is issued by the MHRA on the implementation of the Pregnancy Prevention Programme, setting out the responsibilities and actions that need to be taken by different healthcare professionals involved in the prescribing and dispensing of sodium valproate.

Women receiving methotrexate therapy also need to ensure that they do not get pregnant during treatment and must be counselled regarding pregnancy prevention and planning. Effective contraception must be used during methotrexate treatment and for at least six months thereafter.

Paternal exposure

It is generally thought that there is unlikely to be a significantly increased risk of teratogenicity following paternal exposure to drugs or chemicals – unless the compound is a mutagen with the potential to cause genetic changes to sperm. Theoretically, this might pose an increased risk of adverse effects to the foetus. However, for most medicines, the outcome following paternal exposure has not been studied. Usually, men who are exposed to cytotoxic or mutagenic substances (e.g. methotrexate) are advised to wait about six months (two sperm cycles) before attempting conception. This is thought to allow enough time for regeneration of exposure-free sperm.

UK Teratology Information Service

The UK Teratology Information Service (UKTIS) is commissioned by Public Health England to provide evidence-based information and advice to healthcare professionals in the UK. UKTIS also conducts surveillance on the foetal effects of maternal exposure to medicines and other chemicals during pregnancy. Healthcare professionals should seek advice from UKTIS to ensure safer prescribing in pregnancy.

Activity 6.2

To assess the risks of a medicine or chemical exposure in a pregnant woman, you may decide to contact UKTIS for advice. What information about your patient would be useful to provide in the following scenarios?

1. A medicine is to be used for a therapeutic reason
2. The patient has inadvertently been exposed to a chemical or a drug.

Nutritional supplements

Folic acid

To reduce the risk of neural tube defects (such as spina bifida) occurring in the foetus, pregnant women and those planning a pregnancy are advised to take folic acid supplements before conception and for the first 12 weeks of the pregnancy. The recommended dose is 400 micrograms daily. However, a higher dose of 5mg daily is recommended for women who at higher risk of conceiving an infant with a neural birth defect. Women considered to be in the high-risk group are those who have previously had a child with a neural tube defect, those taking anti-epileptic medicines and those who have diabetes or sickle cell disease (NICE 2019a).

Iron
Iron supplementation should be offered only where indicated and not offered routinely to all pregnant women. It can cause unpleasant maternal side effects and does not benefit the health of the mother or the baby (NICE 2019a).

Vitamin A
All pregnant women should be informed of the teratogenic risk with the intake of vitamin A (above 700 micrograms) and should therefore avoid it. Liver and liver products, in particular, may contain high levels of vitamin A. Consumption of these products should therefore also be avoided (NICE 2019a).

Vitamin D
During pregnancy and breastfeeding, it is important for women to maintain adequate levels of vitamin D for the benefit of their own health as well as their baby's. It is therefore advised that women should take a vitamin D supplement (10 micrograms of vitamin D per day). This should be followed more stringently by those at a greater risk of vitamin D deficiency (NICE 2019a), particularly:

- Women with darker skin (such as those of African, Afro-Caribbean or South Asian family origin)
- Women who have limited exposure to sunlight (e.g. housebound or confined indoors for long periods, or who cover their skin for cultural reasons).

Managing common symptoms and medical conditions during pregnancy

This section covers the management of common symptoms in pregnancy. Non-pharmacological treatment options should be considered first, where possible, to minimise the risks from medicines to the foetus. A medicine should be prescribed only when it is essential. Polypharmacy should be avoided, and women should be advised to seek advice from a healthcare professional before taking any medicine, including medicines bought from a pharmacy or a shop and any herbal remedies. Only a few over-the-counter medicines and complementary medicines have been established as being safe and effective in pregnancy, so these should also be avoided or used as little as possible.

Nausea and vomiting in early pregnancy
Nausea and vomiting are common symptoms in early pregnancy and these symptoms are usually attributed to the effects of the human chorionic gonadotrophin (HCG) hormone produced by the placenta. Women should be advised that most cases of nausea and vomiting resolve spontaneously within 16 to 20 weeks without causing any harm to the pregnancy. Non-pharmacological treatments that have been shown to be effective in reducing symptoms, include (P6) wrist acupressure and ginger. In available studies, ginger was taken as capsules, biscuits, syrup and even tea, with doses

ranging from 0.6g to 2.5g daily for 4–21 days during pregnancies between 12 and 20 weeks gestation. A dose of ≤1.5g is considered adequate for relief of nausea and a maximum dose of 2g per day is considered safe for use in pregnant women (Specialist Pharmacy Service 2019).

Where symptoms are debilitating, and non-pharmacological treatments have failed, antihistamines (such as promethazine or cyclizine) are the drugs of choice, though these can cause drowsiness as a side effect. Prochlorperazine is an alternative first-line antihistamine, but it should be used with caution due to the risk of dystonic reactions in young pregnant women.

Second-line agents include domperidone and metoclopramide. These are not recommended as first-line anti-emetic agents, as there are concerns over potential maternal side effects that can occur with their use. Domperidone is associated with a small increased risk of serious cardiac side effects. Metoclopramide has been used at all stages of pregnancy without evidence of toxicity to the foetus or the embryo. However, it can cause extrapyramidal side effects (such as dystonic-dyskinetic head and neck movements), particularly in young women.

Ondansetron is also limited to second-line use at present. Although there is encouraging data on pregnancy outcomes, further research is required to investigate a possible small increased risk of orofacial cleft palate malformations when it is used during the first trimester and some concerns about possible cardiac and kidney malformations.

Table 6.3: Recommended anti-emetic therapies and dosages (RCOG 2016)

First line	- Cyclizine 50mg PO, IM or IV 8 hourly - Prochlorperazine 5–10 mg 6–8 hourly PO; 12.5mg 8 hourly IM/IV; 25mg PR daily - Promethazine 12.5–25mg 4–8 hourly PO, IM, IV or PR - Chlorpromazine 10–25mg 4–6 hourly PO, IV or IM; or 50–100mg 6–8 hourly PR
Second line	- Metoclopramide 5–10mg 8 hourly PO, IV or IM (maximum 5 days' duration) - Domperidone 10mg 8 hourly PO; 30–60mg 8 hourly PR - Ondansetron 4–8mg 6–8 hourly PO; 8mg over 15 minutes 12 hourly IV
Third line	- Corticosteroids - Hydrocortisone 100mg twice daily IV - Once clinical improvement occurs, switch to prednisolone 40–50mg daily PO, with the dose gradually tapered until the lowest maintenance dose that controls the symptoms is reached

PO: per oral (by mouth); IV: intravenous; IM: intramuscular; PR: per (by) rectal

If oral preparations cannot be tolerated, other administration routes can be used.

Xonvea®, a delayed-release tablet formulation of doxylamine 10mg (an antihistamine) and pyridoxine 10mg (vitamin B6) was marketed in the UK in 2018. It is the first anti-emetic specifically licensed for treatment of nausea and vomiting in pregnancy when conventional management has not worked. However, there is no evidence to show how the safety and efficacy of doxylamine/pyridoxine compares with current first-line treatment options such as antihistamines (NICE 2019c).

Dyspepsia

Dyspepsia occurs in 30–80% of women at some point during their pregnancy, and it is due to gastro-oesophageal reflux involving a combination of mechanical and hormonal factors (CKS 2017). Lifestyle and diet modification advice should be offered to women presenting with symptoms of dyspepsia. This includes:

- Eating smaller meals more frequently (every 3 hours)
- Avoiding eating late at night (less than 3 hours before bedtime)
- Avoiding known irritants (e.g. alcohol, caffeine, carbonated drinks, fatty and spicy food)
- Keeping a food diary to identify triggers
- Raising the head by 10–15cm in bed
- Avoiding medicines that may trigger symptoms where possible (e.g. NSAIDs)
- Stopping smoking (if applicable).

If heartburn remains troublesome, despite lifestyle and diet modification measures, antacids may be offered. Antacid products containing combinations of aluminium and magnesium are recommended on an 'as required' basis. Alginate products (such as Gaviscon® Advance) are particularly useful if symptoms of gastro-oesophageal reflux are dominant. Antacids affect the absorption of many drugs and may damage enteric coatings, so these should not be taken at the same time as other medicines.

If symptoms are severe or persist (despite treatment with an antacid or alginate), an acid-suppressing medicine such as ranitidine (off-label in pregnancy) or omeprazole is recommended. The recommended dose for ranitidine is 150mg twice a day. The standard dose for omeprazole is 20mg daily, although a lower dose of 10mg has been shown to be effective in some people. Therefore, the lowest effective dose should be prescribed in pregnancy (CKS 2017).

Constipation

Women who present with constipation in pregnancy should be offered information regarding diet modification, such as bran or wheat fibre supplementation. They should also be offered advice on fluid intake and activity levels, as appropriate. If these measures are ineffective, or symptoms do not respond adequately, short-term treatment with oral laxatives can be considered. The dose, choice, and combination of laxatives used should be adjusted, depending on the woman's symptoms, their preference, the desired speed of symptom relief and the response to treatment. A bulk-forming laxative (such as ispaghula) is first-line. If stools remain hard, an osmotic laxative (such as lactulose) can be taken. If stools are soft but difficult to pass, or there is a sensation of incomplete emptying, a short course of a stimulant such as senna can be considered. If the response to treatment remains inadequate, a glycerol suppository can be considered to provide relief (NICE 2019a).

Haemorrhoids

There is lack of evidence on the effectiveness of treatments for haemorrhoids in pregnancy. Diet modification and advice to minimise constipation and straining should be given. An increase in daily fluid and fibre intake is advised to promote soft, bulky regular stools, to relieve constipation and reduce straining. If symptoms persist despite these measures, a topical preparation for haemorrhoids can be offered (NICE 2019a).

Varicose veins

Varicose veins are a common symptom of pregnancy and do not cause harm. Compression stockings can ease the symptoms but will not prevent varicose veins from emerging (NICE 2019a).

Vaginal discharge

An increase in vaginal discharge is a common physiological change that occurs during pregnancy. If it is associated with itch, soreness, offensive smell or pain on passing urine, the cause may be an infection and investigation should be considered. If vaginal candidiasis is suspected, a seven-day course of a topical imidazole is an effective treatment. There is uncertainty about the effectiveness and safety of oral treatments for vaginal candidiasis in pregnancy so these treatments should not be offered (NICE 2019a).

Backache

Exercising in water, massage therapy, and group or individual back care classes may help to ease back pain during pregnancy. Paracetamol is generally considered to be safe to use in pregnancy (NICE 2019a).

Diabetes

It is estimated that approximately 5% of pregnant women have either pre-existing diabetes or gestational diabetes. Women with pre-existing diabetes who are planning to get pregnant should establish good blood glucose control before conception and continue this throughout pregnancy to reduce the risk of miscarriage, congenital malformation and stillbirth. Folic acid (5mg daily) should be taken until 12 weeks of gestation to reduce the risk of having a baby with a neural tube defect. The recommended capillary plasma glucose ranges are the same as those for people with type 1 diabetes:

- A fasting plasma glucose level of 5–7mmol/litre on waking
- A plasma glucose level 4–7mmol/litre before meals at other times of the day.

Women should also aim to keep their HbA1c level below 48mmol/mol (6.5%), if this is possible without causing problematic hypoglycaemia (NICE 2015).

All oral anti-diabetic drugs, except metformin hydrochloride, should be discontinued before pregnancy (or as soon as an unplanned pregnancy is identified) and replaced with insulin therapy (NICE 2015). Metformin is a biguanide used in the management of type 2 diabetes or off-licence in pregnant women with type 1 diabetes. It acts by lowering basal and postprandial plasma glucose without stimulating insulin secretion, thereby reducing the risk of hypoglycaemia associated with insulin therapy. The available evidence does not show an increased risk of congenital malformation, or other adverse effects on the foetus, with the use of metformin.

Gestational diabetes can develop during pregnancy and usually disappears after giving birth. It can occur at any stage of pregnancy but is more common in the second or third trimester. It develops as a result of insufficient production of insulin to meet the extra needs in pregnancy. To estimate the risk of women developing gestational diabetes, the following risk factors should be determined (NICE 2015):

- BMI above 30kg/m^2
- Previous macrosomic baby weighing 4.5kg or above
- Previous gestational diabetes
- Family history of diabetes (first-degree relative with diabetes)
- Minority ethnic family origin with a high prevalence of diabetes.

In individuals who have a fasting plasma glucose level below 7mmol/litre at diagnosis, a trial of changes in diet and exercise should be considered first. If blood glucose targets are not met within 1–2 weeks, despite these lifestyle modifications, metformin should be offered. If metformin is not suitable, then insulin should be considered instead (NICE 2015).

In insulin-treated diabetes, the rapid-acting insulin analogues (aspart and lispro) have advantages over soluble human insulin during pregnancy. Women using insulin should be informed of the risks of hypoglycaemia and impaired awareness of hypoglycaemia in pregnancy, particularly in the first trimester. They should therefore always carry with them a fast-acting form of glucose (e.g. dextrose tablets or glucose-containing drinks).

Best practice guidelines should be referred to for further information on the diagnosis and management of diabetes during pregnancy, labour and birth (American Diabetes Association 2020, NICE 2015).

Case study: Pregnancy with diabetes

A 35-year-old woman is planning to get pregnant. She was diagnosed with type 2 diabetes two years ago and is currently taking gliclazide 80mg once a day. Her last HbA1c level was 55mmol/mol (7.2%).

Activity 6.3 (Case study)
What advice would you give this woman, and what changes to her medication would you consider?

Hypertension

Hypertension can present in different ways in pregnancy:
- Chronic – pre-existing hypertension or detected before 20 weeks of gestation
- Gestational – new hypertension presenting after 20 weeks of gestation without significant proteinuria
- Pre-eclampsia – new hypertension presenting after 20 weeks with significant proteinuria
- Eclampsia – occurrence of seizures associated with pre-eclampsia.

Hypertensive disorders occur in 8–10% of all pregnancies. Women are at high risk of developing pre-eclampsia if they have any of the following risk factors (NICE 2019b):
- Hypertensive disease during a previous pregnancy
- Chronic kidney disease
- Autoimmune disease such as lupus erythematosus or antiphospholipid syndrome
- Type 1 or type 2 diabetes
- Chronic hypertension.

Women with one of the above risk factors should be advised to take 75–150mg aspirin daily from 12 weeks gestation until birth. The same advice applies to women who have more than one moderate risk factor from the following (NICE 2019b):
- First pregnancy
- Age 40 years or older
- Pregnancy interval of more than 10 years
- Body mass index (BMI) of $35kg/m^2$ or more at first visit
- Family history of pre-eclampsia
- Multi-foetal pregnancy.

Women with chronic hypertension who are planning a pregnancy should be referred to a specialist in hypertensive disorders to discuss the risks and benefits of treatment. If they are taking angiotensin-converting enzyme (ACE) inhibitors (e.g. ramipril) or angiotensin II receptor blockers (ARBs) (e.g. losartan) or thiazide (e.g. bendroflumethiazide) or thiazide-like diuretics, they should be advised that these drugs carry an increased risk of congenital abnormalities if taken during pregnancy. Alternative treatment should therefore be discussed as appropriate.

If a woman becomes pregnant, ACE inhibitors or ARBs should be stopped within two working days of notification of the pregnancy, and alternative treatments should be offered (NICE 2019b).

Labetalol is the drug of choice when treating chronic hypertension in pregnant women. If labetalol is unsuitable, nifedipine should be offered. Methyldopa is the third-line option if neither labetalol nor nifedipine is suitable. The choice of anti-hypertensive treatment should take into account any pre-existing treatment, side-effect profiles, risks (including foetal effects) and the woman's preference. The target blood pressure is 135/85mmHg, when using medicines to control hypertension in pregnancy (NICE 2019b). This treatment protocol with the pharmacological agents outlined so far also applies in the treatment of gestational hypertension and pre-eclampsia. Best practice guidelines should be referred to for further information on the diagnosis and management of hypertensive disorders during pregnancy, labour and birth (NICE 2019b).

Mental health disorders

The most common mental health disorders encountered in pregnancy are depression and anxiety. Around 12% of women experience depression and approximately 13% experience anxiety at some point, and many women will experience both. These conditions also affect 15–20% of women in the first year after childbirth. It is therefore of the utmost importance that healthcare professionals discuss mental health with all women of childbearing potential who have a pre-existing, new or past mental health problem (NICE 2020). The discussions should include:

- Any plans to get pregnant and the use of contraception
- The effects of pregnancy and childbirth on mental health, including the possibility of relapse
- The effects of treatment for a mental health disorder on the mother, the foetus and the infant
- The effects of mental health disorders and associated treatments on parenting.

The most up-to-date data should be considered when deciding to prescribe psychotropic medicines for women with childbearing potential. Women should be involved in all decisions concerning their care and that of their babies. A multidisciplinary integrated care plan should be developed for any woman with a mental health problem to ensure that interventions are offered in a timely manner in the postnatal period and care provided is effective, with ongoing review. In women who are stabilised on an antidepressant, it may be appropriate to continue their current treatment to minimise the risks associated with destabilisation, especially in cases where there is a high risk of relapse (NICE 2020).

Medicines during breastfeeding

It is widely recognised that breastfeeding provides immunological and nutritional benefits for infants. However, when a mother takes medicines, there are concerns about the possible effects on the infant. There is little evidence available on this. However, the potential for harm to the infant theoretically depends on:

- The amount of drug or active substance that reaches the infant
- The pharmacokinetics of the infant
- The pharmacodynamic properties of the drug in the infant.

The amount of drug transferred to the infant via breast milk is often thought to be insufficient to exert a noticeable effect on the infant. However, a small amount of drug present in breast milk can induce a hypersensitivity reaction.

If a drug is present in a substantial quantity in breast milk it can produce a pharmacological effect on the infant and potentially cause adverse effects. Infants born prematurely, or who have jaundice, are at higher risk of toxicity from drugs in breast milk.

General principles

Knowledge of the extent of a drug's passage into breast milk and its effects in infants is required to assess the benefit and risks of a treatment. When prescribing medicines in breastfeeding mothers, the following principles should be followed (Specialist Pharmacy Service 2017):

- Avoid unnecessary use of medicines and limit the use of over-the-counter products
- Advise breastfeeding mothers to seek guidance on the suitability of any over-the-counter medicines prior to use
- Assess the benefits and risks both to the mother and the infant
- Avoid the use of medicines known to be toxic in adults and/or infants
- Remember that neonates and premature infants are at increased risk from exposure to medicines via breast milk due to the risk of drug accumulation
- Select a regimen and route of administration which exposes the infant to the lowest possible quantity of the drug
- Remember that drugs with a long half-life can increase the risk of accumulation in the infant and increase the risk of adverse effects
- Polypharmacy may pose an increased risk, especially when there are adverse side effects such as drowsiness
- Infants exposed to drugs via breast milk should be monitored for unusual signs or symptoms
- Avoid prescribing new drugs if therapeutically equivalent alternatives that have been more widely used are available.

Case study: Pain relief while pregnant or breastfeeding

A woman was taking codeine infrequently for lower back pain while she was pregnant. She has given birth recently but is still experiencing lower back pain which cannot be managed with paracetamol alone.

She is wondering if she can have more codeine to manage her pain. And, during your consultation, you find out that she is breastfeeding her infant.

Activity 6.4 (Case study)
Describe your approach in managing this case.

Case study:
Blood pressure treatment while breastfeeding
A woman with chronic hypertension has recently given birth. She is worried that she will be unable to breastfeed her baby, as she is taking medication to manage her blood pressure.

Activity 6.5 (Case study)
1. What advice would you give her on the use of anti-hypertensive treatment while breastfeeding?
2. What changes to her treatment and additional monitoring would you consider making?

Answers to activities

Activity 6.1
Taking into consideration the properties of the drugs/agents below, describe whether or not each one is likely to cross the placenta:

1. Enoxaparin
Enoxaparin is a low molecular weight heparin (LMWH) with a mean molecular weight of approximately 4,500 daltons (Da), most drugs with molecular weight >1000 Da do not cross the placenta. LMWHs are therefore agents of choice for antenatal and postnatal thromboprophylaxis as they do not cross the placenta.

2. Diazepam
Diazepam is highly lipid soluble so it can rapidly cross the placenta. This is of particular importance if it is used in high doses near term, as it is associated with a risk of neonatal withdrawal syndrome. Monitoring for withdrawal signs (such as neonatal respiratory depression) is advised. Use of diazepam around term should therefore be avoided unless use can be clinically justified (e.g. for seizure control).

3. Insulin
Insulin has a high molecular weight so it does not cross the placenta. It is a preferred agent for managing diabetes in pregnancy.

4. Alcohol
Alcohol is relatively small and therefore readily diffuses across the placenta. Although it is polar in nature, it is lipophilic to a degree and this also helps it cross the placenta. Alcohol should be avoided in pregnancy as it can cause toxicity in the foetus.

Activity 6.2
To assess the risks of a medicine or chemical exposure in a pregnant woman, you decide to contact UKTIS for advice. What information about your patient would be useful to provide in the following scenarios?

1. A medicine is to be used for a therapeutic reason

2. The patient has inadvertently been exposed to a chemical or a drug.

In both cases the following maternal details would be useful to ascertain:
- Last menstrual period and estimated date of delivery
- Maternal medical history and any medications taken (including herbal and over-the-counter medicines)
- Obstetric history (how many previous pregnancies, any history of miscarriage or malformations)
- Family history.

1. A medicine is to be used for a therapeutic reason:
- Indication for treatment
- Retrospective or prospective use of the medicine
- Drug, dose, frequency, route, duration of treatment if known
- Stage of pregnancy at exposure
- Previous treatments and efficacy.

2. For overdose and chemical exposures:
- Agent/s involved (including route of exposure and estimated dose)
- Date, time and duration of exposure
- Maternal symptoms and treatment received
- Results of relevant investigations and foetal monitoring.

Activity 6.3 (Case study)
A 35-year-old woman is planning to get pregnant. She was diagnosed with type 2 diabetes two years ago and is currently taking gliclazide 80mg once a day. Her last HbA1c level was 55mmol/mol (7.2%).

What advice would you give this woman, and what changes to her medication would you consider?

Appropriate advice, information and support should be provided to women with diabetes to enable them to have a positive experience of pregnancy and childbirth. Establishing good control of blood glucose before conception and maintaining this throughout pregnancy helps to reduce the risk of miscarriage, congenital malformation, stillbirth and neonatal death. Information provided should also cover the following (NICE 2015):

- How nausea and vomiting in pregnancy can affect blood glucose control
- The increased risk of having a baby who is large for gestational age, which increases the likelihood of birth trauma, induction of labour and caesarean section
- The need for assessment of diabetic retinopathy before and during pregnancy
- The need for assessment of diabetic nephropathy before pregnancy
- The importance of maternal blood glucose control during labour and birth and early feeding of the baby, in order to reduce the risk of neonatal hypoglycaemia
- The possibility of temporary health problems in the baby during the neonatal period, which may require admission to the neonatal unit
- The risk of the baby developing obesity and/or diabetes in later life.

Individualised dietary advice should also be provided and, where possible, women should be invited to attend a structured education programme. Women who have a BMI above $27kg/m^2$ should be given advice on how to lose weight. When trying to conceive, women with diabetes should also take folic acid (5mg/day) until 12 weeks of gestation to reduce the risk of having a baby with a neural tube defect. Until good blood glucose control is achieved, women should be advised to use contraception. Monthly monitoring of HbA1c levels should be undertaken in women planning to get pregnant and they should also be self-monitoring their blood glucose (NICE 2015).

Full medication history should be taken, and medicines should be reviewed before and during pregnancy. In this case, the patient is on gliclazide, which is a sulfonylurea. Sulfonylureas should generally be avoided in pregnancy because of the risk of neonatal hypoglycaemia. It would therefore be useful to identify why the patient was not on metformin, as it is the recommended first-line treatment, and whether it is possible to switch her to it. If metformin is not suitable or effective, insulin should be considered.

Activity 6.4 (Case study)

A woman was taking codeine infrequently for lower back pain while she was pregnant. She has given birth recently but is still experiencing lower back pain which cannot be managed with paracetamol alone.

She is wondering if she can have more codeine to manage her pain. And, during your consultation, you find out that she is breastfeeding her infant.

Describe your approach in managing this case.

It is important to manage pain appropriately during pregnancy and postpartum in order to minimise the risk of adverse outcomes for both mother and baby. Inadequately managed pain can lead to anxiety and depression, which can affect the mother's overall physical and psychological well-being, as well as her ability to provide care for her baby. Non-pharmacological interventions should be considered first – for example, adequate rest, hot and cold compresses, massage, acupuncture, physiotherapy, relaxation and exercise. Non-pharmacological remedies are advocated where possible, but in some cases reluctance to prescribe analgesia can inadvertently result in increased use of inappropriate over-the-counter medication or herbal remedies (RCOG 2016).

Paracetamol is considered the analgesic of choice for breastfeeding women as the risk to a breastfed infant is low. The quantity of paracetamol that reaches the milk is very small, representing only a small proportion of a normal therapeutic infant dose.

There is very limited information on the use of NSAIDs and breastfeeding but the preferred NSAID in this situation is ibuprofen. Ibuprofen is considered safe for the breastfed infant as only very small quantities appear to be excreted into breast milk after maternal ingestion. It is therefore the second-line option after paracetamol (RCOG 2016).

If ibuprofen is ineffective or unsuitable or women experience more severe pain and require additional analgesia, then opioid analgesics should be used.

Until recently, codeine was the preferred opioid for use in breastfeeding mothers. However, a fatal case of morphine toxicity in a breastfed infant following maternal use of codeine led the Medicines and Healthcare products Regulatory Agency (MHRA) and European Medicines Agency (EMA) to contraindicate its use in breastfeeding women. There have also been several reports of adverse effects in breastfed infants following maternal use of codeine. These include bradycardia, respiratory depression, lethargy, drowsiness, poor feeding, cyanosis and infant death. Instead of codeine, the weak opioids, dihydrocodeine and tramadol, can be considered. The lowest effective dose should be administered for the shortest duration, and regular use of any opioid beyond three days should always be under close medical supervision (RCOG 2016).

All breastfeeding mothers should be informed of potential problems with opioids and advised to stop breastfeeding if adverse effects develop and to seek medical advice.

Activity 6.5 (Case study)

A woman with chronic hypertension has recently given birth. She is worried that she will be unable to breastfeed her baby, as she is taking medication to manage her blood pressure.

1. **What advice would you give her on the use of anti-hypertensive treatment while breastfeeding?**

2. What changes to her treatment and additional monitoring would you consider making?

Women with hypertension who wish to breastfeed should be advised that their treatment can be adapted to accommodate breastfeeding; and taking anti-hypertensive medication need not prevent them breastfeeding (NICE 2019b).

However, it should be explained to these women that anti-hypertensive medicines can pass into breast milk but usually only at very low levels (NICE 2019b). The amounts taken in by babies are therefore very small and would be unlikely to have any clinical effect. The manufacturer's information may advise against the use of a medicine during breastfeeding, but this is generally because most medicines are not tested in pregnant or breastfeeding women and not because of any specific safety concerns or evidence of harm. Women should be involved in the decisions on their treatment and these decisions should take their preferences into account (NICE 2019b).

As anti-hypertensive medicines have the potential to transfer into breast milk, monitoring the blood pressure of babies should be considered, especially in those born premature. Women should be advised to monitor their babies for drowsiness, lethargy, pallor, cold peripheries or poor feeding.

When treating women with anti-hypertensive medication during the postnatal period, medicines that are taken once daily should be used when possible (NICE 2019b).

Enalapril, which is an ACE inhibitor, is the recommended agent to treat hypertension in women during the postnatal period, with appropriate monitoring of maternal renal function and maternal serum potassium. For women of black African or Caribbean family origin with hypertension during the postnatal period, nifedipine or amlodipine are recommended instead (NICE 2019b).

References and further reading

American Diabetes Association (ADA) (2020). Management of diabetes in pregnancy: Standards of medical care. *Diabetes Care.* **43** (1), S.183–92. https://doi.org/10.2337/dc20-S014 (Last accessed 5 October 2020).

British National Formulary (BNF) (2020). https://bnf.nice.org.uk/ (Last accessed 9 September 2020).

Clinical Knowledge Summary (CKS) (2017). Dyspepsia – pregnancy associated. https://cks.nice.org.uk/topics/dyspepsia-pregnancy-associated/ (Last accessed 9 September 2020).

Clinical Knowledge Summary (CKS) (2019). Antenatal care – uncomplicated pregnancy. https://cks.nice.org.uk/topics/antenatal-care-uncomplicated-pregnancy (Last accessed 9 September 2020).

Clinical Knowledge Summary (CKS) (2020). Nausea/vomiting in pregnancy. https://cks.nice.org.uk/nauseavomiting-in-pregnancy (Last accessed 9 September 2020).

Davey, L. & Houghton, D. (2020). *The Midwives Pocket Formulary,* 4th edn. London: Elsevier.

Department of Health (DH) (1997). The Prescription Only Medicines (Human Use) Amendment Order 1997.

Electronic Medicines Compendium (emc) (n.d.). *Summary of Product Characteristics.* https://www.medicines.org.uk/emc#gref (Last accessed 20 September 2020).

Legislation.gov.uk. 2020. Medicines Act 1968. [online] http://www.legislation.gov.uk/ukpga/1968/67/contents (Last accessed May 2020).

Medicines and Healthcare Products Regulatory Agency (MHRA) (2019a). Medicines with teratogenic potential: what is effective contraception and how often is pregnancy testing needed? https://www.gov.uk/drug-safety-update/medicines-with-teratogenic-potential-what-is-effective-contraception-and-how-often-is-pregnancy-testing-needed (Last accessed 9 September 2020).

Medicines and Healthcare Products Regulatory Agency (MHRA) (2019b). Pregnancy testing and contraception for pregnancy prevention during treatment with medicines of teratogenic potential. https://assets.publishing.service.gov.uk/media/5c936a4840f0b633f5bfd895/pregnancy_testing_and_contraception_table_for_medicines_with_teratogenic_potential_final.pdf (Last accessed 9 September 2020).

National Institute for Health and Clinical Excellence (NICE) (2015). Diabetes in pregnancy: management from preconception to the postnatal period. https://www.nice.org.uk/guidance/ng3 (Last accessed 9 September 2020).

National Institute for Health and Clinical Excellence (NICE) (2018). Depression–antenatal and postnatal. Clinical Knowledge Summary. https://cks.nice.org.uk/depression-antenatal-and-postnatal (Last accessed 9 September 2020).

National Institute for Health and Clinical Excellence (NICE) (2019a). Antenatal care for uncomplicated pregnancies. https://www.nice.org.uk/guidance/cg62 (Last accessed 9 September 2020).

National Institute for Health and Clinical Excellence (NICE) (2019b). Hypertension in pregnancy: diagnosis and management. https://www.nice.org.uk/guidance/ng133 (Last accessed 9 September 2020).

National Institute for Health and Clinical Excellence (NICE) (2019c). Doxylamine/pyridoxine (Xonvea) for treating nausea and vomiting of pregnancy. https://www.nice.org.uk/advice/es20/chapter/Key-messages (Last accessed 9 September 2020).

National Institute for Health and Clinical Excellence (NICE) (2020). Antenatal and postnatal mental health: clinical management and service guidance. https://www.nice.org.uk/guidance/cg192 (Last accessed 9 September 2020).

Nursing and Midwifery Council (NMC) (2019). *Standards of Proficiency for Midwives*. London: Nursing & Midwifery Council.

Nursing and Midwifery Council (NMC) (2020). Practising as a midwife in the UK (2020). London: NMC.

Royal College of Nursing (RCN). (2019). Prescribing in Pregnancy. https://www.rcn.org.uk/clinical-topics/medicines-management/prescribing-in-pregnancy (Last accessed 9 September 2020).

Royal College of Obstetricians and Gynaecologists (RCOG) (2016). The management of nausea and vomiting of pregnancy and hyperemesis gravidarum. https://www.rcog.org.uk/en/guidelines-research-services/guidelines/gtg69/ (Last accessed 9 September 2020).

Royal College of Obstetricians and Gynaecologists (RCOG) (2018). Antenatal and postnatal analgesia. https://obgyn.onlinelibrary.wiley.com/doi/full/10.1111/1471-0528.15510 (Last accessed 9 September 2020).

Royal Pharmaceutical Society (RPS) and Royal College of Nursing (RCN) (2019). Professional Guidance on the Administration of Medicines in Healthcare Settings. https://www.rpharms.com/Portals/0/RPS%20document%20library/Open%20access/Professional%20standards/SSHM%20and%20Admin/Admin%20of%20Meds%20prof%20guidance.pdf?ver=2019-01-23-145026-567. (Last accessed 5 October 2020).

Royal Pharmaceutical Society (RPS) (2016). A Competency Framework for all Prescribers. https://www.rpharms.com/resources/frameworks/prescribers-competency-framework (Last accessed 9 September 2020).

Specialist Pharmacy Service (2017), UKDILAS: General Principles for medicine use during breastfeeding. https://www.sps.nhs.uk/articles/ukdilas-general-principles-for-medicine-use-during-breastfeeding/ (Last accessed 9 September 2020).

Specialist Pharmacy Service (2019), UKMi: How can nausea and vomiting be treated during pregnancy? https://www.sps.nhs.uk/articles/how-can-nausea-and-vomiting-be-treated-during-pregnancy-2/ (Last accessed 9 September 2020).

Stephens, S. & Wilson, G. (2009). Principles in pregnant women: guide to general principles. *Prescriber*. **20**(23/24), 43–46.

Schaefer, C., Peters, P.W.J. & Miller, R.K. (2015). *Drugs During Pregnancy and Lactation*. 3rd edn. London: Elsevier.

UK Teratology Information Service (2020). http://www.uktis.org/ (Last accessed 9 September 2020).

Whittlesea, C. & Walker, R. (2012). *Clinical Pharmacy and Therapeutics*. 5th edn. London: Churchill Livingstone Elsevier.

7

Pharmacological case studies: Children

Jennie Craske
MSc, RN (child),
Clinical Nurse Specialist, Pain and Sedation Service, Alder Hey Children's NHS Foundation Trust

Andrea Gill
MSc, MRPharmS,
Clinical Pharmacy Services Manager and Chair of Safe Medication Practice Committee, Alder Hey Children's NHS Foundation Trust

This chapter:
- Explores the influence of age and immaturity in prescribing analgesia for neonates and infants
- Explains the licensing of medicines in children
- Discusses the different drugs used in acute pain, and the concept of multimodal analgesia
- Outlines the principles of prescribing oral analgesia appropriate to a child's level of pain
- Explains the concepts of weight-related dosing and age-banded dosing in children.

Introduction

Babies and children feel pain in much the same way as adults do, and analgesia should be administered to help relieve their pain. However, when prescribing analgesia for children, the prescriber needs to consider a range of additional factors that are not usually considered when prescribing for adults. These factors include:

- The influence of age and immaturity in prescribing analgesia for neonates and infants
- Dose calculations based on the age and weight of the child
- Dose formulations available and the palatability of medicines
- Any restrictions in the marketing authorisation (MA)/product licence of the medicine.

The terms 'neonate', 'infant' and 'child' describe specific age groups in paediatrics. In common with the BNF, this chapter will define these age groups as:
- Neonate: up to 28 days of life
- Infant: up to one year of age
- Child: up to 12 years of age.

The influence of age and immaturity

The ways drugs are handled by the body develop and mature throughout childhood but especially during the first two years of life. Accurate dosing for neonates and infants must therefore take into account not only differences in weight, but also the patient's age. To distinguish between the stages when age impacts on dosing, Anderson and Holford (2013) used the term 'immature children' to describe neonates and infants, and the term 'small adults' to describe children. For example, doses of paracetamol and morphine vary with age and weight in neonates and infants, whereas doses in children over one year of age only vary with the weight of the child.

Prescribing small doses

Weight-based dosing in babies and infants may result in small volumes of medicine being administered. A recent audit of liquid medications prescribed for babies and children in hospital showed that 1 in 8 of these doses could not be measured in a single syringe (Morecroft *et al.* 2013). When prescribing small doses, the prescriber therefore has a duty to check not only that the dose is correct, but also that it is possible to administer the dose accurately, given the available drug formulation(s).

Licensing of medicines for children

The use of many medicines in children is not licensed. A summary of the information contained in the marketing authorisation/licence is contained in the Summary of Product Characteristics (SPC) available on www.medicines.org.uk. There are two types of prescribing that are not included in this information:
- Unlicensed prescribing
- Off-label prescribing.

Unlicensed prescribing

This term describes prescribing a medicinal product that has not been subject to the UK licensing process overseen by the Medicines and Healthcare Regulatory Agency (MHRA). Products may be licensed in other countries and imported, or manufactured by 'specials' units or by individual pharmacies. Or they may be chemicals or clinical trial preparations. Examples include:

- Tramadol suspension prepared by a hospital pharmacy department
- Paracetamol 30mg suppositories available from a specials manufacturer.

Off-label prescribing

This term describes situations in which a licensed medicinal product is used in a way that was not included in the MA/licence. Examples include:

- Paracetamol oral suspension for a four-week-old baby; this is off-label as this product is licensed for those over two months old
- Diclofenac suppositories in a four-year-old child with post-operative pain; this is off-label as this product is licensed for this age for juvenile chronic arthritis only.

Non-medical prescribers are allowed to prescribe an off-label or unlicensed medicine as long as they are able to justify their case that use is reasonable and there is no suitable licensed alternative. However, information leaflets included in the packaging of medicines can only reflect licensed uses. For this reason, the Royal College of Paediatrics and Child Health and the Neonatal and Paediatric Pharmacists Group have produced additional information leaflets to support unlicensed use of many medicines in children. These leaflets are available at www.medicinesforchildren.org.uk

Prescribing analgesia

When prescribing analgesia for children, it is important to start by assessing the degree of pain the child is experiencing. A range of pain tools exist to score pain in babies and children. Self-report tools are preferred for verbal children. The FACES scale (Wong & Baker 1988) consists of six faces ranging in expression from neutral to distressed, with each representing a different pain score, from 0 to 10. The child is asked to point at the face that best describes their pain. The FACES scale is validated for children from three years of age. In older children, a visual analogue scale may be used. The choice of tool depends on the cognitive level at which the child is functioning, which may be impaired when they are experiencing severe pain or illness. In practice, a sheet containing both tools allows the child to choose the one they prefer.

Behavioural tools can be used to score pain in babies and non-verbal children. FLACC (Merkel *et al.* 1997) and CRIES (Krechel & Bildner 1995) each use five pain behaviours, which are scored from 0 to 2, depending on severity. CRIES is validated in babies from 32 weeks' gestation; FLACC is validated in babies from two months to seven years of age.

The pain tools described above use a 0–10 scale. Scores 1–3 represent mild pain, 4–6 moderate pain and 7–10 severe pain. Using a validated pain tool to score pain prior to giving analgesia and one hour later allows the analgesic efficacy of the chosen prescription(s) to be evaluated.

Analgesic drugs can be split into two main categories – non-opioid and opioid analgesics.

Table 7.1: Common oral analgesics used in children with acute pain

Non-opioid analgesics	Opioid analgesics
Paracetamol NSAIDs: • Diclofenac • Ibuprofen	Dihydrocodeine Morphine Tramadol

The analgesic ladder below shows how severity of pain determines which combination of analgesia should be prescribed. Mild pain may be treated with either paracetamol or ibuprofen, moderate pain with a combination of paracetamol and ibuprofen, and severe pain with a combination of paracetamol, ibuprofen and morphine.

Table 7.2: Analgesic ladder in children with acute pain

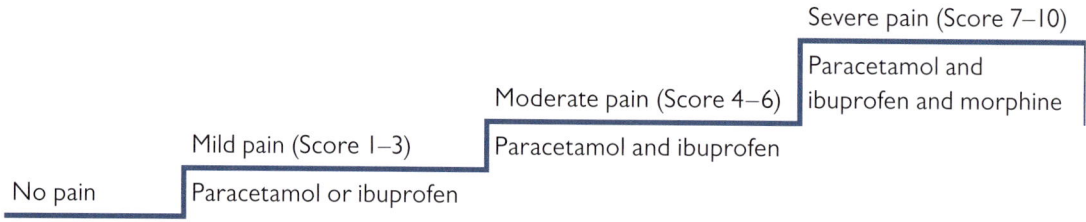

Paracetamol

Licensing
Oral paracetamol preparations are licensed for treatment of mild to moderate pain and as an antipyretic in children from the age of two months, and for the treatment of post-vaccination fever in infants aged two to three months.

Pharmacokinetics
The bioavailability of oral paracetamol is about 80% and onset of action should be within 20 minutes after administration, with maximum effects within 2 hours. Paracetamol is metabolised primarily by the liver but metabolic pathways in younger children may differ from those in adults. One pathway that occurs in both adults and children involves cytochrome P450 and results in a toxic metabolite, N-acetyl-p-benzo-quinone imine (NAPQI). Normally NAPQI is detoxified by glutathione. However, if there is insufficient glutathione, NAPQI will bind to hepatocytes, causing severe liver damage. Thus hepatotoxicity may occur due to excess NAPQI levels (for instance, after a paracetamol overdose) or with 'normal' doses of paracetamol if glutathione levels are depleted as a result of taking liver enzyme-inducing drugs, being malnourished or having a febrile illness (see 'Emergency Treatment of Poisoning' section in the BNFc).

Formulations of paracetamol

Paracetamol is available in a range of child-friendly formulations, as shown in Table 6.3 (below).

Table 7.3: Child-friendly paracetamol formulations

Oral suspension	Soluble tablet	Tablet	Suppository
120mg/5ml 250mg/5ml	120mg 500mg	500mg	30mg, 60mg, 125mg, 250mg, 500mg

Paracetamol dosing

The simplicity gained from the range of formulations is contrasted by the complicated issue of which dose to prescribe. Should the dose be based on the age or the weight of the child?

Weight-related doses of paracetamol

In the BNFc 2013/14, the oral paracetamol dose for severe postoperative pain in children from 1 month to 12 years is 20–30mg/kg as a single dose then 15–20mg/kg every 4–6 hours; maximum 90mg/kg daily in divided doses. The electronic version of BNFc now states a maximum daily dose of 75mg/kg, due to recent evidence which suggests that, while there may be little analgesic benefit to be gained from daily doses greater than 75mg/kg, there is a small possibility of paracetamol toxicity in 'at risk' children given 90mg/kg daily for more than two consecutive days. In contrast, the age-banded doses of paracetamol suspension may be on the conservative side and may not provide adequate analgesia, especially if the child is a reasonable weight for their age (see BNFc for details).

> **Good practice point: Millilitres versus milligrams**
>
> Although the age-banded doses on bottles of paracetamol oral suspension are printed on the bottles in millilitres (ml), it is good practice to prescribe doses in milligrams (mg) in order to reduce the risk of medication error due to administering the correct volume of the wrong strength suspension.

> **Good practice point: Fixed doses and dose ranges**
>
> With some of the age-banded doses printed on bottles of paracetamol oral suspension, a dose range is advised. Although, this may be appropriate for parent-initiated treatment, it is best practice to prescribe a fixed dose from within that range, so that the dose choice is determined by the prescriber, rather than the person administering the medication.

> ### Case study: Paracetamol
> John is 10 years old, a twin, and weighs 25kg. He has chronic renal impairment but does not require dialysis. John's twin brother, James, is fit and well and weighs 33kg. John has occasional headaches, which last for a day but are relieved with regular paracetamol for 24 hours. John's mother asks your advice. She uses the doses printed on the paracetamol bottle for both her sons, but as James weighs more than John (who is small for his age), she is concerned that she may be inadvertently overdosing John. She has brought a bottle of 250mg/5ml paracetamol suspension with her.

> ### Activity 7.1 (Case study)
> What dosing advice will you give the twins' mother?

NSAIDs

There are more than 20 NSAIDs listed in the BNF but most are not recommended for use in children. Aspirin should be avoided in children due to its association with Reye's syndrome. Ibuprofen is licensed for children and has a palatable oral suspension (100mg/5ml), from which doses can be easily measured and is therefore considered as the first-line NSAID for acute pain in children. Diclofenac may be considered as an alternative NSAID, but licensing in children is limited, depending upon the formulation used. If 25mg tablets are unsuitable for the child, because of the dose or the child being unable to swallow tablets, dispersible tablets may be considered. Unfortunately, there is little evidence to suggest that an accurate dose may be gained by dissolving a dispersible tablet in a known volume of water (e.g. 5–10ml) and withdrawing a portion, despite this being common practice in children's hospitals. The remainder of this section will focus on ibuprofen as the NSAID of choice for children's pain.

Ibuprofen

Licensing

Ibuprofen is licensed for children aged from three months (over 5kg) for mild to moderate pain, post-immunisation pyrexia, rheumatic or muscular pain, headache, reduction of fever, sore throat, teething pain, toothache, minor aches and pains, and symptoms of cold and influenza.

Pharmacokinetics

Ibuprofen has analgesic, antipyretic and anti-inflammatory properties. Onset of action occurs within 30 minutes with the maximum analgesic effect occurring 45 minutes after administration if taken on an empty stomach, or after 1–2 hours when taken with food. The mechanism of action of ibuprofen is unclear but may be due to inhibition of cyclooxygenase activity and prostaglandin synthesis. Ibuprofen is excreted in the urine.

Ibuprofen dosing

As with paracetamol, the prescriber must negotiate the age-based versus weight-based dose choice with ibuprofen. The BNFc states both the weight-based and age-banded doses for the 100mg/5ml ibuprofen suspension (see BNFc for details). The weight-based dose is 30mg/kg daily (maximum 2.4g) in 3–4 divided doses.

Activity 7.2

Access a centile weight chart (boys or girls) for ages 0–4 years, which provides the range of children's weights by age. (Centile charts are available on the Internet if you do not have access to a paper copy.) Determine the following weights:

1. A one-year-old on the 2nd centile for weight
2. A four-year-old on the 98th centile for weight

These two weights represent the range of weights for children aged 1–4 years.

3. Identify the age-banded dose of ibuprofen for children aged 1–4 years, from the BNFc. Then calculate the highest and lowest doses in mg/kg for children in this age range. Compare these doses with the recommended weight-based dose of 30mg/kg daily in 3–4 divided doses.

Case study: NSAIDs

Laura is six years old and weighs 20kg. She was diagnosed with tonsillitis this morning by her GP and has started a course of oral antibiotics. Her mother has brought her to the walk-in clinic this evening because her throat remains very sore and she has already had the four doses of paracetamol she is allowed today. Laura's pain is making it difficult for her to eat and drink. Laura is usually fit and well and has a salbutamol inhaler, which she requires occasionally for viral-induced wheeze.

Activity 7.3 (Case study)

What will you suggest for Laura?

Opioid analgesia

Until very recently, codeine was the oral opioid analgesic most frequently used for children. However, in June 2013 the MHRA recommended restrictions on the use of codeine in children, following a review of reports of children in the USA who developed serious adverse effects or died after taking codeine for pain relief. Codeine is converted to morphine in the liver by the CYP2D6 enzyme. There are many genetic variations of CYP2D6 which affect the rate and extent of this conversion and which vary markedly with ethnicity. Most of the cases of serious adverse events or death occurred in children who had evidence of being 'ultra-rapid metabolisers' of codeine. This can result in high levels of morphine in the blood and an increased risk of morphine toxicity, such as respiratory depression. Children undergoing tonsillectomy for obstructive sleep apnoea were found to be at increased risk.

Codeine (alone, or in combination with other products) is now contraindicated in:

- ALL children aged 0–18 years old who undergo tonsillectomy or adenoidectomy (or both) for obstructive sleep apnoea
- ALL patients of any age known to be CYP2D6 ultra-rapid metabolisers.

Codeine is not recommended for use in children whose breathing might be compromised, including those with neuromuscular disorders, severe cardiac or respiratory conditions, upper respiratory or lung infections, multiple trauma or extensive surgical procedures.

Codeine should not be used by breastfeeding mothers because it can pass into breast milk.

Other oral opioids that may be used for children are tramadol, dihydrocodeine, oxycodone and morphine. Tramadol is not licensed for children younger than six years of age and is also not available in a licensed child-friendly formulation, so its use is limited. Dihydrocodeine has been found to have poor analgesic activity in children. Oxycodone use in children tends to be limited to relief of chronic, rather than acute pain.

Morphine is now the preferred opioid analgesic for the treatment of moderate to severe pain in children, which has not responded to optimised doses of paracetamol and ibuprofen.

Morphine

Licensing

Oral morphine is not licensed for children less than one year of age. Below this age, the strength of the licensed liquid preparation (10mg/5ml) means that accurate measurement of small doses is difficult and may lead to 10-fold errors. Because of this, specially manufactured oral solutions may be used for smaller doses (e.g. 100 micrograms/ml or 500 micrograms/ml).

Case study: Prescribing small doses

Chloe is a four-year-old girl who has cerebral palsy and weighs 8kg. She has recently had an extended stay in hospital after orthopaedic surgery and is on a weaning regime of oral morphine. Since obtaining further supplies of morphine from her GP, her mother is concerned that she has become very sleepy. She shows you the label on the bottle: 'Morphine 10mg/5ml. Take 0.05ml every 6 hours'. When you ask her to show you the amount she has been giving on an oral syringe, you realise that she has been giving 0.5ml of this solution.

Activity 7.4 (Case study)

Identify how the mother's error could have been prevented.

Pharmacokinetics

The pharmacokinetics of morphine in children are generally considered similar to those in adults, although clearance from the body is slower (morphine half-life is approximately 2 hours in an adult but up to 10 hours in a pre-term neonate). Slower clearance in younger patients is due to immaturity in both hepatic metabolism and renal clearance.

Dosing

The dose of morphine prescribed should be based upon careful assessment of the severity of the child's pain.

If high doses are given, powerful analgesia will occur but the risk of dose-related side effects (such as nausea/vomiting, constipation, drowsiness and potentially serious respiratory depression and reduction in level of consciousness) will be increased.

If low doses are given, weak analgesia will occur, with a reduced incidence of the above side effects.

The age-related doses in the BNFc are intended for the treatment of moderate to severe pain. In our experience, reducing these doses by half should provide adequate doses for mild to moderate pain in conjunction with paracetamol and ibuprofen.

Case study: Multimodal analgesia

Tommy is three years old (weighs 15kg) and had a tonsillectomy three days ago at the local hospital. His mother has dropped into the GP's surgery where you work for advice on his pain relief and has brought Tommy's painkillers to show you. She's worried that there seems to be an awful lot of pain relief medication. Although he's in pain, she's worried about overdosing him. She's also struggling to get all the doses in while he's awake. She's trying to spread out the pain relief over the course of the day and is only managing to get about two doses of each medicine into him.

You see that Tommy has been prescribed:
  Paracetamol 240 mg QDS
  Ibuprofen 150 mg TDS
  Morphine 1.5 mg QDS

Activity 7.5 (Case study)
Work out a dosing schedule that will support Tommy's mother to optimise his analgesia.

Summary

Effective treatment of children's pain relies on optimal dosing of multi-modal analgesia, alone or in combination, depending on the intensity of pain experienced. For the prescriber, this means bearing in mind the influences of age and immaturity when making drug and dose choices and then matching these to a palatable and measurable drug formulation.

Answers to activities

Activity 7.1 (Case study)

What dosing advice will you give the twins' mother?
Ascertain what dose of paracetamol the mother is administering and at what frequency.
If she is using 375mg (8–10 years pre-printed dose):
- This dose for John equates to dose/body weight = 375/25 = 15 mg/kg 4 times daily.
- This is the correct dose of paracetamol for John.
- This dose for James equates to dose/body weight = 375/33 = 11.4 mg/kg 4 times daily.
- This dose is too small for James.

If the dose is paracetamol 500mg (10–12 years pre-printed dose):
- This dose for John equates to dose/body weight = 500/25 = 20 mg/kg 4 times daily.
- This dose is too high for John.
- This dose for James equates to dose/body weight = 500/33 = 15.1 mg/kg 4 times daily
- This is the correct dose of paracetamol for James.

Activity 7.2

Calculate the highest and lowest doses in mg/kg for children in this age range. Compare these doses to the recommended weight-based dose of 30mg/kg daily in 3–4 divided doses.

1. Using a girl's centile chart, a one-year-old on the 2nd centile weighs 7kg.
2. A four-year-old on the 98th centile weighs 21.5kg.
3. Identify the age-banded dose of ibuprofen for children aged 1–4 years, from the BNFc. Then calculate the highest and lowest doses in mg/kg for children in this age range. Compare these doses with the recommended weight-based dose of 30mg/kg daily in 3–4 divided doses.

- The age-banded ibuprofen dose for children aged 1–4 years is 100mg TDS.
- The highest dose for children in this age range would be the 7kg child.
- This dose equates to dose/body weight = 100/7 = 14.3 mg/kg TDS.
- This equates to a daily dose of 14.3 × 3 = 42.9mg/kg, which exceeds the recommended weight-based daily dose of 30mg/kg by more than 40%.
- The lowest dose for children in this age range would be the 21.5kg child.
- This dose equates to dose/body weight = 100/21.5 = 4.7mg/kg TDS.
- This equates to a daily dose of 4.7 × 3 = 14.1mg/kg, which is less than half the recommended weight-based dose of 30mg/kg.

Activity 7.3 (Case study)

What will you suggest for Laura?

To optimise the paracetamol dose:

- Investigate what dose of paracetamol Laura's mother has administered. Has this dose relieved Laura's pain, and, if so, how long did the effect last? Is there scope to recommend another dose and remain within the maximum daily dose of 75mg/kg/day?
- If Laura's mum has been giving her a paracetamol dose of 250mg (the dose on the bottle), this equates to 250/20 = 12.5 mg/kg/dose. This means that so far today Laura has had 4 doses, which is 12.5 × 4 = 50 mg/kg.
- To maximise Laura's daily dose of paracetamol up to 75mg/kg/day, her weight-related dose would be 75 × 20 = 1500mg/4 = 375mg every 6 hours.
- There is plenty of scope for Laura to have another dose now, at the walk-in clinic, of 375mg (and still remain within the daily limit of 75mg/kg). You can recommend that she takes paracetamol at this higher dose for the next 24–36 hours, by which time the antibiotics should have started to take effect and Laura's pain should be relieved.

Possible cautions regarding ibuprofen:

- Is Laura managing to eat and drink or has she stopped taking anything orally due to pain? If she has stopped taking anything orally, is she dehydrated? NSAIDs should be avoided or used with caution in children who might be dehydrated.
- Laura has viral-induced wheeze. About 2–5% of asthmatics are sensitive to NSAIDs, which causes a worsening of asthma symptoms (Jenkins et al. 2004). Check if Laura's mum has ever given her ibuprofen, and – if so – whether there were any problems.
- If Laura is not dehydrated and has previously had ibuprofen to no ill effect, then recommending ibuprofen 150mg TDS (the dose on the bottle) is a good idea.
- If Laura is not dehydrated but has never had ibuprofen before, you will have to decide whether to administer a dose while she is in the walk-in clinic and monitor the effect. The ibuprofen should be given in addition to paracetamol.

Activity 7.4 (Case study)

Identify how the mother's error could have been prevented.

This error may have happened because:
- The parents were given the wrong instructions or misunderstood how to measure 0.05ml (this is a tiny volume, less than 0.1ml, on the oral syringe and is very difficult to measure, while 0.5ml is labelled on the syringe and is much more visible).
- A different strength of morphine has been provided.
- A prescribing or dispensing error has occurred.

This error could have been prevented by:
- Providing written and verbal information and ensuring that the parents understood the instructions and were able to demonstrate how much to administer. An oral syringe should be marked to indicate the appropriate volume.
- Ensuring the hospital provided information on the strength of the morphine solution being used to the GP, as well as the dose required.
- Ensuring this information was also communicated to the community pharmacist.

Activity 7.5 (Case study)

Work out a dosing schedule that will support Tommy's mother to optimise his analgesia.

You are satisfied that these doses are correct. You are also aware that children usually require analgesia for one week after a tonsillectomy, with a peak in pain occurring about three days post-op. You expect Tommy will require regular dosing of these analgesics for at least another four days.

A preschool child may sleep up to 12 hours at night, so a standard six-hourly dosing regime will inevitably result in missed doses. Tommy's mum should be advised that paracetamol, ibuprofen and morphine can be given at the same time. Tommy could be given a dose of each of his medicines at mealtimes – breakfast, lunch and teatime. His mum should be advised to leave at least four hours between doses. This regime leaves one dose of paracetamol and one dose of morphine remaining from his total daily dose, which can be administered together overnight if he wakes. In this way, you can allay Tommy's mother's fears and optimise Tommy's analgesia.

References and further reading

Anderson, B.J. & Holford N.H.G. (2013). Understanding dosing: children are small adults, neonates are immature children. *Archives of Diseases in Childhood.* **98**, 737–44.

BMJ Group. *BNF for Children 2014–2015.* The Royal Pharmaceutical Society of Great Britain, and RCPCH Publications Ltd, UK.

Jenkins, C., Costello, J. & Hodge, L. (2004). Systematic review of prevalence of aspirin induced asthma and its implications for clinical practice. *British Medical Journal.* **328**, 434.

Krechel, S.W. & Bildner, J. (1995). CRIES: a new neonatal postoperative pain measurement score. Initial testing of validity and reliability. *Pediatric Anesthesia.* **5** (1), 53–61.

Merkel, S.I., Voepel-Lewis, T., Shayevitz, J.R. & Malviya, S. (1997). The FLACC: a behavioural scale for scoring postoperative pain in young children. *Pediatric Nursing.* **23** (3), 293–297.

Morecroft, C.W., Caldwell, N.A. & Gill, A. (2013). Prescribing liquid medication: can the dose be accurately given? *Archives of Diseases in Childhood.* **98** (10), 831–32.

NMC circular 4/2010. Nurse and Midwife independent prescribing of unlicensed medicines: http://www.nmc-uk.org/Documents/Circulars/2010circulars/NMCcircular04_2010.pdf (Last accessed 15 August 2014).

Wong, D.L. & Baker, C.M. (1988). Pain in children: comparison of assessment scales. *Pediatric Nurse.* **14** (1), 9–17.

8

Pharmacological case studies: Sexual health and contraception

Su Everett MSc, BSc (Hons), RN V300 Independent Prescriber.
Senior Lecturer, Senior Teaching Fellow Health and Education, Middlesex University, London

Sophie Molloy BSc (Hons), RN. V300 Independent Prescriber.
Module Leader for Contraception and Sexual Health, Lecturer in Adult Nursing, Health and Education, Middlesex University, London

This chapter:
- Discusses the effects on the body of the hormones used in contraception
- Describes the pharmacokinetics of hormonal contraception
- Discusses the teratogenic effects of hormonal contraception
- Discusses prescribing of contraception and sexual health drugs off label
- Discusses antimicrobial resistance related to the prescribing of common antibiotics in the treatment of sexually transmitted infections
- Discusses human immunodeficiency virus (HIV), pre-exposure prophylaxis (PrEP) and post-exposure prophylaxis after sexual exposure (PEP/PEPSE).

Introduction

When prescribing contraception, it is best practice to refer to The Faculty of Sexual and Reproductive Health (FSRH 2016) *Clinical Effectiveness Unit: United Kingdom Medical Eligibility Criteria* (UKMEC), and current method-specific guidance, alongside the British National Formulary (BNF). It is also essential to hold a recognised contraceptive and sexual health qualification in order to prescribe in this area. The UKMEC offers guidance on the safety of different methods of contraception and whether patients are eligible to have them prescribed. These criteria recognise certain health conditions and offer evidence-based recommendations about the likely safety of each contraceptive method.

Table 8.1: The UKMEC recognises four categories of contraceptive methods, summarised in the table below, according to whether the method can be prescribed for certain medical conditions, ages and weights.

UKMEC	Definition
Category 1	• No restriction on use
Category 2	• The advantages of using the method outweigh the risks
Category 3	• Expert opinion is usually required, as the risks generally outweigh the safety of using this method
Category 4	• The method should not be used in this condition as it poses an unacceptable health risk

Adapted from FSRH 2016

For current guidance on prescribing in sexual health, please refer to the British Association for Sexual Health and HIV website (https://www.bashh.org – last accessed 18 September 2020).

Contraception

Prescribing hormones: the difference between progestogens and oestrogens

Understanding how hormones relate to reproduction is essential to understanding the effects of oestrogens and progesterones on the body. Synthetic oestrogens and progesterones found in contraception are called ethinylestradiol and progestogen.

When there is a persistently elevated level of synthetic ethinylestradiol and progestogen, the normal cyclic menstrual cycle is prevented. Ethinylestradiol and progestogen are used together. As in all methods of combined hormonal contraception (CHC), they suppress the release of follicular stimulating hormone (FSH), which in turn prevents the development of follicles within the ovaries. As there is no follicle, the production of oestrogen is impaired. The combination of the plasma oestrogen levels not rising and negative feedback from progesterone prevents the luteinising hormone (LH) levels from rising. This rise is known as the LH surge and it is essential for ovulation to occur.

Progesterone:
- Thins the lining of the endometrium, which makes it less conducive to implantation
- Has the effect of thickening cervical mucus, thus reducing sperm penetration through the cervix.

Pharmacological case studies: Sexual health and contraception

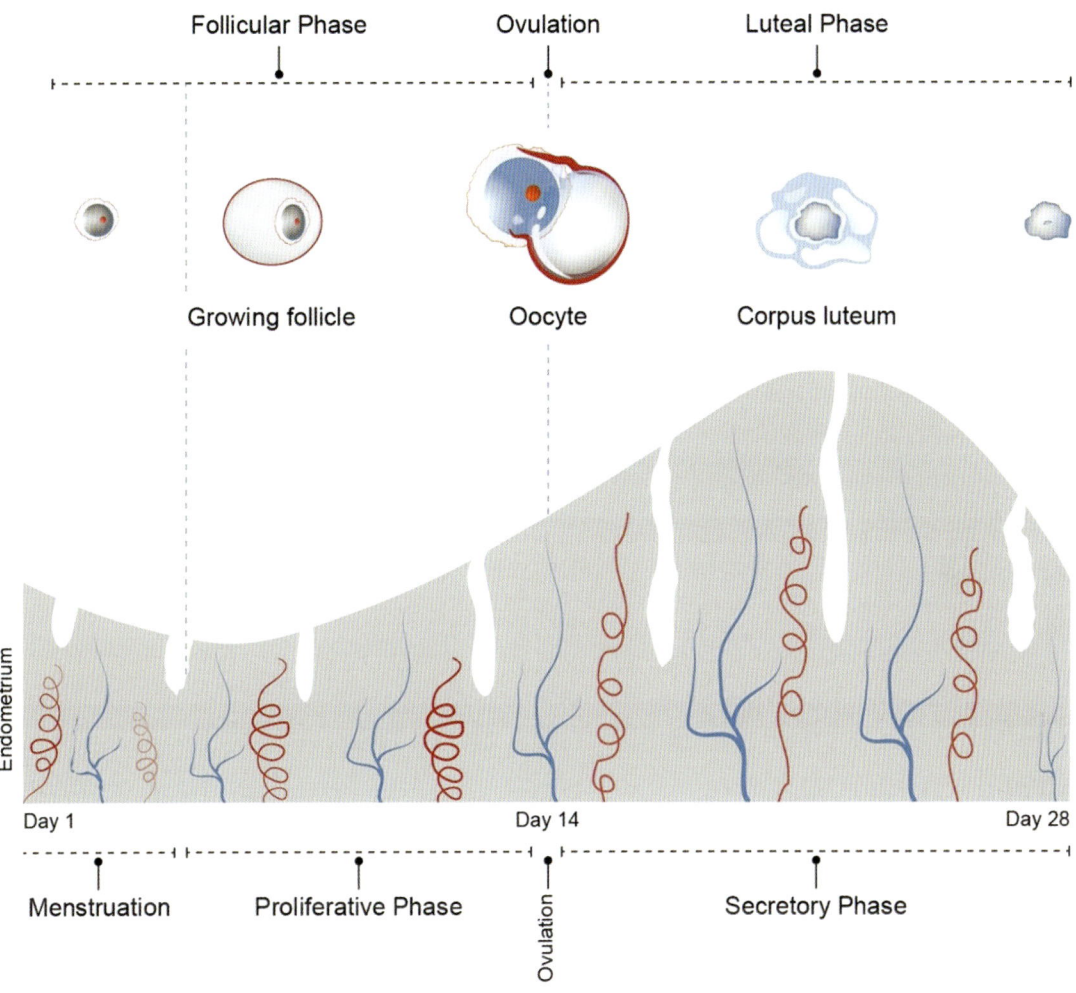

Figure 8.1: The endocrine control of the menstrual cycle

The pharmacokinetics of hormonal contraception

Hormonal contraception comprises either a combination of synthetic ethinylestradiol and progestogen, or progestogen on its own. Methods containing both ethinylestradiol and progestogen in different formulations are referred to as combined hormonal contraception (CHC) and include the combined pill (COC), the combined transdermal patch (CTP), and the combined vaginal ring (CVR). Progestogen-only contraception (POC) includes the progestogen-only pill (POP), the contraceptive injection, the contraceptive implant and the intra-uterine system (IUS).

In the UK, combined oral contraception, the transdermal patch and the vaginal ring contain doses ranging between 20 and 50 micrograms of ethinylestradiol. Mestranol metabolises into ethinylestradiol and can be found in combined pills such as ortho-novum and norinyl.

Once ingested, progestogens are 80–100% bioavailable from the upper small bowel, whilst oestrogen is subject to first-pass metabolism via the hepatic portal vein to the liver. Drugs that are highly metabolised lose much of their effectiveness in the first-pass effect as they travel through the liver (see Chapter 1). For drugs that undergo a high first-pass effect, higher oral doses may be needed to achieve a therapeutic level of circulating drug, and combined hormonal contraception is one of these drugs. The liver metabolises oestrogen into glucuronides, which re-enter the bowel, where bowel flora helps to restore some of the oestrogen for reabsorption. Any increase in the metabolism of oestrogen and progestogen, due to the induction of liver enzymes, will reduce the efficacy of the oestrogen and progestogen.

Factors that affect drug metabolism include:
- Enzyme induction
- Enzyme inhibition
- Genetic polymorphisms
- Age.

P450 cytochrome enzymes and hormonal contraception

Hormones are metabolised by P450 cytochrome enzymes CYP3A4. They metabolise unwanted substances so that they can safely be excreted by the kidneys. Some drugs increase or decrease P450 activity (see Chapter 1).

Table 8.2 Enzyme-inducing drugs and enzyme-inhibiting drugs which affect hormonal contraception (FSRH 2018a)

Enzyme-inducing drugs that reduce hormonal contraception bioavailability, causing reduced efficacy	Enzyme-inhibiting drugs that increase hormonal contraception bioavailability
Anti-epileptics (e.g. carbamazepine, eslicarbazepine, fosphenytoin, oxcarbazepine, phenobarbital, phenytoin, primidone, rufinamide, topiramate)	Antibacterials (e.g. erythromycin)
Antibacterials (e.g. rifabutin, rifampicin)	Antifungals (e.g. fluconazole, itraconazole, ketoconazole, posaconazole, voriconazole)
Antiretrovirals (e.g. ritonavir, ritonavir-boosted protease inhibitors, efavirenz, nevirapine)	Antiretrovirals (e.g. atazanavir)

Antidepressants (e.g. St John's Wort, a herbal preparation)	Immunosuppressants (e.g. tacrolimus)
Others (e.g. modafinil, bosentan, aprepitant)	Non-steroidal anti-inflammatories (e.g. etoricoxib)
	Statins (e.g. atorvastatin, rosuvastatin).
	Vasodilators (e.g. sitaxentan sodium)
	Non-steroidal anti-inflammatories (e.g. etoricoxib)

Advice to women on hormonal contraception taking enzyme-inducing drugs

Once CYP450 enzymes are induced, the pharmacokinetic effect starts within two days but is at maximum by one week. It will take four weeks after cessation for enzymes to return to normal.

Women who need to take an enzyme-inducing drug should be told about the effect on contraception and advised to use intra-uterine or injectable contraception methods, which are not affected by these drugs. If they are taking combined hormonal contraception and do not wish to change, they could be given an increased dose of 50 micrograms of ethinylestradiol and advised to tri-cycle (i.e. take three packets in a row without a pill-free interval) and shorten the pill-free interval to four days. The doubling of contraceptive rings or patches is not recommended (FSRH 2019).

Alternatively, they could use condoms with their normal dose of hormonal contraception. They will need to continue using the condoms and hormonal contraception whilst taking the enzyme-inducing drug and until four weeks after the enzyme-inducing drug has been stopped (BNF 2019).

Activity 8.1
Why might young women take modafinil?

Genetic polymorphism

Around 8% of the population have a faulty expression of CYP2D6 and research is looking at other forms of genetic polymorphism. In a recent study, 3 women out of a sample of 350 had a gene called CYP3A7*1C which is active in foetuses but switched off at birth. These women still had the CYP3A7 enzyme, which has been found to metabolise hormones faster. This may be one reason why some women have unexplained contraceptive failures with the implant (Lazorwitz, Aquilante, et al. 2019).

Interactions with hormonal contraception

No additional contraception is required for non-enzyme-inducing antibiotics (FSRH 2019). However, hormonal contraception efficacy may be reduced by severe diarrhoea and vomiting, and women should be advised to use extra precautions if they experience these symptoms.

The effects of hormonal contraception on other drugs

Hormonal contraception can affect how other drugs work. For instance, women taking lamotrigine should be warned that combined hormonal contraception may reduce the serum levels of lamotrigine and they may therefore have reduced seizure control or there may be a risk of lamotrigine toxicity (FSRH 2019). Oestrogen in combined hormonal contraception may reduce sodium valproate levels, causing increased seizures (FSRH 2018a).

Ulipristal acetate emergency contraception (UPA-EC) is a progestogen-receptor modulator. This means that, if hormonal contraception is commenced immediately after taking it, the effectiveness of the emergency contraception may be reduced (FSRH 2018a). This may also apply to Esmya, a drug used to treat fibroids, but there is currently limited research on this.

Combined hormonal contraception can increase tacrolimus concentration and serum levels should therefore be monitored. Both oestrogen and progestogen can increase the levels of the immunosuppressant ciclosporin and ulipristal acetate may increase everolimus and sirolimus concentrations. Oestrogen and progestogens can increase the dopaminergic selegiline, causing an increased risk of toxicity. Ropinirole elimination has been shown to reduce with oestrogen. Plasma concentrations of melatonin can be increased by oestrogen (FSRH 2018a).

Advice to women taking teratogenic drugs

Some drugs are known to be teratogenic (e.g. methotrexate, some anti-epileptic drugs and retinoids). If women are prescribed these drugs and they are at risk of pregnancy, they should be advised to use highly effective methods of contraception and be given specialist advice on this (FSRH 2018a, 2018b). These women should also be advised on how soon it is safe to get pregnant after discontinuing these medications. A pregnancy prevention plan should be in place so that the patient and medical team can plan ahead to avoid the risk of conception. Further information on teratogenic drugs is available from the UK Teratology Information Service (UKTIS) website, http://www.uktis.org (last accessed 21 September 2020).

First, second, third and fourth generation pills

The first contraceptive pills were developed in the 1960s. Since then the pill has evolved and dosages have been lowered to ensure that women take the safest, most effective pills with minimal unacceptable side effects. The table below shows the different generations of pills.

Table 8.3 Generations of pills

Generation of pill	Estradiol	Progestogen
First generation	Mestranol	Norethindrone or norethnodrel
Second generation	Ethinyl estradiol	Levonorgestrel and norithesterone
Third generation	Ethinyl estradiol	Desogestrel and gestodene
Fourth generation		Drospirenone or a different oestrogen – 17 beta-estradiol (a natural oestrogen) with nomegestrol acetate or estradiol valerate (a natural oestrogen) and dienogest

Activity 8.2

Write down all the combined oral contraceptives you know and put them into second, third and fourth generation groups. Please refer to the BNF for the most up-to-date hormonal contraception preparations.

Risks associated with combined hormonal contraception

There are minor risks associated with combined hormonal contraception which must be discussed with all women considering these methods.

Venous thromboembolism (VTE)

There is a small increased risk of venous thromboembolism with the use of combined hormonal contraception (CHC) but it is important to acknowledge that the risk is small – and lower than during and immediately after pregnancy (FSRH 2019). The level of risk associated with CHC depends on progestogen type and oestrogen dose.

According to the European Medicines Agency (2014), the risk for a woman not using any hormonal contraception is around 2 per 10,000 women per year (FSRH 2019, BNF 2019). The risk is higher when just starting combined hormonal contraception or when restarting after a break of a month or more (FSRH 2019). The stopping and starting of combined hormonal contraception are discouraged for this reason.

The risk also varies according to the type of progestogen. The risk for combined hormonal contraception containing levonorgestrel, norethisterone or norgestimate (second generation progestogens) is 5–7 per 10,000 women per year. For combined hormonal contraception containing etonogestrel or norelgestromin, it is 6–12 per 10,000 women per year; and for combined hormonal contraceptions containing drospirenone, gestodene or desogestrel (third generation progestogens) it is 9–12 per 10,000 women per year (FSRH 2019).

Progestogen type may also affect the risk of venous thromboembolism. A higher risk is associated with third generation combined oral contraception, such as those containing gestodene and desogestrel (FSRH 2019).

Myocardial infarction (MI)

Women taking combined hormonal contraception have a small increased risk of myocardial infarction and ischaemic stroke, and this risk is higher with higher doses of oestrogen. Although users should be informed of this small increased risk, it is important to note that it is extremely rare. However, those with additional risk factors for arterial disease should be advised to avoid combined hormonal contraception (FSRH 2019).

Migraine and risk of ischaemic stroke

The use of combined hormonal contraception in women who suffer migraine with aura is classified as UKMEC 4. For migraine sufferers without aura it is classified as UKMEC 2. Evidence suggest that users who experience migraine with aura have an increased risk of ischaemic stroke; compared to users without migraine (FSRH 2019).

Cervical cancer

Women using combined hormonal contraception for more than five years have a small increased risk of cervical cancer which reduces after stopping combined hormonal contraception (FSRH 2019). The use of condoms will significantly reduce this risk. It is important to note that few studies have considered the risk of cervical cancer for combined hormonal contraceptive users who have tested positive for human papillomavirus (HPV).

Breast cancer

Large observational studies have identified an increased breast cancer risk in women currently using combined hormonal contraception. This risk disappears over time after stopping – and 10 years after stopping the risk is no longer significant (FSRH 2019).

Activity 8.3
Name three different types of progesterone in progestogen-only pills.

Case study: Choosing a combined pill
Ellie is a 25-year-old woman who has taken Dianette since she was 15 years old. She was originally put on Dianette because of acne but since she turned 18 she has used it as a contraceptive. Ellie is fit and well – she has a normal BP of 110/70 and a BMI of 23. She does not take any other medications and is not allergic to anything. She has had no operations or illnesses and does not suffer from migraines. Her father is 51 years old and has raised blood pressure and her mother is well and healthy.

Activity 8.4 (Case study)
1. Why should Ellie be advised to change from Dianette?
2. What type of combined pill would you change Ellie to, and why?

Off-label prescribing guidance

When a drug is prescribed outside the terms of its licence, this is known as unlicensed or off-label prescribing. In the field of contraception and sexual health, there are many situations where prescribing off-label is in the best interests of the patient and expert opinion would endorse off-label prescribing. In these situations, you should involve the individual in the decision, discuss why you are suggesting this course of treatment, and give information about the drug, including serious and common adverse reactions, so that they are able to give informed consent.

This prescribing practice is in line with the Royal Pharmaceutical Society Prescribing Framework (RPS 2016). As the prescriber, you will be taking responsibility for monitoring this patient and submitting any suspected adverse reactions through the Yellow Card system. You should also have enough evidence and experience of using the drug to show its safety and efficacy and be able to justify your proposed course of treatment (BNF 2019).

Case study: Off-label contraceptive prescribing

Aisha has been taking Microgynon 30 for one year. She is 17 years old and suffers from painful and heavy periods. The combined pill has improved her periods, but they are still heavy, and she is about to do a school trip and has exams coming up. Aisha has a boyfriend who is the same age, and there are no signs of grooming. She has no illnesses, operations and is not taking medications. You discuss her options with Aisha – she could change to another method (like the injectable) or have an intra-uterine system fitted which would help her heavy periods. However, Aisha is happy taking Microgynon 30. She does not want to change things too much, with her exams coming up, and does not like the thought of an intra-uterine system. You suggest that she tri-cycles Microgynon 30, which means taking three months of pills in a row and then having her pill-free interval. The Faculty of Sexual and Reproductive Healthcare clinical guidelines endorse this practice, but it is outside the product licence of Microgynon 30 and would therefore be unlicensed or off-label prescribing (FSRH 2019).

Aisha likes the idea of tri-cycling because it means she will have four periods in a year (instead of 12) during this busy time in her life. It will also give her a chance to reflect on her other choices and maybe change in the future to another method when she feels the time is right. You explain to her why you think this off-label use of Microgynon is a good idea, and the expert advice surrounding this practice. Aisha understands and says she is happy to tri-cycle Microgynon 30.

Storing and administering contraception

Contraceptive pills should be stored at room temperature, not in direct sunlight, away from moisture and away from children. However, the contraceptive vaginal ring requires cold chain prior to it being issued to patients. Cold chain is the refrigeration transport and storage of a drug at 2–8 degrees centigrade before it is prescribed and issued. Once it has been issued by the prescribing clinician, it can be used without loss of effectiveness within 4 months, stored at 25 degrees centigrade. It is therefore important that users are informed by the prescriber at the time of issuing of the lifespan of the contraceptive vaginal ring, to guard against loss of effectiveness and possible contraceptive failure.

Advice to patients using the contraceptive vaginal ring

Patients are advised they do not need to keep their contraceptive vaginal ring in the fridge. This also effects how many months' supply can be issued to a patient at each clinic visit (3 months' supply). Some clinics adopt the policy of issuing 3 months' supply and a further 3 months' supply in the form of a written prescription which can be collected from their local pharmacist.

> **Activity 8.5**
> What could be the impact of supplying 6 months of NuvaRing?

Sexual health

Antimicrobials and drug resistance

There has been a steady increase in the incidence of sexually transmitted infections, including chlamydia, syphilis, gonorrhoea and HIV, in the UK. With this increase in sexually transmitted infections there has also been an increase in resistance to antibiotics and this has been clearly seen with gonorrhoea. Gonorrhoea is a gram-negative intracellular diplococci bacterium. The cell walls of gram-negative bacteria have a thin layer of peptidoglycan sandwiched between two membranes. Therefore, gram-negative bacteria are more resistant to antimicrobial drugs because their cell structure is more complex.

Public Health England keep data on gonorrhoea incidence and antibiotic resistance in the Gonococcal Resistance to Antimicrobials Surveillance Programme (GRASP) (Public Health England 2018). Health professionals need to ensure they are up to date with gonorrhoea resistance and changes in treatment and management guidelines developed by the British Association of Sexual Health and HIV (BASHH 2019).

> **Case study: Prescribing for gonorrhoea**
>
> Josh is a 19-year-old man who says he has had a discharge from his penis for two days. He feels unwell but has no other medical health issues. Josh has a partner of three months who is female, he does not use barrier contraception and he had unprotected sexual intercourse with another female partner four days ago. He did not use a condom and had oral and vaginal sex. He has not had a sexually transmitted infection before, he has no allergies, and he was last screened one year ago.
>
> Josh is examined and his discharge is confirmed under microscopy as gonorrhoea. A sample is sent for culture to ensure that treatment will be successful. Josh is also screened for chlamydia, HIV and syphilis. He is treated with ceftriaxone 1gm intramuscularly and advised not to have sexual intercourse until he returns in two weeks for a test of cure (BASHH 2019). By this time, the culture result will have been returned and should confirm any sensitivities and resistance. All partners will need to be treated and advised to abstain from sexual intercourse until test of cure has been completed. Your discussion with Josh focuses on how gonorrhoea has been contracted and how this can be avoided in future.
>
> Josh is an example of a case where we do need to prescribe but it is important to acknowledge that there are cases where we do not prescribe. The over-prescribing of antibiotics has led to antibiotic resistance and the following case study is an example where prescribing antibiotics is unnecessary.

> ### Case study:
> ### Not prescribing for vaginal infection
>
> Elizabeth has attended the clinic requesting cervical screening, having received a recall letter from her GP practice. A full sexual health history is taken. Elizabeth reports that she is not sexually active, and her last sexual intercourse was more than six months ago, with a condom. On examination, a thin white homogenous discharge is noted to be covering the walls of the vagina, accompanied by a strong fishy odour, although Elizabeth has not reported any symptoms. The pH is noted as 7 and a full sexual health screen is carried out to exclude infection.
>
> The likely diagnosis is bacterial vaginosis (BV), a vaginal infection Elizabeth has reported and been treated for in the past. Approximately 50% of women with this condition are asymptomatic. BV can be diagnosed following Amsel's criteria, which requires three of the following criteria to be present (BASHH 2012):
>
> - Thin, white, homogenous discharge
> - Clue cells on microscopy of wet mount
> - pH of vaginal fluid >4.5
> - Release of a fishy odour.
>
> After discussion, you reach a shared decision not to treat with antibiotics, as bacterial vaginosis will resolve without therapeutic treatment. You advise Elizabeth on avoiding triggers such as bubble bath, vaginal douching, use of shower gel and use of antiseptic agents or shampoo in the bath. You also advise her that if she becomes symptomatic, she can return to the clinic for treatment and that it may take time for her symptoms to resolve.

Human immunodeficiency virus (HIV)

HIV is a retrovirus that enters the immune system via the CD4 cells, and kills these cells by using the host's own metabolic process, resulting in the release of more virus. Viruses are quite complex structures, often replicating rapidly and before the host has experienced any symptoms. As viruses replicate so rapidly, many drugs and vaccines are useless. In HIV, once the T cells have been reduced considerably, the host becomes increasingly susceptible to infection, which can prove fatal.

HIV medication works by reducing the amount of virus in the blood to undetectable levels. For someone recently diagnosed and started on antiretroviral therapy (ART), it usually takes about six months for the virus to be reduced to an undetectable level. At this stage, the virus cannot be passed on. This is what is described as having an undetectable viral load. According to the British HIV Association (https://www.bhiva.org, last accessed 24 September 2020): Undetectable = untransmittible (U=U).

It is important that treatment is adhered to – otherwise there is a risk of treatment resistance.

Treatment of HIV

Currently there is no cure for HIV. However, antiretroviral drugs can lower the number of virus particles and slow the progression of HIV. The treatment consists of at least three drugs and some formulations include 2–3 medications in a single dose. ART works by blocking steps in the viral replication process in order to achieve an undetectable viral load. This can be done in two ways:

- The viral enzyme reverse transcriptase can be inhibited by drugs called reverse transcriptase inhibitors, which block the conversion of viral RNA into viral DNA in the host cell
- Proteases, which are viral proteins. Protease inhibitors block the action of protease enzymes. Protease is an enzyme in the body that's important for HIV replication. Protease inhibitors work by disrupting the life cycle of HIV and stopping it from multiplying.

The use of antivirals is indicated as soon as HIV diagnosis is confirmed; and there are three main types of inhibitors, which are listed in Tables 8.4, 8.5 and 8.6.

Table 8.4 Nucleoside reverse transcriptase inhibitors

Action	Adverse effects	Contraindications
The enzyme reverse transcriptase is fooled into incorporating the drug into the strand of growing viral DNA which prevents the reaction continuing and prevents further replication. Examples include abacavir, didanosine, emtricitabine, tenofovir and zidovudine.	• Nausea, headaches and muscle pain • Bone marrow suppression	

Table 8.5 Non-nucleoside reverse transcriptase inhibitors

Action	Adverse effects	Contraindications
Interfere with the action of viral reverse transcriptase. Examples are efavirenz and nevirapine.	• Side effects of efavirenz include rash, abnormal dreams, dizziness, impaired concentration and insomnia • Nevirapine has similar side effects • Liver toxicity can also be a problem	• Efavirenz is contraindicated when breastfeeding • Use with caution in patients with hepatic impairment and pregnancy • Nevirapine is contraindicated when breastfeeding and in patients with severe hepatic impairment

Table 8.6 Protease inhibitors

Action	Adverse effects	Contraindications
Inhibits viral proteases which are needed for the formation of viral proteins. Examples include ritonavir, amprenavir, atanzanavir and saquinavir.	• Nausea, vomiting and diarrhoea, hepatic impairment • Use with caution in patients with renal problems	• Contraindicated when breastfeeding • Ritonavir is contraindicated in patients with hepatic impairment

Post-exposure prophylaxis

If there is a risk of HIV exposure, post-exposure prophylaxis (PEP) can be given to reduce the risk of infection. This is also sometimes referred to as post-exposure prophylaxis after sexual exposure (PEPSE). Research indicates that there is a period just after exposure to HIV when antiretroviral treatment can be used to inhibit viral replication and stop the integration of the virus into the host DNA. Once HIV crosses a mucosal barrier, it may take 48–72 hours before HIV can be detected within regional lymph nodes and up to five days before HIV can be detected in the blood (BASHH 2015).

To be effective this treatment must be started within 72 hours, and preferably within 24 hours of contact with the virus. It is recommended for high-risk exposure – for example, where a partner is known to be HIV positive. Treatment is recommended for 28 days and side effects (such as nausea, headaches and fatigue) may occur. Adherence to treatment is paramount to ensure that drug plasma levels are maintained above therapeutic levels throughout the treatment period.

Treatment used is a single dose of truvada and 2 tablets of raltegravir (BASHH 2015). Oral contraceptives and the contraceptive implant may have reduced effectiveness and alternative contraception may therefore be needed.

To find out whether PEP is needed, you can access an online risk assessment through the Terrence Higgins Trust (https://www.tht.org.uk).

Pre-exposure prophylaxis

Pre-exposure prophylaxis (PrEP) is a drug for HIV-negative people, taken before possible exposure to HIV. It can block HIV if it enters the body. It consists of a tablet containing tenofovir and emtricitabine. This treatment is not available to everyone as it is currently part of a trial which started in September 2017. Further information is available on the PrEP Impact Trial website (https://www.prepimpacttrial.org.uk).

Activity 8.6

Using the HIV drug interaction checker available at https://www.hiv-druginteractions.org check for any possible interactions between the following HIV medications and hormonal contraception:

1. Efavirenz with desogestrel (POP), etonogestrel (implant) or medroxyprogesterone (contraceptive injection)
2. Atazanavir with gestodene (POP), etonogestrel (vaginal ring) or medroxyprogesterone (contraceptive injection)
3. Truvada and ulipristal acetate (ellaone).

Answers to activities

Activity 8.1

Why might young women take modafinil?

There have been reports of young women taking the 'smart drug' modafinil to enhance cognitive function. As it is an enzyme-inducing drug, women should be warned that this may reduce the efficacy of hormonal contraception, excluding intra-uterine and injectable contraception (FSRH 2018a).

Activity 8.2

Write down all the combined oral contraceptives you know and put them into second, third and fourth generation groups. Please refer to the BNF for the most up-to-date hormonal contraception preparations.

Combination and dosage of monophasic COCs	Brand names	Generation of Pill
Ethinylestradiol 20 micrograms Desogestrel 150 micrograms	Gedarel 20/150, Mercilon	Third generation
Ethinylestradiol 20 micrograms Gestodene 75 micrograms	Femodette, Millinette 20/75, Sunya 20/75	Third generation
Ethinylestradiol 20 micrograms Norethisterone acetate 1mg	Loestrin 20	Second generation

Ethinylestradiol 30 micrograms Desogestrel 150 micrograms	Gedarel 30/150, Marvelon	Third generation
Ethinylestradiol 30 micrograms Drospirenone 3mg	Yasmin	Fourth generation
Ethinylestradiol 30 micrograms Gestodene 75 micrograms	Femodene, Millinette 30/75, Katya 30/75	Third generation
Ethinylestradiol 30 micrograms Levonorgestrel 150 micrograms	Levest, Microgynon, Ovranette, Rigevedon	Second generation
Ethinylestradiol 30 micrograms Norethisterone acetate 1.5mg	Loestrin 30	Second generation
Ethinylestradiol 35 micrograms Norgestimate 250 micrograms	Cilest	Second generation
Ethinylestradiol 35 micrograms Norethisterone 500 micrograms	Brevinor	Second generation

Activity 8.3

Name three different types of progesterone in progestogen-only pills.

Type of progesterone	Common brand names
Desogestrel 75 micrograms	Cerelle, Zelletta, Feanolla, Aizea, Cerazette, Nacrez, Desorex, Desomono
Levonorgestrel 300 micrograms	Norgeston
Norethisterone 350 micrograms	Noriday

Activity 8.4

1. Why should Ellie be advised to change from Dianette?

Dianette contains co-cyprindiol and has a similar risk of venous thrombo-embolism as third-generation combined pills (FSRH 2019). Co-cyprindiol may have an increased risk of cardiovascular disease and is a second-line treatment for acne and should not be used solely for contraception (BNF 2019).

2. What type of combined pill would you change Ellie to, and why?

The best combined contraceptive pill would be a second-generation combined pill containing 30mg of ethinylestradiol and levonorgestrel. This would give Ellie the lowest risk of venous thrombo-embolism, with an incidence of 5–7 per 10,000 women (FSRH 2019). However, for women with acne, a third-generation combined pill is often used, such as Marvelon. Marvelon contains the progestogen desogestrel, which has an incidence of venous thrombo-embolism of 9–12 per 10,000 women (FSRH 2019). It is also very effective in resolving acne. However, Ellie needs to understand the risks linked to each type of pill and be involved in the decision. Often women have no recurrence of acne with a second-generation combined pill so it may be worth starting her on a pill like Microgynon and changing if her skin worsens.

Activity 8.5

What could be the impact of supplying 6 months of NuvaRing?
NuvaRing is a cold chain drug (which means it can be stored for 40 months between 2 and 8 degrees centigrade). Once it has been dispensed to the user, it must be used within 4 months and stored at 25 degrees centigrade, avoiding direct sunlight. The effectiveness of NuvaRing used after 4 months is likely to be reduced. Supplies should therefore not exceed 3 months at a time.

Activity 8.6

Using the HIV drug interaction checker available at https://www.hiv-druginteractions.org check for any possible interactions between the following HIV medications and hormonal contraception:

1. Efavirenz with desogestrel (POP), etonogestrel (implant) or medroxyprogesterone (contraceptive injection)

Efavirenz and desogestrel and etonogestrel – do not co-administer medroxyprogesterone, no interaction expected.

2. Atazanavir with gestodene (POP), etonogestrel (vaginal ring) or medroxyprogesterone (contraceptive injection)

Atazanavir with gestodene (POP) – potential interaction, Etonogestrel (vaginal ring) – potential weak interaction, medroxyprogesterone (contraceptive injection) – no interaction expected. Atazanavir may increase hormone levels.

3. Truvada and ulipristal acetate (ellaone)

Truvada and ulipristal acetate (ellaone) – no interaction expected. Efavirenz and nevirapine reduce the bioavailability of progestogens by inducing glucuronidation. They may therefore decrease contraceptive efficacy.

References and further reading

British Association for Sexual Health and HIV (BASHH) (2012). UK National Guideline for the Management of Bacterial Vaginosis. https://www.bashhguidelines.org/media/1041/bv-2012.pdf (Last accessed 25 September 2020).

British Association for Sexual Health and HIV (BASHH) (2015). UK guideline for the use of HIV Post-Exposure Prophylaxis Following Sexual Exposure. https://www.bashhguidelines.org/media/1027/pepse-2015.pdf (Last accessed 25 September 2020).

British Association for Sexual Health and HIV (BASHH) (2019). British Association for Sexual Health and HIV national guideline for the management of infection with Neisseria gonorrhoeae. https://www.bashhguidelines.org/media/1208/gc-2019.pdf (Last accessed 25 September 2020).

British HIV Association (BHIVA) (2020). https://www.bhiva.org/ (Last accessed 25 September 2020).

British National Formulary (BNF) (2019). Contraceptives, interactions. https://bnf.nice.org.uk/treatment-summary/contraceptives-interactions.html (Last accessed 25 September 2020).

Electronic Medicines Compendium (EMC) (2020). https://www.medicines.org.uk/emc (Last accessed 25 September 2020).

European Medicines Agency (EMA) (2014). Press release; Benefits of combined oral contraceptives (CHCs) continue to outweigh the risks. https://www.ema.europa.eu/en/news/benefits-combined-hormonal-contraceptives-chcs-continue-outweigh-risks-chmp-endorses-prac (Last accessed 25 September 2020).

Faculty of Sexual and Reproductive Healthcare (FSRH) (2016). Clinical Effectiveness Unit: United Kingdom Medical Eligibility Criteria. London: FSRH.

Faculty of Sexual and Reproductive Healthcare (FSRH) (2017). CEU Statement; Response to study Contemporary Hormonal Contraception and the Risk of Breast Cancer. London: FSRH.

Faculty of Sexual and Reproductive Healthcare (FSRH) (2018a). Clinical Guidance: Drug Interactions with Hormonal Contraception. London: FSRH.

Faculty of Sexual and Reproductive Healthcare (FSRH) (2018b). CEU Statement: Contraception for women using known teratogenic drugs or drugs with potential teratogenic effects. London: FSRH.

Faculty of Sexual and Reproductive Healthcare (FSRH) (2019). FSRH Guideline. Combined Hormonal Contraception. London: FSRH.

Faculty of Sexual and Reproductive Healthcare (FSRH) (2020). https://www.fsrh.org.uk (Last accessed 25 September 2020).

HIV Drug Interactions (2020). https://www.hiv-druginteractions.org (Last accessed 25.9.2020).

Lazorwitz, A., Aquilante, C.L., Oreschak, K., Sheeder, J., Guiahi, M. & Teal, S. (2019). Influence of genetic variants on steady state etonogestrel concentrations among contraceptive implant users. *Obstetrics and Gynaecology*. Doi 10.1097/AOG0000000000000003189

Medicines Complete (2020). https://about.medicinescomplete.com (Last accessed 25 September 2020).

PrEP Impact Trial Website (2020). www.prepimpacttrial.org.uk (Last accessed 25 September 2020).

Public Health England (PHE) (2018). Surveillance of antimicrobial resistance in Neisseria gonorrhoeae in England and Wales Key findings from the Gonococcal Resistance to Antimicrobials Surveillance Programme (GRASP). https://assets.publishing.service.gov.uk/government/uploads/system/uploads/attachment_data/file/746261/GRASP_2017_report.pdf (Last accessed 25 September 2020).

Royal Pharmaceutical Society (2016). Prescribing Specials: Guidance for the prescribers of Specials. https://www.rpharms.com/Portals/0/RPS%20document%20library/Open%20access/Support/toolkit/professional-standards---prescribing-specials.pdf (Last accessed 16 February 2021).

Terrence Higgins Trust (THT) (2020). https://www.tht.org.uk (Last accessed 25 September 2020).

UK Teratogenic Information Service (UKTIS) (2020). http://www.uktis.org (Last accessed 25 September 2020).

9

Pharmacological case studies: Stable angina

Donna Scholefield MSc, BSc (Hons), RN, PGDip HE; Cardiac Nursing (254);
Senior Lecturer, Health and Education, Middlesex University, London

Raquel Rosales MA in HE, BSc (Hons), RN
Lecturer, Health and Education, Middlesex University, London

This chapter:

- Discusses the incidence and prevalence of cardiovascular diseases such as coronary heart disease
- Explains the causes and pathophysiology of atheromatous plaque
- Assesses the pharmacological basis for the use of the major drug groups in the management of stable angina
- Applies knowledge of some of the main drugs used to treat angina in clinical practice case studies.

Introduction

Deaths from cardiovascular disease (CVD), which is any disease of the heart and circulatory system, have been falling successively in the UK since the 1970s. Nevertheless, despite this welcome decline, compared with other Western European countries (such as France and Italy), mortality rates remain high, contributing to 180,000 deaths in 2010. Coronary heart disease (CHD) and stroke are the two main types of CVD and were responsible for a total of 80,000 and 50,000 deaths respectively in the UK in 2010. Indeed, CHD is the most common cause of death in both sexes (BHF 2012).

The aim of this chapter is to discuss the pharmacological management of one of the most common manifestations of CHD, stable angina, with well over 95,000 cases being diagnosed each year. The pathophysiology, clinical manifestation and major drug groups will be explored, and three case studies will be used to illustrate the pharmacological management of this condition.

Classification of coronary heart disease (CHD)

The two main forms of CHD are conditions broadly known as angina pectoris (from the Latin word *pectus* meaning 'chest'), commonly known as angina, and myocardial infarction. More specifically, the clinical manifestation of CHD includes silent myocardial ischaemia, stable angina, unstable angina, myocardial infarction (MI), heart failure and sudden death.

CHDs, as the name implies, are diseases of the coronary arteries, which are mainly caused by the build-up of atheromatous plaques, a lipid material, in the lining (intima) of the coronary arteries (see Figure 9.1, p. 153). This material accumulates over a period of time, resulting in narrowing of the coronary arteries. Due to increasing deposition of atheromatous plaques, the coronary arteries eventually become so narrow that, when the individual exercises or makes increased effort, the blood flow to the myocardium is insufficient to meet demand. The ischaemic myocardium will produce the classic symptoms of angina, which can be described as chest pain or constricting discomfort that radiates to areas such as the jaw, arms and neck. However, these classic symptoms are not always present in every patient and atypical presentations are not uncommon (see case studies on pp. 153 and 157).

The pathogenesis of atherosclerosis

Atherosclerosis is the thickening and hardening of arteries as a result of the disease process called atheroma (from a Greek word *athere* meaning 'porridge'). Atheroma itself is the build-up of lipid-rich substances in the intima of arteries. These lesions are known as plaques and histologically consist of lipids (rich in cholesterol), muscle cells, collagen and macrophages that contain lipids (foam cells). The processes involved in the accumulation of these lesions are complex and are thought to involve lipid retention, oxidation and modification, which stimulate chronic inflammation at susceptible sites in large and medium-sized arteries. The main complications of atherosclerosis are, as discussed above, narrowing of the lumen of vessels such as the coronary arteries, reducing blood flow, rupture which could initiate thrombus, and aneurysm formation (see Figure 9.2, p. 154).

Atheroma has been identified in the arteries of early teenagers as lipid streaks that, with ageing, develop into fibrous plaques. The process of plaque development is the same regardless of race, sex or ethnicity, but it is accelerated by diseases such as hypertension, diabetes and lifestyle factors (such as smoking, obesity or a high-cholesterol diet). Fortunately, a number of clinical trials have shown unequivocally that the size of these plaques can be reduced by the administration of lipid-lowering drugs such as statins.

In summary, atherosclerosis is a disease of the intima layer of arteries that can progress to involve the media as well. These lipid-rich plaques are the cause of a number of clinical conditions such as angina and myocardial infarction. Symptoms, like angina, are produced by myocardial ischaemia, which is due to a build-up of toxins and a reduction in oxygen supply to the myocardium.

Angina can be further classified into stable and unstable angina. Stable angina, the focus of this chapter, is the most common manifestation of CHD in Western Europe. As described earlier, it occurs when physical activity increases the heart's demand for blood that is rich in oxygen but the supply is limited by the narrowed coronary arteries. In short, the pain occurs on physical exertion.

When the symptoms worsen with less strenuous physical activity and/or occur at rest, the condition is known as unstable angina. Other associated clinical signs and symptoms (such as shortness of breath, clamminess and nausea) may also be present. The underlying aetiology in unstable angina is caused by a disruption in the atherosclerotic plaque, whereby the plaque may rupture and/or erode with overlying thrombus (see Figure 9.2, p. 154). If unstable angina is not managed immediately, irreversible damage to the myocardium can result.

Unstable angina belongs to a spectrum of clinical conditions known as acute coronary syndrome (ACS), which also includes ST segment elevation myocardial infarction (STEMI – the ST segment of the ECG is elevated with raised cardiac enzymes and troponin levels) and non-ST segment elevation (NSTEMI). However, the ECG often demonstrates depression of the ST segment but no new Q waves. In fact the older term for this category of myocardial infarction was non-Q wave myocardial infarction. It is differentiated from unstable angina by a rise in both troponin and cardiac enzyme levels.

In a few individuals, narrowing of the coronary arteries can be due to spasm of the smooth muscles lining the arteries rather than atherosclerosis. For example, in Prinzmetal's angina, an uncommon condition, spasms can cause severe ischaemia at rest. In addition, recreational drugs such as cocaine can cause severe spasms of the coronary arteries due to excessive adrenergic stimulation. This is one reason why it is important to obtain a thorough drug history from the patient on admission.

Activity 9.1

Can you suggest two other conditions that can cause angina?

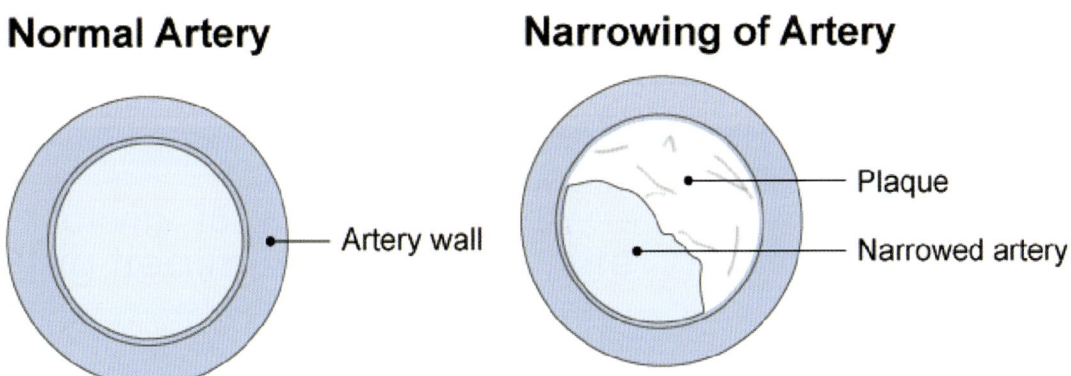

Figure 9.1: Coronary artery occlusion by an atheromatous plaque

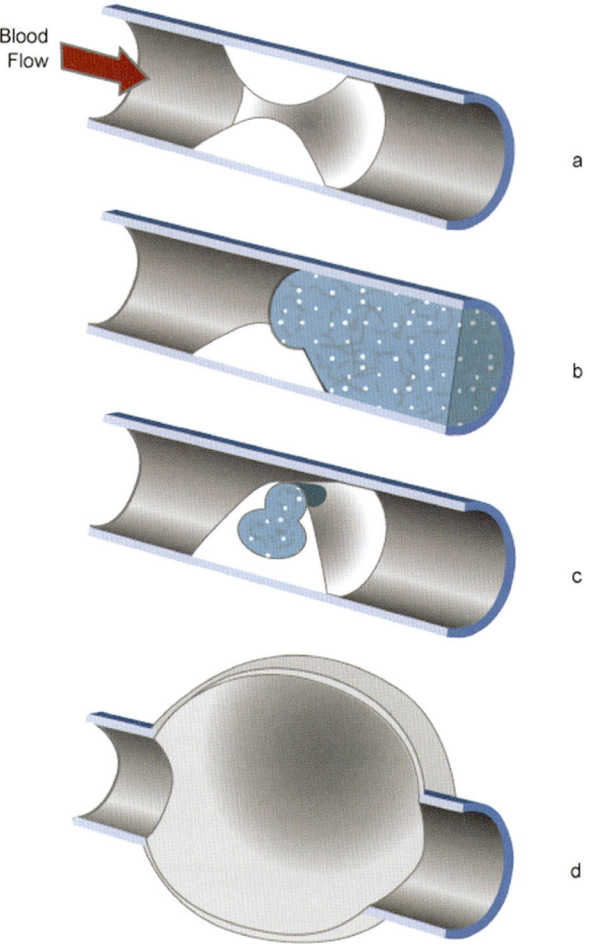

Figure 9.2: Complications of arterial atheroma: a) Narrowing of the artery;
b) Thrombus on plaque; c) Bleed into plaque; d) Aneurysm.
From Stevens & Lowe (1995) Pathology (Reproduced by kind permission of Elsiever Ltd).

General approach to managing angina

The diagnosis of stable angina is based on the presenting symptom, which is essentially chest pain on exertion relieved by rest. However, as mentioned earlier, symptoms may be typical or atypical (see case studies on pp. 156 and 157). Patient-centred care should be implemented, in which the patient is treated individually and their preferences taken into account. For example, age alone should not constitute a barrier to treatment. In addition, the relevant advice and information about self-managing their condition should be incorporated into their care pathways (see Good practice point below).

Pharmacological case studies: Stable angina

> ### Good practice point: Patient education and angina
> - Include the person's family or carers in discussions when appropriate.
> - Explain stable angina, the factors provoking it, and its long-term course and management.
> - Encourage questions and provide opportunities for the person to discuss concerns, ideas and expectations about their condition, prognosis and treatment.
> - Explore and address any misconceptions about stable angina and its implications for daily activities, heart attack risk and life expectancy.
> - Discuss the purpose, risks and benefits of treatment.
> - Assess the need for lifestyle advice and psychological support. Offer interventions as necessary.
> - Explore and address issues such as self-management skills, concerns about the impact of stress, anxiety or depression on angina and physical exertion including sex.
> - Advise the person to seek professional help if their angina suddenly worsens.
> - Pain management: do not offer transcutaneous electrical nerve stimulation (TENS), acupuncture or enhanced external counter pulsation (EECP).
>
> Source: National Institute for Health and Care Excellence (2011a). 'CG 126 Management of stable angina'. Manchester: NICE. Available from www.nice.org.uk/CG126. Reproduced with permission.

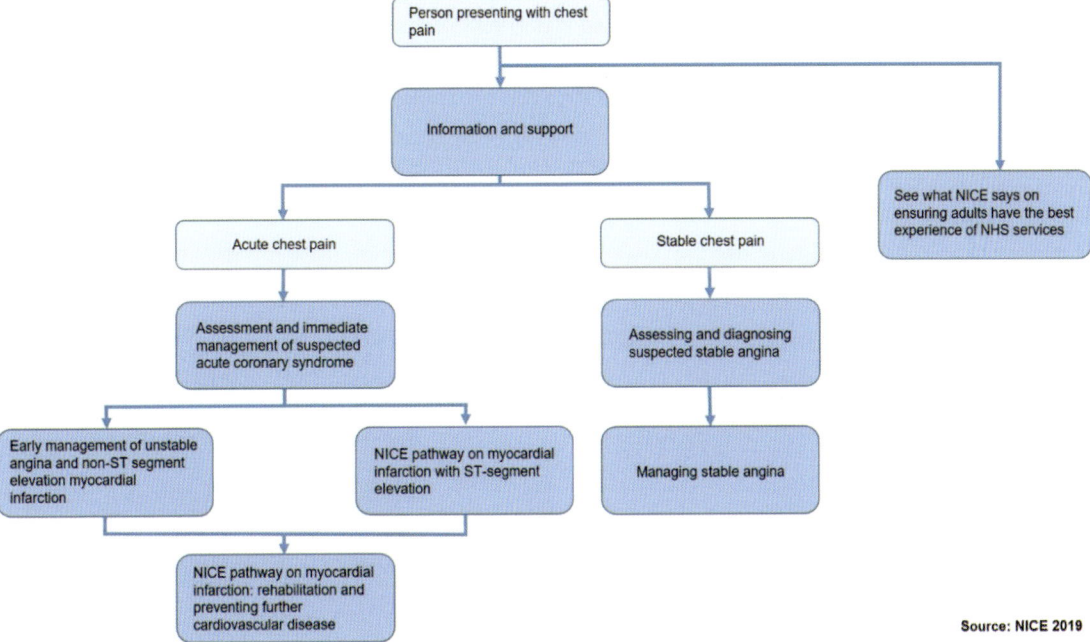

Figure 9.3: The National Institute for Health and Care Excellence (2020) provides an interactive, regularly updated flowchart, incorporating various NICE guidelines on management of chest pain.

This is the March 2020 update of the flowchart. © NICE [2020] Recent-onset chest pain of suspected cardiac origin: assessment and diagnosis. Available from https://pathways.nice.org.uk/pathways/chest-pain All rights reserved. Subject to notice of rights. Reproduced with permission.

Atypical presentation of coronary artery disease

As discussed in the previous sections, the presentation of coronary artery disease is not always typical, as demonstrated by the following scenarios, which are based on real-life case studies. They also show the importance of obtaining a good history.

Case study:
Atypical presentation of coronary artery disease 1

Mr O'Connor is a 62-year-old man who loves walking. He comes to the rapid chest pain clinic with a four-week history of breathlessness, brought on by walking uphill. He has noticed that he is becoming short of breath even walking on a flat surface after 1 or 2 miles. Mr O'Connor has experienced no chest pain either on exertion or at rest. He has a past medical history of type 2 diabetes, hypertension and cholesterol of 5.0mmol/l. His current medication is simvastatin 40mg nocte, metformin 500mg tds, aspirin 75mg daily and Lantus insulin 39 units daily. On examination, he appears well, with no shortness of breath (SOB), chest clear, heart sounds – early systolic murmur (ESM), no peripheral oedema, pulse rate 81bpm, BP 156/86 mmHg and his ECG demonstrated normal sinus rhythm.

Activity 9.2 (Case study)

1. Based on Mr O'Connor's history, what diagnosis would you suspect?

2. Suggest a pharmacological management plan for Mr O'Connor based on the above case study.

Note: You may find this activity easier if you first read the 'Drug management' section later in this chapter.

Case study:
Atypical presentation of coronary artery disease 2

Mr Smith is a 54-year-old gentleman with a presenting symptom of a dry throat. This usually occurs within about 5 minutes after walking and is relieved with rest. He has no chest pain at rest, no radiation of the pain to left arm or jaw, or any associated SOB on exertion. Mr Smith has a past medical history of type 2 diabetes and hypertension, which were managed with metformin 500mg tds, gliclazide 80mg twice daily and amlodipine 5mg daily respectively. He was also taking aspirin 75mg od and simvastatin 40mg nocte. His cholesterol level was 5.2mmol/l. On examination, he appears generally well with no SOB, chest clear, no peripheral oedema, BP 112/60, normal heart sounds and heart rate 91 beats per minute. Nevertheless, although his ECG demonstrated normal sinus rhythm, there was T wave inversion in leads V3–V6.

Activity 9.3 (Case study)

1. What evidence in Mr Smith's history would make you suspect that CHD may be present?
2. What adjustments would you initially make to Mr Smith's medication?

Note: You may find this activity easier if you first read the 'Drug management' section later in this chapter.

Drugs used in the treatment of stable angina

Once a diagnosis of stable angina has been established, optimal drug therapy should be implemented to control the symptoms. Optimal drug therapy is 'one or two anti-anginal drugs as necessary plus drugs for secondary prevention of cardiovascular disease' (NICE 2011a). Studies have shown that optimal drug therapy improves mortality and controls the symptoms of angina effectively.

Previously, percutaneous coronary intervention (PCI) was also believed to reduce mortality rates but the COURAGE study (Boden *et al.* 2007) demonstrated this was not the case. PCI is therefore now mainly used to manage the symptoms of stable angina that are not fully controlled by drug therapy. Calcium channel blockers and beta-blockers are the first-line drugs used in the management of stable angina. The decision as to which of these drugs should be used depends on several factors including individual preference, any contraindication and the presence of any comorbidities. If monotherapy does not control the symptoms, the two drugs can be used together. However, if this combination is not tolerated, NICE (2011a) suggests using either a long-acting nitrate such as isosorbide dinitrate or one of the newer anti-anginals such as ivabradine, nicorandil or ranolazine. Again, the choice of drug will be based on the individual's preference, comorbidities, contraindications and the cost of the drug.

Short-acting nitrates such as glyceryl trinitrate (GTN) are offered for episodes of angina but healthcare professionals must ensure that the person is given clear advice regarding administration and when to seek medical help.

Drugs such as aspirin and statins, as well as preventing myocardial infarction and strokes, are also an established part of the management of stable angina. These will be reviewed later.

Table 9.1: Summary of drugs used in the management of angina

Drug group	Mechanism of action	Clinical benefits in angina	Examples
Nitrates	• Peripheral vasodilation of smooth muscles in veins and coronary arteries, due to the formation of nitric oxide and cGMP • Effects include pooling of blood in veins which leads to reduced venous return and reduction in preload	• Pain relief • Reduces myocardial oxygen demand • Reduced heart size • Increased coronary blood flow	• Glyceryl trinitrate • Isosorbide dinitrate, mononitrate
*Calcium-channel blockers	• Blocks the entry of L-type voltage sensitive calcium in cardiac muscles and smooth muscles of blood vessels • Reduces contractility of the heart • Vasodilates smooth muscles in arteries, which reduces peripheral vascular resistance in blood vessels	• Pain relief and reduces heart's workload • Reduced BP due to reduction in cardiac output and peripheral vascular resistance (afterload) • Reduced myocardial oxygen demand • Increased coronary blood flow	• Nifedipine • Diltiazem • Amlodipine
*Beta-Adrenoceptor antagonist	• Beta-antagonists dampen down the sympathetic nervous system on the heart as a result of exercise, thus reducing heart rate and contractility	• Used prophylactically to prevent, rather than treat, angina attacks. Prevent over-activity of the heart	• Bisoprolol • Atenolol • Metoprolol

Newer drugs	• Acts on the sinoatrial node to reduce heart rate and myocardial oxygen demand It also improves coronary blood flow	• Relieves pain, reduces the heart's workload and improves coronary blood flow	• Ivabradine
	• Activates potassium channels and dilates coronary arteries and veins (reduces preload)	• Relieves pain, reduces the heart's workload and improves coronary blood flow	• Nicorandil
	• Alters sodium-dependent calcium channels, preventing calcium overload, which is thought to contribute to myocardial ischaemia	• Reduces angina pain • Increases exercise tolerance	• Ranolazine

*NICE (2012) guidelines give equal weighting to beta-blockers and calcium channel blockers. The newer drugs (such as ivabradine, nicorandil and ranolazine) are considered as second-line treatments. See next section for information relating to other key drugs such as statins (Table 9.4, p. 163) and anti-platelets.

Nitrates

These drugs have been used in the treatment of angina since Dr William Murrel used nitroglycerin to relieve the pain of patients suffering from angina in 1878. After his findings were published in *The Lancet* the following year, the name was changed to glyceryl trinitrate (GTN) to avoid the association with the dangerous explosive, and the use of nitrates to manage this condition soon became commonplace.

Nitrates cause vasodilation of smooth muscles in the vascular system by stimulating the production of nitric oxide via the second messenger cyclic guanosine monophosphate (cGMP). This prevents calcium entering the muscle cells, causing relaxation. The overall clinical effect in patients with angina is pain relief by increasing coronary blood flow and reducing myocardium oxygen demand. Three nitrates are commonly used in the treatment of angina; these include GTN, isosorbide mononitrate and dinitrate.

Glyceryl trinitrate

This is a short-acting nitrate, with rapid onset action, and is very effective in treating angina attacks. GTN has a high first-pass metabolism and its oral bioavailability is therefore poor. It is administered via a number of different routes, such as sublingual tablets or spray, buccal tablets, transdermal patches and intravenously. The sublingual route is the most rapid but its effects are short-lived.

The transdermal and buccal route are longer-acting and can be used for prevention. When used sublingually for acute chest pain, patients should be advised to use the first dose and repeat after 5 minutes if necessary. If there is no response after the second dose then they should seek medical attention. Patients should be informed that they may experience headaches and light-headedness.

Activity 9.4

What do the terms 'high first-pass metabolism' and 'low bioavailability' mean and why do you think GTN is not taken orally? Refer to Chapter 1 (How the body affects drugs) and the BNF. Alternatively, consult one of the pharmacology texts listed under 'References and further reading' on p. 170, such as McFadden, R. (2013). *Introducing Pharmacology for Nursing and Healthcare*.

Isosorbide dinitrate and mononitrate

These are longer acting and generally more stable nitrates than GTN, with effects lasting for a number of hours, depending on the formulation. They are widely used in the treatment of angina, mainly to prevent an attack, although isosorbide dinitrate can be used in its sublingual form to treat an angina attack that has already started. With regard to the pharmacokinetics of isosorbide dinitrate, absorption can be variable and it is metabolised extensively in the liver to the active ingredients isosorbide-2-mononitrate and isosorbide-5-mononitrate, with half-lives of 2 and 4 hours respectively. It is generally administered more than once per day. Isosorbide mononitrate, on the other hand, does not undergo first-pass metabolism. The slow-release formulation is given once a day and is therefore better for patient compliance.

Tolerance

Tolerance to nitrates (especially the longer-acting preparations described above) can sometimes develop, but this is usually resolved when the drug is stopped for a period of time. The chances of developing tolerance are reduced if long-acting nitrates are dosed asymmetrically, with the second dose being given 6–8 hours after the first dose (i.e. 8am and 2pm), rather than every 12 hours.

Activity 9.5

Define the term 'tolerance' and explain why asymmetric dosing of isosorbide dinitrate does not produce tolerance.

Table 9.2: Adverse effects of nitrates

- Headaches
- Flushing
- Syncope due to fall in blood pressure, especially with long-acting nitrates
- Palpitations
- Tachycardia
- Less common: nausea, vomiting, methaemoglobinaemias – patient may appear cyanosed
- Major interaction (e.g. sudden reduction in BP) occurs with phosphodiesterase inhibitors such as sildenafil (Viagra®).

Beta-blockers

In the management of angina, beta-blockers (such as atenolol and metoprolol) are generally used prophylactically to prevent the pain associated with angina, rather than treat it. That said, studies have demonstrated that perfusion of the myocardium is more effective at lower heart rates, and some guidelines such as the Scottish Intercollegiate Guidelines Network (2007) use beta-blockers as a first-line treatment for stable angina. Furthermore, the American College of Cardiology guidelines (Gibbons 2002) have set a target heart rate of 55–60bpm using beta-blockers in controlling the symptoms of angina. Beta-blockers block beta-1 receptors in the heart, toning down the effects of the sympathetic nervous system on the heart during exercise, reducing the heart rate, blood pressure and workload, and thereby preventing myocardial ischaemia. However, beta-blockers are also associated with a number of side effects (see Table 9.3 below) and are contraindicated in asthmatics, as they can cause bronchospasm and induce an asthmatic attack.

Table 9.3: Adverse effects of beta-blockers

- Bronchospasm
- Reduced myocardial contractility (can worsen heart failure)
- Cold extremities (reduce cardiac output, leading to reduced blood flow to peripheries)
- Masks hypoglycaemic symptoms in diabetes
- Lethargy

Activity 9.6

Briefly explain why beta-blockers can induce bronchospasm.

Calcium channel blockers and newer antianginals

Calcium antagonists, such as nifedipine and diltiazem, are also commonly used in the management of angina. They produce their effect by blocking the L-type voltage-sensitive calcium channels in the smooth muscles of arteries. The overall effect is vasodilation, which reduces peripheral vascular resistance (afterload) and thus the workload of the heart. In addition, they relax and dilate the coronary arteries and are therefore valuable in Prinzmetal's angina (spasm of the arteries is a cause of angina pain).

NICE (2011a) guidelines suggest that if a calcium antagonist is not tolerated then a beta-blocker should be considered, or vice versa. If neither of these drugs is effective in controlling the symptoms then either a long-acting nitrate or one of the newer drugs (such as ivabradine, nicorandil or ranolazine) should be used. As outlined in Table 9.1 (p. 158), the principal action of ivabradine is to block the calcium channels in the sinoatrial node, thus lowering the heart rate. Support for the value of a lower heart rate in controlling the symptoms of angina comes from studies using ivabradine (Tardif et al. 2005). Furthermore, in the ASSOCIATE study (Tardif et al. 2009), when ivabradine was added to a beta-blocker it was shown to improve symptoms further. Both nicorandil and ranolazine are effective in relieving angina pain.

Statins

Cholesterol, as discussed above, forms a significant component of the atheromatous plaques that narrow and occlude coronary arteries, leading to complications such as angina. Many epidemiological studies have confirmed the strong link between high-plasma low density lipoprotein (LDL) cholesterol levels and atherosclerosis. LDLs are the main type of cholesterol responsible for the development of atherosclerosis. Meanwhile, high density lipoproteins (HDLs) have been shown to be protective, as they remove cholesterol from the artery walls, and the cholesterol is then returned to the liver.

Cholesterol is made in the liver and the enzyme HMG CoA reductase has an integral role in this process. Statins, such as simvastatin and pravastatin, are HMG CoA reductase inhibitors. By inhibiting the production of this liver enzyme, they block the synthesis of cholesterol. The reduced levels of cholesterol cause increased production of LDL receptors, which clears more cholesterol than normal from the blood plasma. Many studies have demonstrated the effectiveness of these drugs in reducing cholesterol levels.

More specifically, there is a direct link between lowering cholesterol and reducing coronary events and the associated mortality rates. Of course, other lipid-lowering drugs (such as fibrates, anion exchange resins and ezetimibe) reduce cholesterol levels by other mechanisms (see Table 9.4 below) but statins are very effective, widely used and have better outcome data, which is why they are generally the drug of choice. More recent studies (Blake & Ridker 2000) have also shown that statins not only reduce cholesterol levels but also have anti-inflammatory properties. As the inflammatory process is also a major part of the pathophysiology of atherosclerosis, these findings provide further support for the important role of statins in preventing coronary events.

Indeed NICE (2014a), in their draft guidelines on lipid modification, have recently recommended that statins should be prescribed more widely, to include people who have only a 10% risk (using the QRISK 2 risk assessment tool) of cardiovascular disease over a 10-year period. Nevertheless, studies have shown that the relative potency of statins is associated with a few adverse effects.

Table 9.4: Examples of lipid-lowering drugs

Name	Action	Adverse effects
Statins, e.g. simvastatin pravastatin	• HMG CoA inhibitors – reduce production of cholesterol in liver.	• Myopathy and myositis are rare but can progress to rhabdomyolysis. • Affects liver function tests.
Bile acid sequestrants, e.g. colestyramine, colestipol	• These drugs bind bile acids. Bound bile acids are excreted and this promotes conversion of cholesterol to bile acids.	• Mainly gastrointestinal because the resins are not absorbed, e.g. abdominal discomfort, diarrhoea, constipation, bloating, hypertriglyceridaemia.
Fibrates, e.g. bezafibrate, fenofibrate	• Mainly reduce triglycerides synthesis by stimulating lipoprotein lipase, which transports fat particles to muscles for energy and fat storage in adipose tissue. Fibrates also have a small effect on reducing LDL and increasing HDL.	• Sometimes causes muscle pain, dyspepsia, tiredness. • Combination with statins increases risk of myotoxicity.
Intestinal cholesterol absorption inhibitors, e.g. ezetimibe (fairly new drug)	• Reduces intestinal cholesterol reabsorption of cholesterol and LDL cholesterol. • Used in combination with statins or alone.	• Can cause headaches, muscle pain, gastrointestinal disturbances, fatigue, hypersensitivity reaction.
Nicotinic acid – can be used in combination with statins (can increase risk of rhabdomyolysis), in the management of dys-lipidaemia or solely if the patient is unable to tolerate statins	• Inhibits the production and secretion of very low density lipoprotein. • Lowers triglycerides and LDL cholesterols. • Increases HDL.	• Gastrointestinal symptoms, e.g. nausea, vomiting, dyspepsia, diarrhoea. • Can also lead to a range of other less common symptoms (see BNF).

Activity 9.7

Why are statins generally administered at night?

Anti-platelets

Exposure of collagen in damaged blood vessels is a potent stimulator of platelet aggregation. With this aggregation, the platelets self-activate the release of a number of substances, such as thromboxane A2 (TXA2), adenosine diphosphate (ADP), 5-hydroxytryptamine (5HT) and noradrenaline, which stimulate further platelet aggregation, constriction and activation of the clotting cascade.

Aspirin is now widely used in the management of patients with CVD. Indeed, many studies have shown that it reduces mortality rates in patients who have had a myocardial infarction, prevents acute myocardial infarction in patients with unstable angina, and reduces the incidence of stroke in patients who have suffered transient ischaemic attacks.

Aspirin produces its effect by inhibiting thromboxane A2 formation and release by platelets, thus preventing platelets clumping together to form clots. It achieves this by irreversibly inhibiting platelet cyclooxygenase (COX). Under normal circumstances, thromboxane A2 is a potent inducer of platelet aggregation (clumping). By inhibiting COX, aspirin alters the normal balance between thromboxane A2 (which normally stimulates platelet aggregation) and prostaglandin (PGI2), which inhibits platelet aggregation. Although small doses of aspirin will inhibit TXA2, it does so without significantly reducing PGI2, thereby shifting the balance more towards the anti-aggregation path. Adverse effects of aspirin include gastrointestinal bleeding.

Other commonly used anti-platelets include clopidogrel, which irreversibly inhibits adenosine diphosphate (ADP) mediated platelet aggregation. Clopidogrel is used if aspirin is contraindicated, or not tolerated. It is licensed to be used in combination with aspirin in STEMI and NSTEMI, as well as in revascularisation, to enhance the anti-platelet effect of aspirin. This is an example of a synergistic effect (see Chapter 3). Adverse effects of clopidogrel include diarrhoea and rashes. Clopidogrel is also a prodrug, which must be converted to its active metabolite. This means its onset of action is slower, achieving steady state platelet inhibition within about 2–4 hours after a loading dose of 600mg.

Fish oils are gaining prominence because they not only reduce production of prostaglandins (which are natural promoters of inflammation and clotting), but they also increase production of prostacyclins, which have an anti-inflammatory effect.

Newer, more potent anti-platelet drugs used in the management of acute coronary syndrome include prasugrel and ticagrelor, which are sometimes used to address some of the adverse effects of clopidogrel, but they do have some limitations (NICE 2011b).

Case study 9.3: Chest pain

This is a typical case that a chest pain specialist nurse manages on a regular basis.

Mr David Jones is a 67-year-old retired bus driver who was referred by his GP to the rapid access chest pain clinic (RACPC) with a three-month history of chest pain on exertion, particularly when walking up an incline. He has no chest pain when resting. Mr Jones also has type 2 diabetes, is hypertensive with raised cholesterol levels (total 5.5 mmols/l, HDL 1.0 and LDL 3.4) and is allergic to aspirin. He states that the first time he took aspirin his face swelled. His current medications are metformin 500mg twice a day, enalapril 20mg once daily and simvastatin 40mg nocte.

On assessment in the RACPC, Mr Jones is not distressed or experiencing any pain. His vital signs are temperature: 36.8°C, pulse rate 80bpm, regular; ECG normal sinus rhythm and BP 145/85mmHg. Based on Mr Jones' clinical history and presenting symptoms, he was rated as being at high (97%) risk of having coronary artery disease (NICE 2010). He was commenced on medical therapy for his presenting symptoms and recommended for a coronary angiogram as well as a number of investigations including a full blood count, urea and electrolytes, blood glucose and liver function tests.

Activity 9.8 (Case study)

1. Imagine you are the clinical nurse specialist caring for Mr Jones as a non-medical prescriber. List three drug groups (or types of drugs) you would consider prescribing.
2. Anti-platelets, such as aspirin, are essential in the management of stable and unstable angina. Explain how aspirin produces its effect.
3. What are the key questions you would ask before prescribing an anti-platelet for Mr Jones? Would aspirin be your choice of anti-platelet for Mr Jones? If not, can you say why, and suggest an alternative.

Pharmacology case studies for nurse prescribers

4. Why would you assess Mr Jones' liver function and consider changing his statin?
5. The main aim in the pharmacological treatment of angina is to reduce the workload of the heart and, in doing so, the amount of oxygen it demands. Briefly outline how nitrates would achieve this aim.
6. Glyceryl trinitrate (GTN) spray, two puffs sublingually, was prescribed for Mr Jones. Why is GTN administered by this route? Suggest two other routes of administration.

Activity 9.9 (Case study)

Beta-blockers are one of the drug groups used in the first-line treatment of stable angina.

1. Outline how beta-blockers would reduce Mr Jones' angina attacks.
2. Mr Jones was prescribed a cardioselective long-acting beta-blocker. Can you suggest two types of beta-blockers that would be suitable?
3. List some important checks that you would perform before commencing him on beta-blockers.
4. Explain why beta-blockers (even selective ones) can induce an asthmatic attack.
5. If Mr Jones developed acute asthma induced by beta-blockers, explain why he might not respond to being treated by a drug such as salbutamol.
6. Can you suggest another type of drug that could be added if Mr Jones remained symptomatic and did not tolerate an increase in his beta-blocker dose?

Mr Jones' drug treatment

Mr Jones was prescribed GTN spray, clopidogrel 75mg od, bisoprolol 2.5mg od (GP to review in 1–2 weeks) and simvastatin was replaced with atorvastatin 40mg. Alteration in the drug regime will depend on Mr Jones' response to the current management and his consultant's choice of the recommended drugs, as well as the results of Mr Jones' angiogram report.

Summary

CHD is a major cause of mortality and morbidity rates in the UK. Stable angina is the most common symptom of CHD, and for the majority of patients it is treated effectively by optimal medical treatment and lifestyle changes. This chapter has given some insight into the pathophysiology and pharmacological management of this condition. Furthermore, by completing the activities in the chapter, it is hoped that nurse practitioners will appreciate the importance of having a sound knowledge of pharmacological principles in order to manage patients with coronary heart disease safely and effectively.

Answers to activities

Activity 9.1

Can you suggest two other conditions that can cause angina?

Apart from atherosclerosis, angina can be caused by hypertrophic cardiomyopathy, cardiac syndrome X or anaemia.

Activity 9.2 (Case study)

1. Based on Mr O'Connor's history, what diagnosis would you suspect?

Suspect coronary artery disease, based on presenting symptoms, e.g. shortness of breath on exertion but no chest pain. Beware of exertional breathlessness in diabetic patients and past medical history of type 2 diabetes and hypertension.

2. Suggest a pharmacological management plan for Mr O'Connor based on the above case study.

To manage his symptoms, Mr O'Connor should be commenced on a beta-blocker – bisoprolol 5mg once a day; GTN spray and his statin should be changed to atorvastatin to reduce total cholesterol levels to 4 mmol/l or less.

Activity 9.3 (Case study)

1. What evidence in Mr Smith's history would make you suspect that CHD might be present?

Although atypical features suspect probable coronary artery disease based on presenting symptoms, i.e. shortness of breath, ischaemic changes on ECG in leads V3–V6; past medical history, type 2 diabetes and hypertension but no chest pain.

2. What adjustments would you initially make to Mr Smith's medication?

Mr Smith should be commenced on atenolol 25mg od and GTN spray, and his statin should be changed to atorvastatin 40mg nocte.

Mr Smith's coronary angiogram later confirmed coronary heart disease, demonstrating occlusion to the left anterior descending artery (LAD). Primary coronary intervention was carried out to the LAD and he made a good recovery.

Activity 9.4

What do the terms 'high first-pass metabolism' and 'low bioavailability' mean and why do you think GTN is not taken orally?

If GTN is swallowed whole, it loses its effectiveness. This is because it undergoes significant metabolism in the liver (high first-pass effect) before it reaches the systemic circulation; very little of the drug is therefore available to produce an effect (low bioavailability).

Activity 9.5

Define the term 'tolerance' and explain why asymmetric dosing of isosorbide dinitrate does not produce tolerance.

Tolerance to a drug means there is reduced responsiveness to the drug, both in terms of efficacy and/or duration of action. Tolerance does not occur with asymmetric dosing of isosorbide dinitrate, as mentioned above, possibly because the overnight rest rapidly restores sensitivity to the drug. This is commonly referred to as the 'nitrate-free interval', which most reference sources suggest should be at least 10–12 hours long. The mechanism for tolerance to the effects of nitrates is not fully understood (Rang, Dale et al. 2012).

Activity 9.6

Briefly explain why beta-blockers can induce bronchospasm.

Most beta-blockers (even cardio-selective ones such as atenolol and metoprolol) may also block beta-2 receptors in the bronchioles, thus precipitating a bronchospasm and an asthmatic attack. Stimulation of beta-2 receptors leads to bronchodilation; blocking them would lead to bronchospasms.

Activity 9.7

Why are statins generally administered at night?

The synthesis of cholesterol is highest during the night.

Activity 9.8 (Case study)

1. Imagine you are the clinical nurse specialist caring for Mr Jones as a non-medical prescriber. List three drug groups (or types of drugs) you would consider prescribing.

Anti-platelet, nitrate and beta-blocker, and consider changing the statin Mr Jones is currently taking.

2. Anti-platelets, such as aspirin, are essential in the management of stable and unstable angina. Explain how aspirin produces its effect.

Aspirin irreversibly binds to the enzyme cyclooxygenase (COX), which prevents the formation of thromboxane A2. This substance normally promotes platelet aggregation. Reducing TXA2 formation will prevent platelets adhering to each other and thus reduce the chance of clots forming.

3. What are the key questions you would ask before prescribing an anti-platelet for Mr Jones? Would aspirin be your choice of anti-platelet for Mr Jones? If not, can you state why and suggest an alternative?

Questions to ask: Allergy to aspirin or intolerance, NSAIDs, history of asthma, bleeding from GIT, gastric ulcers, any bleeding or clot disorders? Aspirin would not be the first choice for Mr Jones, as his history suggests he is aspirin-intolerant. An alternative drug would be clopidogrel. Mr Jones should also be informed of the side effects of clopidogrel such as rashes and severe itching.

4. Why would you assess Mr Jones' liver function and consider changing his statin?

Mr Jones' cholesterol levels do not appear to be well controlled with the simvastatin. They are still above the recommended levels. Total cholesterol should be <4mmol/l (Mr Jones has diabetes and hypertension) and his LDL is >2mmol/l. Statins can cause liver impairment, and liver enzymes such as alanine aminotransferase (ALT) and aspartate aminotransferase (AST) may become elevated. Although there is limited research evidence to support liver damage, NICE (2014a) recommends monitoring liver function tests for patients taking statins. Mr Jones was commenced on atorvastatin, as studies have shown that it is more effective than simvastatin in reducing total cholesterol and LDL.

5. The main aim in the pharmacological treatment of angina is to reduce the workload of the heart and, in doing so, the amount of oxygen it demands. Briefly outline how nitrates would achieve this aim.

GTN is a short-acting nitrate and one of the first-line drugs used in the management of angina. It reduces the heart's workload through peripheral vasodilation. This causes pooling of the blood in the veins, reducing venous return and the volume of blood in the left ventricle. If there is less distension of the heart, then oxygen demand will be reduced.

6. Glyceryl trinitrate (GTN) spray, two puffs sublingually, was prescribed for Mr Jones. Why is GTN administered by this route? Suggest two other routes of administration.

GTN is given sublingually to avoid hepatic first-pass metabolism. If swallowed, the liver would break it down significantly, resulting in low bioavailability. GTN can also be administered intravenously or transdermally – both methods would avoid first-pass metabolism. It is indicated for use during an attack and can be used prophylactically if angina symptoms are anticipated – for example, when walking up a hill or climbing stairs. Important advice regarding the use of GTN should be given to Mr Jones, such as the need to use a second dose after 5 minutes if symptoms recur. If he fails to respond to a repeated dose within 5 minutes, he should seek immediate medical attention. He should also be advised that sublingual GTN is likely to induce a headache and may make him feel light-headed. These symptoms tend to settle with repeated use.

Activity 9.9

1. Outline how beta-blockers would reduce Mr Jones' angina attacks.

Beta-blockers reduce the heart rate and contractility of the myocardium, thus reducing myocardial oxygen demand and preventing further angina attack by protecting the heart from over-activity. A reduction in heart rate also increases the proportion of time that the heart remains in diastole, resulting in better perfusion of the myocardium.

2. Mr Jones was prescribed a cardioselective long-acting beta-blocker. Can you suggest two types of beta-blockers that would be suitable?

Two examples of suitable cardioselective beta-blockers are bisoprolol or atenolol.

3. List some important checks that you would perform before commencing beta-blockers.

Important checks: heart rate (ensure >55bpm – this will determine start dose of beta-blocker); blood pressure; history of asthma; ECG exclude second- and third-degree heart block.

4. Explain why beta-blockers (even selective ones) can induce an asthmatic attack.

Even selective beta-1 blockers could cause an asthmatic attack by binding to a proportion of beta-2 receptors in the lungs, thus inducing bronchospasm.

5. If Mr Jones developed acute asthma induced by beta-blockers, explain why he might not respond to being treated by a drug such as salbutamol.

Because of competition for binding sites, the beta-blocker may prevent salbutamol binding to beta-2 receptors in the lungs and the patient may not respond to the salbutamol.

6. Can you suggest another type of drug that could be added if Mr Jones remained symptomatic and did not tolerate an increase in his beta-blocker dose?

Nicorandil is a nitric acid donor and is also a potassium channel activator. The effects of this are vasodilation of veins and arteries. It is used for the prevention and treatment of stable angina.

References and further reading

Baigent, C., Blackwell, L., Emberson, J. et al. (2010). Cholesterol Treatment Trialists' (CTT) Collaboration. Efficacy and safety of more intensive lowering of LDL cholesterol: a meta-analysis of data from 170,000 participants in 26 randomised control trials. *The Lancet.* **376**, 1670–81.

Blake, G.J. & Ridker, P.M, (2000). Are statins anti-inflammatory? *Current Control Trials Cardiovascular Medicine.* **1** (3), 161–65.

Boden, W.E., O'Rourke, R.A. & Teo, K.K. (2007). COURAGE Trial Research Group. Optimal medical therapy with or without PCI for stable coronary disease. *New England Journal of Medicine.* **15**, 1503–16.

British Heart Foundation (2012). *Coronary Heart Disease Statistics.* London: BHF.

Eikelboom, J.W., Connolly, S.J., et al. for the COMPASS Investigators European Society of Cardiology (2016). 2016 European Guidelines on cardiovascular disease prevention in clinical practice. *European Heart Journal.* **37**, 2315–81. doi:10.1093/eurheart/ehw106.

Fox, K., Ford, I., Steg, P.G., Tardif, J-C., Tendera, M. & Ferrari, R. (2014). Ivabradine in stable coronary artery disease without clinical heart failure. *Journal of Medicine.* **371** (12), 1091–99.

Gibbons, R.J. (chair) (2002). ACC/AHA Practice Guidelines. *Circulation.* **106**, 1883–92.

IONA Study Group (2002). Effect of nicorandil on coronary events in patients with stable angina: the Impact of Nicorandil in Angina (IONA) randomised trial. *Lancet.* **359**, 1269–75.

Joint Formulary Committee (2014). *British National Formulary.* 67th edn. London: British Medical Journal Group and Pharmaceutical Press.

McFadden, R. (2013). *Introducing Pharmacology for Nursing and Healthcare.* 2nd edn. Harlow: Pearson Education Limited.

Marsh, N. & Marsh, A. (2000). A short history of nitroglycerine and nitric oxide in pharmacology and physiology. *Clinical Experimental Pharmacology Physiology.* **27** (4), 313–19.

Medicines and Healthcare Products Regulatory Agency (MHRA) (2014). *Ivabradine: carefully monitor for bradycardia.* https://www.gov.uk/government/organisations/medicines-and-healthcare-products-regulatory-agency (Last accessed 21 February 2020).

National Institute for Health and Care Excellence (NICE) (2010). Chest pain of recent onset. *Consensus guidelines for the management of symptomatic stable angina in primary care* (CG95). London: NICE.

National Institute for Health and Care Excellence (NICE) (2011a). *Management of Stable Angina* (CG126). London: NICE (Last updated 2016). Available at https://www.nice.org.uk/guidance/cg126/history (Accessed: December 2020).

National Institute for Health and Care Excellence (NICE) (2011b). *Ticagrelor for the treatment of acute coronary syndromes. Technology appraisal guidance* (TA236). London: NICE.

National Institute for Health and Care Excellence (NICE) (2014a). *Lipid modification: Cardiovascular risk assessment and the modification of blood lipids for the primary and secondary prevention of cardiovascular disease* (CG181). London: NICE.

National Institute for Health and Care Excellence (NICE) (2014b). *Prasugrel with percutaneous coronary intervention for treating acute coronary syndromes. Technology appraisal guidance* (TA317). London: NICE.

National Institute for Health and Care Excellence (NICE) (2019). *Rivaroxaban for preventing atherothrombotic events in people with coronary or peripheral artery disease. Technology appraisal guidance* (TA607). London: NICE.

National Institute for Health and Care Excellence (NICE) (2020). *Chest pain overview.* Available online: https://pathways.nice.org.uk/pathways/chest-pain. (Last accessed 10 May 2020).

Neal, M.J. (2012). *Medical Pharmacology at a Glance*. 6th edn. Chichester: Wiley Blackwell.

Rang, H.P., Dale, M.M., Ritter, J.M., Flower. R.J. & Henderson, G. (2012). *Rang and Dale Pharmacology*. Edinburgh: Churchill Livingstone.

Scottish Intercollegiate Guidelines Network (2007). *Management of stable angina*. Clinical guideline 96. http://www.SIGN.ac.uk (Last accessed 1 October 2020).

Stevens, A. & Lowe, J. (1995). *Pathology*. London: Mosby.

Tardif, J.C., Ford, I., Tendera, M., Bourassa, M.G. & Fox, K. (2005). Efficacy of ivabradine, a new selective I(f) inhibitor, compared with atenolol in patients with chronic stable angina. *European Heart Journal*. **26**, 2529–36.

Tardif, J.C., Ponikowski, P. & Kahan, T. (2009). Efficacy of the If current inhibitor ivabradine in patients with chronic stable angina receiving beta-blocker therapy: a 4-month, randomized, placebo-controlled trial. *European Heart Journal*. **30**, 540–48.

Wilson, S.R., Scirica, B.M., Braunwald, E., Murphy, S.A., Karwatowska-Prokopczuk, E., Buros, J.L., Chaitman, B.R. & Morrow, D.A. (2009). Efficacy of ranolazine in patients with chronic angina observations from the randomised, double-blind, placebo-controlled MERLIN-TIMI (Metabolic Efficiency with Ranolazine for Less Ischemia in Non-ST-Segment Elevation Acute Coronary Syndromes) 36 Trial. *Journal of American College of Cardiology*. **53**, 1510–16.

Wright, P. & Antoniou, S. (2013). Acute coronary syndrome: potent oral anti-platelets. *Nurse Prescribing*. **11** (8), 397–400.

10

Pharmacological case studies: Hypertension

Donna Scholefield
MSc, BSc (Hons), RN, PGDip HE; Cardiac Nursing (254);
Senior Lecturer, Health and Education, Middlesex University, London

This chapter:

- Gives an insight into the prevalence and consequences of high blood pressure
- Outlines the key variables that determine blood pressure
- Discusses the major drug groups used in the management of hypertension
- Explains the pharmacology of key drugs used to manage hypertension
- Applies knowledge of anti-hypertensive drug pharmacology to practice-based case studies.

Introduction

In the UK, the British Heart Foundation (BHF 2020) states that there are over 15 million people in the UK with a diagnosis of hypertension and of these there is an estimated 5 million that are undiagnosed. Furthermore, Public Health England (PHE 2017) estimate that in England alone there are over 11.8 million adults (aged 16 and above) that are known to have hypertension which equates to just over a quarter of the population suffering from this disorder. These figures are of significant concern given major co-morbidities such as diabetes, stroke, CHD, and chronic kidney disease associated with hypertension.

Effective management of hypertension is extremely important, as it is a significant risk factor for cardiovascular disease (CVD) such as strokes, heart failure, ischaemic heart disease and chronic renal disorders. In addition, high blood pressure and its associated morbidities can be prevented by making lifestyle changes. Indeed, the European Society of Hypertension and European Society of Cardiology (ESH & ESC 2018) and NICE clinical guidelines (2019) have emphasised the importance of lifestyle changes such as increasing physical activity, reducing weight and eating a healthy diet with reduced salt and alcohol intake, reduced saturated fats, and increased fruit and vegetables.

Nevertheless, despite growing evidence supporting the effectiveness of lifestyle intervention and effective drug regimes, the ESH/ESC (2018) report raised concerns about the poor level of BP control and its consequences both globally and across many European countries. It is hoped that the pragmatic approach adopted by these guidelines (ESH/ESC 2018 and NICE 2019), guided by recent results from several large clinical trials such as the Systolic Blood Pressure Intervention Trial (SPRINT 2015), will enable practitioners to improve their detection and management of hypertension worldwide.

This chapter aims to provide an overview of the physiology and current pharmacological management of blood pressure. Two case studies will be used to give an insight into the application of this knowledge, as well as the complexities involved in the pharmacological management of hypertension.

Defining hypertension

Like many physiological variables, blood pressure in the population has a normal distribution. The ESH/ESC (2018) recommends that normal BP be subdivided and classified as optimal, normal and high normal (see Table 10.1).

Table 10.1 Normal blood pressure classification

Category	Systolic BP (SBP)	Diastolic BP (DBP)
Optimal	<120	<80
Normal	120–129	80–84
High normal	130–139	85–89

'Hypertension is defined as office SBP values ≥140mmHg and/or diastolic BP (DBP) values ≥90mmHg.' (ESH/ESC, 2018, p. 10).

A lower level (of 135/85) is used to determine hypertension when measurements are taken by ambulatory BP monitoring (ABPM) or home BP monitoring (HBPM), as indicated by Table 10.2. However, if the patient has other associated conditions (such as type 1 diabetes) then hypertension is diagnosed at a level of 130/80mmHg or greater.

In the UK, national guidelines such as NICE (2019) and the British and Irish Hypertension Society (2019) state that stage one hypertension exists if the clinic blood pressure measurement is 140/90mmHg or above. Indeed, both ESH/ESC (2018) and NICE (2019) are in agreement that this value should be the recommended treatment threshold. However, the ESH/ESC has extended its recommendation to reduce the BP in under-65s to a SBP in the range of 120–129 if tolerated (McCormack, Boffa, et al. 2019).

Table 10.2 Classification of hypertension NICE (2019)

Stage 1 hypertension	Clinical BP of 140/90 to 159/99 and subsequent ABPM daytime average of HBPM BP ranging from 135/85mmHg to 149/94* mmHg.
Stage 2 hypertension	Clinic blood pressure is 160/100mmHg or higher, but less than 180/120mmHg, and subsequent ABPM daytime average or HBPM average BP of 150/59 or higher.
Severe hypertension	Clinic systolic blood pressure of 180mmHg or higher, or clinic diastolic blood pressure 120mmHg or higher.

*In people aged over 80 years old the target is <150/90mmHg. The ESC/ESH (2018) recommend a less conservative approach in elderly patients ≥80 who are active and demonstrating no signs of frailty, suggesting BP targets of <130–139mmHg.

Activity 10.1

Although primary hypertension, which is blood pressure due to unknown causes, accounts for 95% of hypertension cases, high blood pressure can also occur due to other disorders. It is then termed secondary hypertension.

Can you identify 2–3 causes of secondary hypertension?

Activity 10.2

1. Reflect on a patient you have recently cared for with hypertension.

How was the diagnosis arrived at? For example, was it based on several clinic BP readings, ABPM or HBPM? Was it taken in both arms?

2. NICE guidelines recommend that the diagnosis of hypertension should be based on the clinic measurements as well as ABPM. Indeed, the ESH/ESC (2018) report also recommended that the role of ABPM and HBPM should be expanded, as they are better predictors of outcomes.

However, if your patient was unable to tolerate ABPM, refused it or ABPM was unavailable, can you suggest another recommended adjunct to clinic blood pressure to confirm the diagnosis?

3. Automated BP devices are often used to assess blood pressure and pulse levels.

If your clinic did not have access to a manual device, how would you ensure that the reading was accurate?

> **4.** There are different requirements when measuring BP in certain patients.
> In what position should BP be taken in type 2 diabetic patients, patients >80 years and individuals with a history of postural hypotension?

Prevalence of hypertension

Although there has been a slight reduction in the level of primary hypertension in the UK since 1998, the prevalence in the general population remains high, with 31% of men and 29% of women being either diagnosed with, or having treatment for, hypertension. Indeed, the ESC/ESH (2018) guidelines for the management of arterial hypertension state that the estimated worldwide prevalence of hypertension is 1.13 billion, with well over 150 million in Central and Eastern Europe.

As mentioned in the introduction, the British Heart Foundation (BHF 2016) and Public Health England (2017) estimate that over 16 million adults in the UK have hypertension – and 7 million of these remain undiagnosed. Furthermore, with trends such as an ageing population, increased obesity and an increasingly sedentary lifestyle, the global figures outlined above are predicted to increase by up to 20% by 2025 (ESC/ESH 2018).

Prevalence increases significantly with the age and lifestyle choices of the individual, despite national and international guidelines on screening and treatment. The fact that primary hypertension is symptomless until organ damage has occurred contributes significantly to these figures. This is why screening for hypertension is an important way of reducing its prevalence. To this end, NICE (2019) has advocated that all adults should have their blood pressure taken every five years until they reach the age of 80, even if hypertension is not diagnosed. If a patient's BP is nearer the 140/90mmHg level, more frequent measurements should be carried out. Type 2 diabetic patients should have, as a minimum, their BP measured annually. Screening will increase early detection of primary hypertension in all groups. However, there are other important contributory factors to the high prevalence of hypertension and these will be discussed later in this chapter.

> ### Activity 10.3
> Can you suggest other approaches that could be used by the healthcare professional to address factors contributing to the prevalence of high blood pressure?

Factors determining blood pressure

Knowledge of the physiological factors that determine blood pressure is essential in order to appreciate how anti-hypertensive drugs produce their pharmacological and clinical effects as well as their undesirable effects.

Blood pressure is defined as the pressure that the blood exerts against the arterial vessel wall and it is determined by many factors. These include the peripheral vascular resistance (PVR), cardiac output, volume and viscosity (thickness) of the blood. If any of these variables change, the blood pressure will also change.

Alteration in the PVR has the greatest effect on blood pressure and blood flow. This resistance is mainly determined by the arterioles, which contain thick muscular walls consisting of circular smooth muscles with some elastic tissue. They control the blood flow from arteries into the capillaries and their diameter is controlled by the sympathetic nervous system. When the sympathetic nervous system is stimulated, it releases noradrenaline, which interacts with receptors on the blood vessel wall, causing them to constrict. The effect of vasoconstriction is to increase peripheral vascular resistance (afterload) and, as a result, BP. The increased resistance, which the heart now has to pump against, results in the heart having to work harder. Many other chemicals, such as angiotensin, anti-diuretic hormones, adrenal medulla hormones and endothelium-derived factor, also narrow the walls of the blood vessels, increasing PVR. Reduced sympathetic stimulation to the arterioles would produce vasodilatation, reducing PVR and lowering BP.

The cardiac output is determined by both heart rate and stroke volume so, again, altering either of these variables will increase or decrease the blood pressure. For example, sympathetic nerve stimulation would release noradrenaline in the heart, which would interact with beta receptors, which would increase stroke volume via an increase in both heart rate and contractility. Blood volume and viscosity are controlled by the kidneys. The kidneys act (both directly and indirectly) on long-term control of blood pressure. The direct action is on renal mechanisms that alter blood volume, and the indirect mechanisms involve the renin-angiotensin-aldosterone system. Aldosterone is a hormone that is released from the cortex of the adrenal glands. It acts on the nephron to retain salt and water, thus increasing blood volume and thereby increasing stroke volume. The following equation offers a simple but useful way of remembering the key variables controlling BP:

Blood pressure (BP) = cardiac output (CO) × peripheral vascular resistance (PVR)

Activity 10.4

Before reviewing the next section, use the information about the physiology of blood pressure control to briefly outline how key drugs, such as ace-inhibitors, beta-blockers and diuretics, reduce blood pressure. You may wish to consult a physiology text, such as Tortora & Derrickson (2017), to review the physiology of blood pressure control.

Drugs used to manage primary hypertension

As discussed previously, high BP is not only one of the main causes of premature death, but also of disability in England (Global Burden of Disease 2017). Furthermore, medication for treatment of hypertension is estimated to have cost the NHS over 2 billion pounds in 2018 (BHF 2018). Drugs and lifestyle interventions are currently the two main approaches used to manage hypertension in the UK. Although evidence of the effectiveness of a range of device-based therapies such as carotid baroreceptor stimulation and renal denervation is emerging, these therapies are not yet recommended by any of the guidelines for the routine management of hypertension until further studies have been carried out to demonstrate their safety and efficacy (ESC/ESH 2018).

Drug treatment therefore remains the primary strategy for the treatment of hypertension in the UK. As illustrated in Table 10.2, NICE suggests that drug therapy should commence if the BP is 140/90mmHg or greater. However, the level at which treatment commences also depends on other factors such as age and multi-morbidities (e.g. diabetes).

Healthcare professionals should also be mindful of the fact that successful management of hypertension is directly associated with the patient's level of involvement in decisions related to their care. The more involved patients are in the decision-making process, the more empowered they will feel, and the more likely they are to adhere to their plan of care (NICE 2009).

Many of the drugs used in the treatment of hypertension work by acting on the physiological variables that control BP, as outlined in the previous section. They produce their effects by reducing peripheral vascular resistance and/or decreasing cardiac output, both of which result in a decrease in blood pressure. Table 10.3 outlines some of the key drugs used in the management of hypertension and their mode of action.

Monitoring treatment and blood pressure targets

Over the last three years, international hypertension guidelines (Unger et al. 2020, ESC/ESH 2018, NICE 2019) committees have revised their guidelines to reflect the findings of studies such as the Systolic Blood Pressure Intervention Trial (SPRINT 2015). This study demonstrated conclusively that treating high blood pressure to a lower target BP had significant benefits – reduction in cardiovascular events and death rates.

These three international guidelines to a large extent both inform and shape clinical practice worldwide. Nevertheless, although they agree on a number of approaches there are many differences (McCormack, Boffa, et al. 2019). In Europe the two major guidelines (ESC/ESH 2018 and NICE 2019) are in agreement on some aspects, such as the diagnosis threshold for hypertension (≤140/90mmHg), but there are also notable differences. For example, the ESC/ESH (2018) has a lower target BP than NICE, recommending that clinicians should aim for a lower target BP in most patients, provided they are tolerant of the treatment and for people under the age of 65 an SBP of 120–129mmHg (McCormack, Boffa, et al. 2019). Go to the following link for a summary of the key changes made to the recent NICE (2019) guidelines for management of hypertension in adults: https://bihsoc.org/guidelines/hypertension-management/

Table 10.3: Drugs used in the management of hypertension

Drug group	Effects	Examples of drugs used in hypertension
• ACE-inhibitors (ACEi)	• Reduce blood volume by blocking salt- and water-retaining effects of aldosterone	• Ramipril, perindopril and enalapril
• Angiotensin II receptor blockers (ARBs)	• Block the effects of angiotensin II on ATI receptors in blood vessels and other tissues, producing a similar overall effect to ACEis	• Losartan, valsartan
• Alpha blockers – used in resistant hypertension if diuretic therapy is ineffective (stage 4)	• Block the vasoconstrictor effects of catecholamines such as adrenaline and noradrenaline at alpha-1 receptors, producing vasodilation and a reduction in peripheral vascular resistance	• Prazosin, doxazosin
• Calcium channel blockers	• Block calcium channel in smooth muscle cells, leading to dilatation of both coronary and peripheral arteries and arterioles • Also exhibit varying degrees of both negative inotropic and chronotropic effects	• Nifedipine, diltiazem, amlodipine
• Thiazide-like diuretic 1st option	• Inhibit sodium reabsorption in the kidney tubules and increase water loss, resulting in reduced blood volume	• Chlortalidone, indapamide
• Thiazide diuretics	• Actual mechanism of action in reducing blood pressure is unknown	• Bendroflumethiazide, hydrochlorothiazide
• Potassium-sparing diuretics and aldosterone antagonists – for resistant hypertension (unlicensed)	• Aldosterone antagonist acting at the distal renal tubule to increase sodium and water loss	• Spironolactone – low dose
• Beta-blockers – used in special situations, e.g. for younger patients, and those who are intolerant of ACEis and ARBs	• Dampen down the effect of the sympathetic nervous system, reducing CO and PVR	• Atenolol, bisoprolol, metoprolol

Table 10.3 summarises the main ways that drugs can lower blood pressure: 1. Reducing total peripheral vascular resistance (PVR) 2. Reducing cardiac output, blood volume or 3. body sodium stores.

The following sections will provide more detail about the pharmacology of the drugs in Table 10.3 (above).

Angiotensin-converting enzyme inhibitors (ACEis)/ Angiotensin receptor blockers (ARBs)

ACEis are the first-line drugs indicated in the management of hypertension for people who have diabetes, or who are under 55 and Caucasian. By blocking the conversion of angiotensin I to angiotensin II, which is a powerful vasoconstrictor, ACEis reduce the peripheral vascular resistance in blood vessels, thus reducing the BP (see Figure 10.1 below). They are one of the best-tolerated groups of drugs used to lower BP but can cause a dry cough, which can be troublesome, especially at night. If this cough becomes a problem, an angiotensin II receptor antagonist (ARB), such as losartan, can be used. The ARBs block the effects of angiotensin II on angiotensin I receptors and have a similar pharmacological effect to ACEis.

ACE-inhibitors are less suitable for patients over the age of 55 years or those of African or Afro-Caribbean origin. Calcium channel blockers are the preferred first-line treatment in this population. Other less common adverse effects of ACEis include precipitation of renal failure in bilateral renal artery stenosis. Renal function tests, such as urea, electrolytes, eGFR and creatinine, should therefore be carried out when initially prescribing an ACEi and titrating the dose upwards.

Activity 10.5
1. Outline in more detail the mechanism of action of ACE-inhibitors.
2. Which receptor do the angiotensin II receptor antagonists act on?
3. List some of the key adverse effects of the ACE-inhibitors. Which of them is the most common and how would you address this if it was an issue for one of your patients?
4. What type of drug interaction could occur with a diuretic and an ACE-inhibitor?

Pharmacological case studies: Hypertension

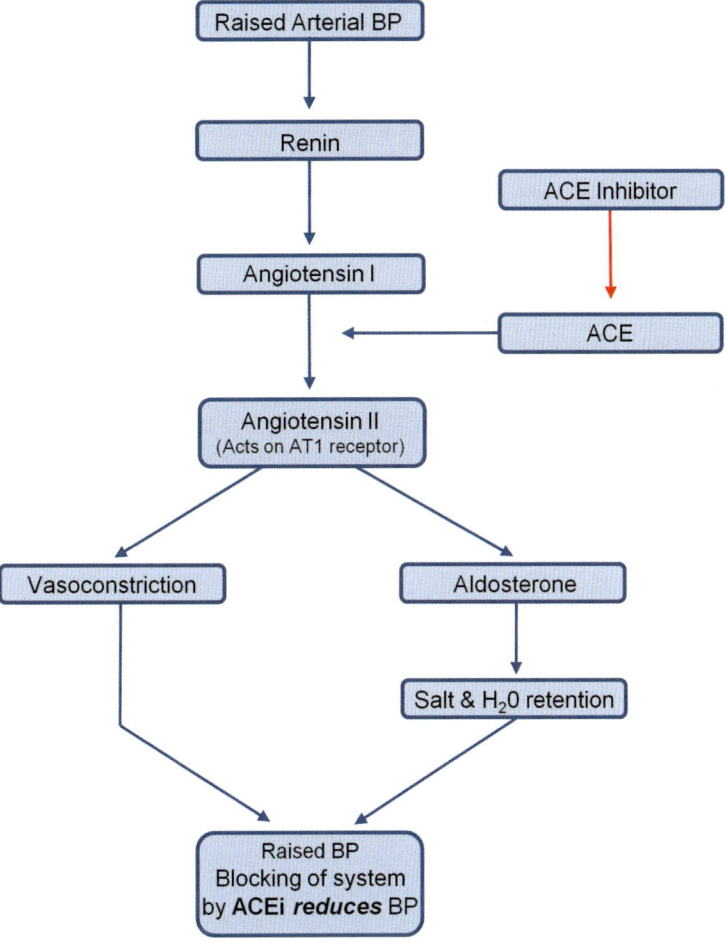

Figure 10.1: BP is reduced through inhibition of the renin-aldosterone-angiotensin system by ACE-inhibitors blocking the action of the angiotensin-converting enzyme, which prevents angiotensin I from being converted to angiotensin II. The effect is a reduction in blood volume and vasoconstriction and therefore a decrease in arterial blood pressure.

Calcium channel blockers (CCBs)

Examples of CCBs include nifedipine and amlodipine. These block the voltage-dependent L-type calcium channels in smooth muscle cells. The effect of this is to prevent the entrance of calcium, causing vasodilatation and a reduction in blood pressure. For non-diabetic patients over the age of 55 years, or of African or Afro-Caribbean origin of any age, a long-acting CCB is recommended as the first drug of choice (see Figure 10.2 on p. 184). This recommendation is supported by findings from studies such as the ALLHAT report (ALLHAT 2002), which showed that stroke and heart disease were more common in those participants who were randomised to the lisinopril group versus those receiving chlortalidone. If long-acting CCBs are prescribed, then prescribers should state the specific brand name selected to ensure bioequivalence and avoid either loss of efficacy or potential adverse effects.

> ## Activity 10.6
> 1. List the common side effects of CCBs.
> 2. If your patient was prescribed both cimetidine and nifedipine, what type of drug interaction could occur?
> 3. Why are the CCBs recommended as first-line therapy in people who are of African or Afro-Caribbean family origin?
> 4. Using the BNF, look up one brand of long-acting diltiazem and compare the different formulations available, with regard to dosing and frequency of administration.

Diuretics

Thiazide-like diuretics are recommended as part of step 2 (NICE 2019) in managing hypertension. The main drug used in the UK is indapamide, although others (such as chlortalidone) are sometimes prescribed.

These diuretics act on the nephron and increase the excretion of sodium and water, thus reducing blood volume and hence cardiac output. However, it is not known exactly how diuretics reduce blood pressure. One theory is that the reduced sodium in muscles reduces the intracellular calcium, which in turn reduces the muscle's response to endogenous vasoconstrictors. Patients whose blood pressure is well controlled on the more conventional types of thiazides (such as bendroflumethiazide or hydrochlorothiazide) should continue with these.

In those with resistant hypertension, provided the potassium level is less than 4.5mmol/l and renal function is satisfactory, low-dose spironolactone can be added, though it is not currently licensed for use as an anti-hypertensive and the patient must be informed of this. As mentioned previously, spironolactone, is a competitive antagonist of aldosterone receptors at the distal segment of the nephron. The overall impact of this blockade is an increase in the excretion of sodium and water but also a reduction in the excretion of potassium. This is why aldosterone antagonists are known as potassium-sparing diuretics.

Alpha-1 adrenoreceptor antagonists

These drugs (primarily doxazosin) block alpha-1 receptors on blood vessels, thus producing vasodilation, reducing peripheral vascular resistance and lowering BP. The latest NICE guidelines recommend that these drugs should only be considered if optimal treatment with the three main groups (ACEis/ARBs, diuretics and CCBs) fails to adequately control BP (see Figure 10.2 on p. 184).

Beta-blockers

Beta-blockers produce their effect by blocking the stimulating effects of the sympathetic nervous system, lowering cardiac output and reducing BP. Examples of beta-blockers include bisoprolol and atenolol. Because adverse effects (such as tiredness, cold peripheries, reduced exercise tolerance and impotence) are common, beta-blockers are no longer recommended as first-line treatment in hypertension. They have also been shown to increase the risk of strokes, and the combination of beta-blockers and diuretics such as bendroflumethiazide may raise the likelihood of patients developing type 2 diabetes. Indeed, the ASCOT (Sever 2012) study demonstrated that the development of diabetes was higher in the atenolol/bendroflumetiazide group compared with the amlodipine/perindopril group.

Nevertheless, beta-blockers are still considered an important treatment option. Furthermore, they are recommended in some groups, such as younger patients of childbearing age, and those who have an enhanced sympathetic drive or are unable to tolerate ARBs and ACEis. However, the ALLHAT study (ALLHAT 2002) showed that in other patient groups (such as people of Afro-Caribbean origin) beta-blockers appear to be less effective when used as monotherapy than calcium channel blockers.

Activity 10.7
Briefly outline the effect of sympathetic nervous stimulation on the blood vessels.

What would be the effect of blocking alpha-1 receptors?

Summary of anti-hypertensive drug treatment

Having discussed some of the anti-hypertensive drugs used in the management of hypertension, the flow chart (NICE 2019) in Figure 10.2 summarises the recommended approach for the pharmacological management of hypertension. It is a useful quick reference guide for practitioners. It is interesting to note that the ESH/ESC (2018) guidelines on drug treatment emphasise an individualised approach, based on patients' comorbidities, which is less hierarchical than Figure 10.2 suggests.

Pharmacology case studies for nurse prescribers

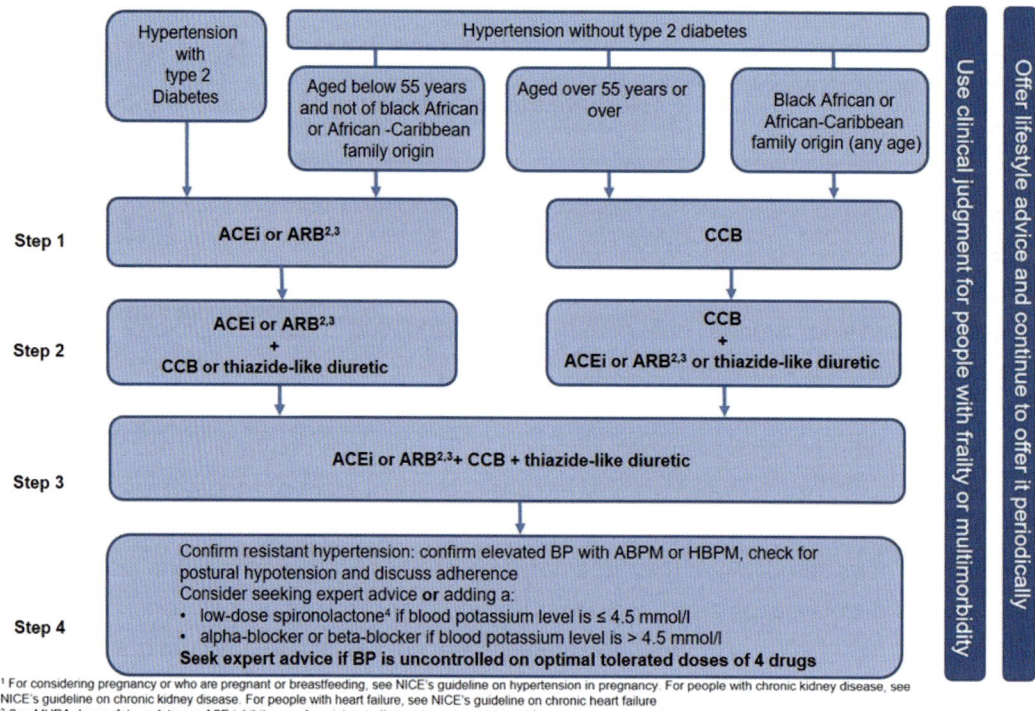

Figure 10.2 Choice of anti-hypertensive drug.
© NICE [2019] Hypertension in adults: diagnosis and treatment. Available from https://www.nice.org.uk/guidance/ng136/resources/visual-summary-pdf-6899919517 All rights reserved. Subject to Notice of rights. Reproduced with Permission.

Case study: Hypertension 1

Mr Smythe is a 68-year-old gentleman who attends a planned appointment at the hypertension clinic. He has had a history of hypertension for the last two years, which is managed with nifedipine slow-release 10mg twice a day and perindopril 8mg daily. The perindopril was increased from 4mg to 8mg on his last visit to the clinic a month ago, to improve control of his BP. Mr Smythe also has type 2 diabetes, which is being managed with diet and lifestyle changes.

His presenting complaint is a swollen mouth, which he developed a few days ago. He was seen at the Accident and Emergency Department and by his GP, who prescribed prednisolone tablets for five days to reduce the swelling. Mr Smythe was advised that the swelling might be caused by his tablets but was not informed which of them were responsible.

On examination, Mr Smythe appears generally well, except for a swollen mouth, and his vital signs are within the normal range. Blood pressure is assessed manually as 134/80mmHg. However, on further discussion, Mr Smythe also reveals that he has slight swelling of his penis.

Activity 10.8 (Case study)

1. Outline the mechanism of action of perindopril.
2. List the adverse effects of perindopril. What do you think could be the cause of Mr Smythe's swollen mouth and penis?
3. What adjustments do you think the clinical nurse specialist and cardiologist will make to Mr Smythe's drug regime?

As indicated previously, BP increases with age. Indeed, studies have shown that there is a high prevalence of hypertension in this age group, with a significant proportion of the elderly having a blood pressure of well over 140/90mmHg. Treating hypertension in the elderly has been shown to be very beneficial in reducing morbidities as well as mortality. There is no particular age where treatment is not advocated, provided the patient is well and not too frail to tolerate the medication. The target is to treat so that BP is less than 150/90mmHg (NICE 2019) but always taking into consideration frailty and multimorbidity (see Figure 10.2).

Many large-scale trials have shown the efficacy of calcium channel blockers and thiazide-like diuretics as well as ACEis. Indeed, Mr Smythe's blood pressure appears to be well controlled on the perindopril and nifedipine. However, the elderly are more susceptible to adverse effects, such as postural hypotension, so sitting and standing blood pressure should be monitored.

Case study: Hypertension 2

Mrs Nidal is a 50-year-old nurse of Afro-Caribbean descent who presents at your clinic with watery, itchy eyes, runny nose and sneezing. Mrs Nidal has no significant past medical history except asthma as a child, cold and influenza. However, she does smoke 15 cigarettes per day and drinks alcohol socially.

On examination, and further history taking, you conclude that Mrs Nidal has hay fever and is allergic to pollen. Apart from the presenting symptoms, she is well but does appear overweight. She states that she feels she has a healthy diet overall, but 'does love her Jamaican patties'. On examination, her vital signs are within the normal limits except her blood pressure, which is 154/94mmHg in her left arm. The second measurement is 150/92 and the final measurement 152/96mmHg. She is 162cm tall and her weight is 75kg.

Activity 10.9 (Case study)

Which blood pressure reading would you record and what further actions would you take?

Mrs Nidal's ABPM results indicate stage 1 hypertension. The results from most of the investigations (including renal) are within the normal range except for serum cholesterol, which is 5.9mmol/l. In addition, the 12-lead ECG and echocardiogram results showed evidence of mild LVH (left ventricular hypertrophy) changes, which may be secondary to the hypertension. The results from Mrs Nidal's formal assessment of cardiovascular risk were used as a basis to discuss her prognosis as well as her healthcare options. She was placed on the appropriate pharmacological therapy and provided with lifestyle advice that was specific to her needs, i.e. on exercise, diet (especially salt intake), smoking and alcohol intake. Further support was made available by referring her to specialist programmes in these areas.

Activity 10.10 (Case study)

1. List the other investigations that you would have requested for Mrs Nidal.
2. How would you manage Mrs Nidal's stage 1 hypertension pharmacologically? Would you prescribe CCBs rather than ACEis/ARBs?
3. Outline the mechanism of action of nifedipine and simvastatin.
4. What advice would you offer Mrs Nidal about the medication in order to reduce non-adherence to treatment?

Approach to management

The use of anti-hypertensive treatment is essential in preventing the morbidities associated with hypertension outlined earlier. Unfortunately, all these drugs have potentially dangerous adverse effects and have to be carefully titrated to the individual needs of the patient. Fortunately, the latest NICE guidelines provide clear and practical recommendations not only for the management of different levels and type of blood pressure but also for 'initiating and titrating antihypertensive drug treatment' (see Figure 10.2, p. 184).

Other equally important aspects of management are preventing adverse effects and encouraging adherence to prescribed medication. Non-adherence to medication contributes significantly to uncontrolled hypertension (see Chapter 5). Healthcare professionals should therefore spend time helping patients understand their condition. Patients should be enabled to make choices based on sound evidence. Discussions about their drug regime should be followed up with written guidance for both the patient and their family. In order to facilitate patient self-management, NICE (2019) has produced a useful patient decision aid which can be accessed via the following link: https://www.nice.org.uk/guidance/ng136/resources/how-do-i-control-my-blood-pressure-lifestyle-options-and-choice-of-medicines-patient-decision-aid-pdf-6899918221

In addition, practitioners should discuss openly some of the side effects that may be experienced and how to address or minimise them. Furthermore, patients should be encouraged to get actively involved in their drug regime – identify where to get additional information about their condition, monitor their blood pressure, record when medicine is to be taken and how they feel about their condition. They should be encouraged to join a suitable group that will offer support and insight into living with hypertension. Group support may enable them to make lifestyle changes such as adapting their diet (reducing salt and saturated fats and increasing fresh fruit and vegetables), joining smoking cessation programmes and reducing stress levels by increasing physical activity. There is increasing evidence demonstrating the correlation between stress and cardiovascular events such as heart attack and stroke.

In a recent systematic review, Mostofsky, Penner and Mittleman (2014) provided convincing evidence of a link between frequent episodes of anger and an increased risk of these cardiovascular events occurring within a short time (2 hours) after these episodes. Furthermore, NICE (2014) has recently published guidelines about exercise referral schemes to increase physical activity in adults. This is timely, as an international report in the *Lancet* (Ng, Fleming *et al.* 2014) identified the UK as having the third-highest obesity rate in Western Europe, with over two-thirds of men (67%) and over half of women (57%) being either overweight or obese. Experts are calling for urgent action at both national and individual level.

Finally, a team-based approach (which includes experienced and appropriately qualified healthcare professionals including specialist nurses) has been shown to improve success rates (ESH/ESC 2013) when compared to standard care. See NICE (2015) medicine optimisation guidelines and patient decision aid (2019) at the following links:

- https://pathways.nice.org.uk/pathways/medicines-optimisation
- https://www.nice.org.uk/guidance/ng136/resources

Summary

Hypertension is a major cause of premature death and disability globally. However, with early detection and effective patient-centred management the global burden of this condition can be significantly reduced. Two important approaches in successfully managing this condition are lifestyle interventions and sound pharmacological management by healthcare professionals working in collaboration with patients, service users, carers and other healthcare professionals. We hope this chapter has provided some insights into current pharmacological management and the application of this approach.

Answers to activities

Activity 10.1

Although primary hypertension, which is blood pressure due to unknown causes, accounts for 95% of hypertension cases, high blood pressure can also occur due to other disorders. It is then termed secondary hypertension. Can you identify 2–3 causes of secondary hypertension?

Causes of secondary hypertension include: phaeochromocytoma (tumour of the adrenal glands, which causes increased production of adrenaline and noradrenaline); renal disease; diabetes; pregnancy; Cushing's syndrome (clinical signs and symptoms caused by high levels of cortisol hormones); hyperthyroidism; coarctation of the aorta (usually a congenital abnormality caused by narrowing of the aorta but can also be due to trauma leading to hypertension in the upper body); drug-induced (e.g. cocaine).

The healthcare professional should exclude these possible causes by taking a full history, performing a physical examination, and carrying out relevant investigations if appropriate.

Activity 10.2

1. Reflect on a patient you have recently cared for with hypertension. How was the diagnosis arrived at? For example, was it based on several clinic BP readings, ABPM or HBPM. Was it taken in both arms?

There is no correct answer, as this activity is based on individual experience. However, despite guidance, anecdotal experience suggests that BP is still being diagnosed on clinic blood pressure readings only, and adjunct monitoring (such as ABPM and HBPM) is either not always utilised or access is limited. It is important to note, however, that both NICE and the latest EHS/ECS (2018) guidelines have placed greater emphasis on the use of both ABPM and HBPM. NICE (2019) guidelines recommend that if the healthcare professional believes a patient could be hypertensive then BP should be measured in both arms. If there is a difference of >15mmHg, the measurement should be repeated. If the measurement remains greater than 15mmHg on the second reading, the BP should be measured in the arm with the higher pressure.

2. NICE guidelines recommend that the diagnosis of hypertension should be based on the clinic measurements as well as ABPM. NICE (2019) and ESH/ESC (2018) recommend that the role of ABPM and HBPM should be expanded, as they are better predictors of outcomes. However, if your patient was unable to tolerate ABPM, refused it or ABPM was unavailable, can you suggest another recommended adjunct to clinic blood pressure to confirm the diagnosis?

NICE suggest using HBPM if patients are intolerant of ABPM.

3. Automated BP devices are often used to assess blood pressure and pulse rate. How would you ensure the pulse reading was accurate?

Automated devices may exclude irregularities in pulse rate. It is therefore good practice to palpate the brachial/radial pulse to exclude irregularities in pulse rate before measuring the BP using such devices. Furthermore, it is important that pulse rate is taken manually to exclude irregular rhythms such as atrial fibrillation, which is responsible for approximately 20% of ischaemic strokes (Stroke Association 2019). If pulse irregularity is detected, then measure BP manually (BIHS 2019). NICE (2019) suggest that healthcare professionals in primary care should use a validated device such as WatchBP Home A to 'opportunistically' detect atrial fibrillation during the process of diagnosing and monitoring hypertension.

4. There are different requirements when measuring BP in certain patients.

In what position should BP be taken in type 2 diabetic patients, patients >80 years and individuals with a history of postural hypotension?

One of the additions to the latest NICE (2019) guideline on the management of hypertension in adults is the inclusion of the approach that should be taken in the management of patients with type 2 diabetes. According to NICE (2019), the threshold for measuring BP and diagnosing hypertension for adults is the same as for those with type 2 diabetes. In addition NICE (2019) recommend that standing and seated BP should be taken not only in type 2 diabetic patients but also in elderly people over the age of 80 years and any individuals with a history of hypertension. If there is a fall in BP, the treatment target should be based on their standing measurements. NICE also states that adult patients with type 2 diabetes who are not hypertensive or have renal disease must have their BP measured yearly or more.

Activity 10.3

Can you suggest other approaches that could be used by the healthcare professional to address factors contributing to the prevalence of high blood pressure?

Discuss:
- Strategies for adherence to medication
- Lifestyle changes reinforced with written/audiovisual material
- Relevant specialist/organisation if appropriate to support lifestyle changes, e.g. dietician, smoking cessation programmes, patient support groups.

The following links will support your discussion.

https://www.nice.org.uk/guidance/NG136 (see p. 9 on Lifestyle interventions, and p. 25 on rationale for deleting the recommendation on relaxation therapies.

https://www.nice.org.uk/about/nice-communities/nice-and-the-public/public-involvement/making-decisions-about-your-care/your-care

https://pathways.nice.org.uk/pathways/medicines-optimisation

Activity 10.4

Before reviewing the next section, use the information about the physiology of blood pressure control to briefly outline how key drugs, such as ACE-inhibitors, beta-blockers and diuretics, reduce blood pressure. You may wish to consult a physiology text, such as Tortora & Derrickson (2017), to review the physiology of blood pressure control.

Beta-blockers block sympathetic stimulation of the heart, reducing both heart rate and stroke volume; diuretics reduce blood volume and also reduce blood pressure by means of an unknown effect on the kidneys; ACEis reduce blood pressure by blocking the pressor effect of angiotensin and they reduce blood volume by blocking production of aldosterone.

Activity 10.5

1. Outline in more detail the mechanism of action of ACE-inhibitors.

They inhibit the formation of angiotensin II. This reduces the vasoconstrictor effect of angiotensin II on the blood vessels, thus reducing afterload and blood pressure. It also inhibits the release of aldosterone, increasing the excretion of sodium and water and thus reducing blood volume and blood pressure. A useful equation to remember is: blood pressure = cardiac output × peripheral vascular resistance

2. Which receptor do the angiotensin II receptor antagonists act on?

Angiotensin receptor blockers (ARBs) prevent angiotensin II from binding to its main receptor, the AT1 (on blood vessels), thus blocking the pressor effect of angiotensin II. They have similar clinical effects to ACE-inhibitors but fewer adverse effects such as the dry cough. They are indicated if ACE-inhibitors are not well tolerated (e.g. if the patient has a persistent dry cough).

They can be used as add-on therapy to ACEis in heart failure patients who are intolerant of beta-blockers, under specialist supervision. ACEis and ARBs are never used in combination for the treatment of hypertension.

3. List some of the key adverse effects of the ACE-inhibitors. Which of them is the most common, and how would you address this if it was an issue for one of your patients?

Adverse effects of ACE-inhibitors include: first-dose hypotension, precipitation of renal failure in renal artery stenosis, persistent dry cough, chest pain, palpitations, angioedema, electrolyte depletion and renal impairment. One of the most common adverse effects is persistent dry cough: consider ARBs if the dry cough does not improve with treatment. ACEis increase bradykinin levels in the lungs, and studies have shown that this may be the cause of the cough.

4. What type of drug interaction could occur with a diuretic and an ACE-inhibitor?

ACE-inhibitors can interact with a number of drugs, such as diuretics, NSAIDs and lithium.

In a synergistic reaction (see Chapter 3), one drug interacts with another drug and enhances the effect.

Although the use of ACE-inhibitors and diuretics is not contraindicated, diuretics can potentiate some of the potential adverse effects of ACE-inhibitors, causing significant electrolyte depletion, leading to collapse or even death. More specifically, they can lead to hyponatraemia and hyperkalaemia – remember ACE-inhibitors promote sodium loss and retention of potassium, especially if combined with spironolactone and other potassium-sparing diuretics, which also promote potassium retention.

Activity 10.6

1. List the common side effects of CCBs.

Common adverse effects of calcium channel blockers include: headaches, flushing, ankle oedema, depression of myocardial contractility – careful monitoring needed in patients with heart failure and/or those taking beta-blockers. Diltiazem is never given together with beta-blockers unless this is under specialist supervision.

2. If your patient was prescribed both cimetidine and nifedipine, what type of drug interaction could occur?

Cimetidine inhibits the liver enzymes that metabolise nifedipine, thus increasing blood levels, which could lead to toxicity. Care required: cimetidine can be brought over the counter. If an H2 antagonist is required, ranitidine can be used.

3. Why are the CCBs recommended as first-line therapy in people who are of African or Afro-Caribbean family origin?

Studies have shown that some black patients may have reduced activity of the renin-angiotensin-aldosterone system so ACE-inhibitors may be less effective. One randomised controlled trial (RCT) demonstrated that calcium antagonists were much more effective than ACEis in reducing risk of stroke and other cardiovascular disorders in these patients (ALLHAT 2002).

4. Using the BNF, look up one brand of long-acting diltiazem and compare the different formulations available, with regard to dosing and frequency of administration.

Looking at Tildiem®, two different long-acting formulations are available for mild to moderate hypertension:

- Tildiem Retard® – given twice a day, initially 90mg or 120mg twice daily; increased if necessary to 360mg daily in divided doses
- Tildiem LA® – given once a day, initially 200mg once daily before or with food, increased if necessary to 300–400mg daily, maximum 500mg daily.

As can be seen, the different formulations are not equivalent in dosing so full brand-name prescribing is necessary, including the Retard and LA portion of the brand name.

Activity 10.7

Briefly outline the effect of sympathetic nervous stimulation on the blood vessels. What would be the effect of blocking alpha-1 receptors?

The sympathetic nervous system releases the neurotransmitter noradrenaline from nerve endings and also from the adrenal glands (adrenaline and noradrenaline). These substances stimulate alpha-1 receptors that are located on arterioles and small arteries, resulting in vasoconstriction of the blood vessels. Remember that contraction of the muscles in the walls of the arterioles is one of the key determinants in the regulation of blood pressure. Drugs like prazosin and doxazosin block alpha-1 receptors, causing vasodilatation of the blood vessels, thus reducing peripheral vascular resistance and therefore blood pressure.

Activity 10.8 (Case study)

1. Outline the mechanism of action of perindopril.

Perindopril is an ACE-inhibitor and acts by inhibiting the conversion of angiotensin I to angiotensin II. By inhibiting the formation of angiotensin II, it reduces vasoconstriction and blood volume, thus lowering blood pressure (see Figure 10.1, p. 181). Perindopril is indicated in hypertension and heart failure.

2. List the adverse effects of perindopril. What do you think could be the cause of Mr Smythe's swollen mouth and penis?

Adverse effects include: angioedema, dry irritating cough, headaches, dizziness, and rarely jaundice, reduced GFR in people with renal artery stenosis and the elderly. The swelling is likely to be a reaction to the perindopril. Angioedema is a known adverse effect of ACEis and ARBs. Other more common clinical signs and symptoms of angioedema include swelling of the hands, eyes and feet. Airway obstruction may occur if laryngeal oedema is involved, in which case this would be a medical emergency.

3. What adjustments do you think the clinical nurse specialist and cardiologist will make to Mr Smythe's drug regime?

Mr Smythe's perindopril was discontinued and his nifedipine was increased to 20mg twice daily (modified release). The cardiologist also advised discontinuing the prednisolone prescribed by the GP, as it was probably unnecessary and may well have increased Mr Smythe's blood glucose levels. Mr Smythe was advised to monitor the swelling and contact his GP or the clinic directly if he had any concerns.

Activity 10.9 (Case study)

Which blood pressure reading would you record and what further actions would you take?

The mean of the readings is recorded as the clinical BP. This would be repeated for both arms.
- Arrange for ambulatory blood pressure monitoring (ABPM) to establish a diagnosis of hypertension.
- Request investigations such as urine (albumin: creatinine ratio, haematuria) and bloods (glucose, urea and electrolytes, creatinine, cholesterol levels, 12-lead ECG).
- Clinical assessment should include a formal CVS risk assessment, using a tool such as QRISK 2 or 3 and assessment of the fundi for hypertensive retinopathy.
- Offer initial and at intervals lifestyle advice: diet (salt, fat, green veg and fruit, sugar intake), smoking, exercise, alcohol intake. When discussing lifestyle advice, suggest support groups and relaxation therapies.

Activity 10.10

1. List the other investigations that you would have requested for Mrs Nidal.

Urine (albumin creatinine ratio); blood (blood glucose, urea and creatinine, eGFR); examination of the fundi for hypertensive retinopathy.

2. How would you manage Mrs Nidal's stage 1 hypertension pharmacologically? Would you prescribe CCBs rather than ACEis/ARBs?

Select a CCB such as nifedipine LA once a day because ACEis/ARBs are less effective in patients of Afro-Caribbean descent. Simvastatin to reduce cholesterol in line with recommended levels.

3. Outline the mechanism of action of nifedipine and simvastatin.

Nifedipine is a calcium channel blocker. Calcium ions are needed for contraction of muscles. These drugs block calcium entering the smooth muscle cells of arteries, relaxing the vessels, thus reducing peripheral vascular resistance and consequently blood pressure.

Simvastatin belongs to a group of drugs called the statins. They block the enzyme HMG-CoA reductase, which is important in cholesterol production, thus lowering cholesterol levels.

4. What advice would you offer Mrs Nidal about the medication in order to reduce non-adherence to treatment?

Discuss the potential adverse effects of the drugs and how to administer the medication. For example, simvastatin is taken at night because this is when cholesterol production is at its highest. Ask her to report any adverse effects. Over-the-counter (OTC) drugs that can interact with her medication (such as nifedipine and OTC NSAIDs) can potentiate renal toxicity and reduce the hypotensive effect of the drug by increasing sodium and water reabsorption, blocking the positive inotropic effect of prostaglandin on the myocardium. She should avoid drinking fruit juices such as grapefruit, which is a known enzyme inhibitor that increases plasma levels of nifedipine and statins like simvastatin. This can lead to toxicity of both drugs. In the case of nifedipine, this is hypotension and heart block. Myalgia, arthralgia, liver toxicity and other side effects are associated with simvastatin.

References and further reading

ALLHAT Collaborative Research Group (2002). Major outcomes in high-risk hypertensive patients randomized to angiotensin-converting enzyme inhibitor or calcium channel blocker vs. diuretic: the anti-hypertensive and lipid lowering treatment to prevent heart attack trial (ALLHAT). *Journal of the American Medicine Association.* **288** (23), 2981–97.

Bailey, D.G. & Dresser, G.K. (2004). Interactions between grapefruit juice and cardiovascular drugs. *American Journal of Cardiovascular Drugs.* **4**, 281–97.

Beckett, N.S., Peters, R. & Fletcher, A.E. (2008). Treatment of hypertension in patients 80 years of age or older. *New England Journal of Medicine.* **336**, 1117–24.

British Heart Foundation (BHF) (2020). BHF analysis: UK estimate based on England figures. Hypertension prevalence estimates for local populations (2016) Public Health England using updated figures in: Blood pressure: how can we do better. https://www.bhf.org.uk/for-professionals/healthcare-professionals/commissioning-and-services/service-innovation/bp-how-can-we-do-better (Last accessed 7 October 2020).

British and Irish Hypertension Society (BIHS) (2011). BP measurement in atrial fibrillation. https://bihsoc.org/resources/bp-measurement/bp-measurement-atrial-fibrillation/ (Last accessed 7 October 2020).

British and Irish Hypertension Society (BIHS) (2019). NICE hypertension in adults: diagnosis and management guideline (NG136) BIHS statement. https://bihsoc.org/wp-content/uploads/2019/12/BIHS-Statement-on-NG136-FINAL.doc.pdf (Last accessed 7 October 2020).

Dahlöf, B., Sever, P.S., Poulter, N.R., et al. (2005). Prevention of cardiovascular events with an antihypertensive regimen of amlodipine adding perindopril as required versus atenolol adding bendroflumethiazide as required, in the Anglo-Scandinavian Cardiac Outcomes Trial-Blood Pressure Lowering Arm (ASCOT-BPLA): a multicentre randomised controlled trial. *Lancet.* **366**, 895–906.

European Society of Hypertension/European Society of Cardiology (ESH/ESC) (2018). Guidelines for the management of arterial hypertension. The Task Force for the management of arterial hypertension of the European Society of Hypertension (ESH) and of the European Society of Cardiology (ESC). https://www.portailvasculaire.fr/sites/default/files/docs/2018_esc_esh_guidelines_hta.pdf (Last accessed 7 October 2020).

Global Burden of Disease (2017). GBD Disease and Injury Incidence and Prevalence Collaborators: Global, regional, and national incidence, prevalence, and years lived with disability for 354 diseases and injuries for 195 countries and territories, 1990–2017: a systematic analysis for the Global Burden of Disease Study 2017 (2018). *Lancet.* **392** (10159), 1789–858.

Hansson, L., Lindholm, L.H. & Ekbom, T. (1999b). Randomized trial of old and new anti-hypertensive drugs in elderly patients: cardiovascular mortality and morbidity in the Swedish Trial in Old Patients with hypertension-2 study. *Lancet.* **534**, 1751–56.

Joint Formulary Committee (2014). *British National Formulary* 67. London: BMJ Group and Pharmaceutical Press.

McCormack, T., Boffa, R.J., Jones, N.R., Carville, S. & McManus, R.J. (2019). The 2018 ESC/ESH hypertension guideline and the 2019 NICE hypertension guideline, how and why they differ. *European Heart Journal.* **40**, 3456–458. doi:10.1093/eurheartj/ehz681.

Messerli, F., Williams, B. & Ritz, E. (2007). Essential hypertension. *Lancet.* **370**, 591–603.

Mostofsky, E., Penner, E.A. & Mittleman, M.A. (2014). Outbursts of anger as a trigger of acute cardiovascular events: a systematic review and meta-analysis. *European Heart Journal.* doi: 10.1093/eurheartj/ehu033

Ng, M., Fleming, T., Robinson, M. et al. (2014). Global, regional, and national prevalence of overweight and obesity in children and adults during 1980–2013: a systematic analysis for the Global Burden of Disease Study 2013. *Lancet.* doi:10.1016/S0140-6736(14)60460-8

National Institute for Health and Care Excellence (NICE) (2009). Medicines adherence. London: NICE. https://www.nice.org.uk/Guidance/CG76 (Last accessed 7 October 2020).

National Institute for Health and Care Excellence (NICE) (2014). Exercise referral schemes to promote physical activity consultation draft. London: NICE. https://www.nice.org.uk/guidance/ph54/documents/exercise-referral-schemes-draft-guideline2 (Last accessed 7 October 2020).

National Institute for Health and Care Excellence (NICE) (2015). Medicines optimisation guidelines. https://pathways.nice.org.uk/pathways/medicines-optimisation (Last accessed 7 October 2020).

National Institute for Health and Care Excellence (NICE) (2019). Hypertension in adults: diagnosis and management. NICE guidelines 136. https://www.nice.org.uk/guidance/ng136 (Last accessed 7 October 2020),

Peters, R., Beckett, N., McCormack, T., Fagard, R., Fletcher, A. & Bulpitt, C. (2013). Treating hypertension in the very elderly: benefits, risks and future directions, a focus on the hypertension in the very elderly trial. *New England Journal of Medicine*. doi: 10.1093/eurheartj/eht464.

PROGRESS Collaboration Group (2001). Randomised trial perindopril-based blood pressure lowering regimen among 6105 individuals with previous stroke or transient ischaemic attack. *Lancet*. **358**, 1033–41.

Public Health England. Health matters: combating high blood pressure (2017). https://www.gov.uk/government/publications/health-matters-combating-high-blood-pressure/health-matters-combating-high-blood-pressure (Last accessed 7 October 2020).

Sever, P.S. (2012). The Anglo-Scandinavian Cardiac Outcomes Trial (ASCOT) Implications and further outcomes. *Hypertension*. **60**, 248–59. doi:10.1161HYPERTENSION AHA.111 187070

Stroke Association (2019). Atrial fibrillation and stroke. https://www.stroke.org.uk/what-is-stroke/are-you-at-risk-of-stroke/atrial-fibrillation (Last accessed 7 October 2020)

Systolic Blood Pressure Intervention Trial (SPRINT) Research Group (2015). A randomized trial of intensive versus standard blood-pressure control. *New England Journal of Medicine*. **373**, 2103–116. doi: 10.1056/NEJMoa1511939.

Tortora, G.J. & Derrickson, B. (2017). *Principles of Anatomy and Physiology*. 15th edn. New Jersey: John Wiley & Sons.

Unger, T., Borghi, C., Charchar, F., Khan, N.A., Poulter, N.R., Prabhakaran, D., Ramirez, A., Schlaich, M., Stergiou, G.S., Tomaszewski, M., Wainford, R.D., Williams, B., & Schutte, A.E. (2020). American College of Cardiology (ACC) & American Heart Association (AHA). Hypertension. **75**: 1334-1357. https://doi.org/10.1161/HYPERTENSIONAHA.120.15026

Available at: https://www.ahajournals.org/doi/10.1161/HYPERTENSIONAHA.120.15026 (Accessed 12 February 2021).

Whelton P.K., Carey R.M., Aronow W.S., *et al.* (2018) 2017 ACC/AHA/AAPA/ABC/ACPM/AGS /APhA/ASH/ASPC/NMA/PCNA guideline for the prevention, detection, evaluation, and management of high blood pressure in adults: executive summary: a report of the American College of Cardiology/American Heart Association (ACC/AHA) Task Force on Clinical Practice Guidelines. *Journal of the American College of Cardiology*. **71**, 2199–269.

Williams, B., Poulter, N.R., Brown, M.J., Davis, M., McInnes, G.T., Potter, J.P., Sever, P.S. & Thom, S.M. (2004). The BHS Guidelines Working Party Guidelines for Management of Hypertension: Report of the Fourth Working Party of the British Hypertension Society, 2004, - BHS IV. *Journal of Human Hypertension*. **18**, 139–85.

Pharmacological case studies: Heart failure

Donna Scholefield
MSc, BSc (Hons), RN, PGDip HE; Cardiac Nursing (254);
Senior Lecturer, Health and Education, Middlesex University, London

Hiba Yusuf
BSc (Hons), RN,
Clinical Nurse Specialist in Heart Failure, Harefield Hospital.

This chapter:
- Gives an overview of the function of the heart
- Outlines the pathophysiology of heart failure and key clinical symptoms
- Considers the pharmacology of key drugs used for prescribing in heart failure
- Applies knowledge of drugs used in the treatment of heart failure to practice-based case studies.

Introduction

It is estimated that over 920,000 people in the UK have been diagnosed with heart failure (NICE 2018) and this figure is likely to increase in the coming years due to the ageing population and improvement in acute care for patients with cardiovascular disease. Indeed, studies have shown that both the incidence and prevalence of heart failure increase with age. Furthermore, hospitalisation due to decompensated heart failure will cause an increasing economic burden. The prognosis for patients with heart failure is very poor without treatment. The aim of this chapter is to discuss current pharmacological management of heart failure patients and illustrate approaches through the use of two case studies.

Overview of the function of the heart

The cardiovascular system consists of the heart and blood vessels. Its main function is to pump blood to the tissues to meet their metabolic needs by supplying them with oxygen and nutrients as well as removing carbon dioxide and other waste products. The heart is the muscular pump that drives blood through the circulation. It consists of four chambers that act as individual pumps but each of these must work in a co-ordinated manner to produce an effective cardiac output. To do this, the heart has an internal wiring called the conduction system that allows it to fill, pump and empty in a co-ordinated sequence. If part of the conduction system fails, there are 'pacemakers' throughout the myocardium that will stimulate the heart to continue pumping. There are also external nerves (namely the sympathetic and parasympathetic nerve) that will adjust the performance of the pump according to the body's physiological needs. Finally, to fine-tune the performance of the pump even further, there are receptors in the heart that will alter its function in response to its changing workload.

The cardiac output

The cardiac output is the amount of blood that is pumped out by both ventricles in 1 minute. The cardiac output (CO) can be calculated using the following equation:

$$CO = SV \times HR$$

where HR is heart rate (and in a resting adult this is approximately 75 bpm) and SV is stroke volume (which is the volume of blood ejected by the ventricles during each contraction). This is approximately 70ml in an adult at rest.

> ### Activity 11.1
> Using the figures given above for stroke volume (SV) and heart rate (HR), calculate the cardiac output.

Cardiac output depends on a number of factors:
- If the heart rate increases, the cardiac output will increase in the healthy heart. However, in the failing heart, an increase in rate will reduce cardiac output.
- The filling pressure depends on venous return (preload). If venous return increases, cardiac output will increase within normal limits, then drop off according to Starling's law (see Figure 11.1).
- The contractility of the cardiac muscle also affects cardiac output.

- The afterload is the resistance against which the heart must pump. If the resistance in the arterial circulation is too high, as in hypertension, the heart needs to work harder against this increased pressure to push blood through the circulation. To cope with this increased work, the ventricles will gradually stiffen and become enlarged (hypertrophic). If the hypertension remains uncontrolled, heart failure will develop.
- If any of these factors is compromised, cardiac output will be adversely affected and heart failure may result.

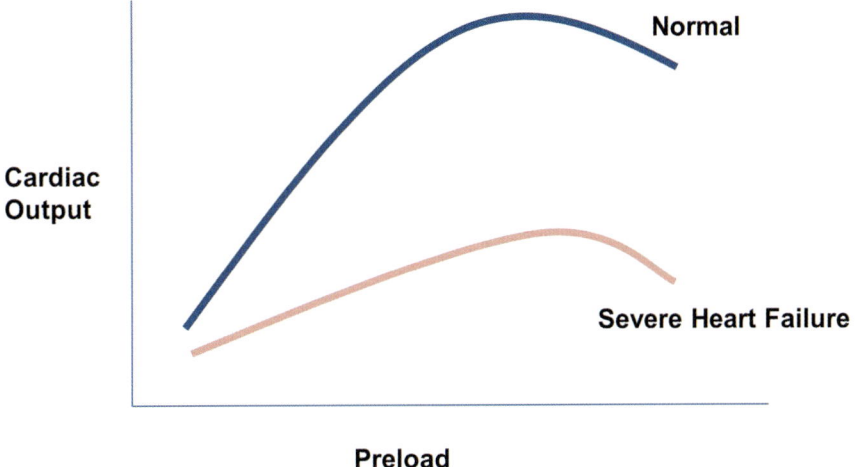

Figure 11.1: Frank-Starling curve in a normal heart and a failing heart. The curves show the relationship between cardiac output (stroke volume) and preload. In summary, the more the muscle fibre is stretched (within limits) by end diastolic filling (preload), the greater the contraction and hence cardiac output. In left ventricular failure, the end diastolic pressure increases significantly and the damaged left ventricle is unable to cope so cardiac output is reduced.

Heart failure

Heart failure occurs when the pumping heart fails to such an extent that it is unable to meet the metabolic requirements of the tissue. In other words, it is unable to sustain an adequate circulation for the needs of the body (see Figures 11.1 and 11.2). This failure will lead to a number of clinical symptoms such as dyspnoea, fatigue, decreased exercise tolerance and oedema. These clinical symptoms are a manifestation of reduced contractile force, cardiac output and tissue perfusion and increased peripheral vascular resistance (PVR). There are many causes of heart failure but some key ones include coronary artery disease, hypertension, cardiomyopathy, respiratory disease, congenital heart disease and valvular disease. In the UK, coronary heart disease and hypertension are the main causes of heart failure, with many patients having a past history of myocardial infarction.

Types of heart failure

Heart failure can be subdivided into several different types. It can be acute (sudden onset of pathology) or chronic (gradual onset) or categorised according to the chamber that has failed (i.e. left or right ventricular failure). Some patients have heart failure due to left ventricular systolic dysfunction which is associated with reduced left ventricular ejection fraction (EF), also known as heart failure with reduced ejection fraction (HFrEF). Others have heart failure with a preserved ejection (HFpEF), which was previously referred to as diastolic heart failure (see Table 11.2, p. 201). HFpEF is a clinical entity characterised by signs and symptoms of heart failure with low normal to normal left ventricular ejection fraction and no significant valvular abnormalities (i.e. no significant aortic stenosis or mitral regurgitation). The exact pathophysiology of HFpEF remains uncertain, although impaired isovolumetric relaxation, decreased ventricular compliance and increased left ventricular stiffness have been reported frequently in patients. Nearly half of all patients with heart failure have normal ejection fraction.

Table 11.1: NYHA classification of heart failure symptoms (grading of severity)

Class I	Asymptomatic left ventricular dysfunction is included in this category; without limitation of physical activity – ordinary physical activity does not cause fatigue, breathlessness or palpitation.
Class II	Symptomatically 'mild' heart failure; light limitation of physical activity. Such people are comfortable at rest. Ordinary physical activity results in fatigue, palpitation, breathlessness or angina pectoris.
Class III	Symptomatically 'moderate' heart failure; marked limitation of physical activity. Although people are comfortable at rest, less than ordinary physical activity will lead to symptoms.
Class IV	Symptomatically 'severe' heart failure; inability to sustain any physical activity without discomfort. Symptoms of cardiac failure are present even at rest.

Note: This classification is commonly used in clinical practice as well as research but does not always reflect what occurs in reality – in the sense that a patient can have severe heart failure but with few symptoms, or have few symptoms and have severe pathology. The Criteria Committee of the New York Heart Association (1994).

Pharmacological case studies: Heart failure

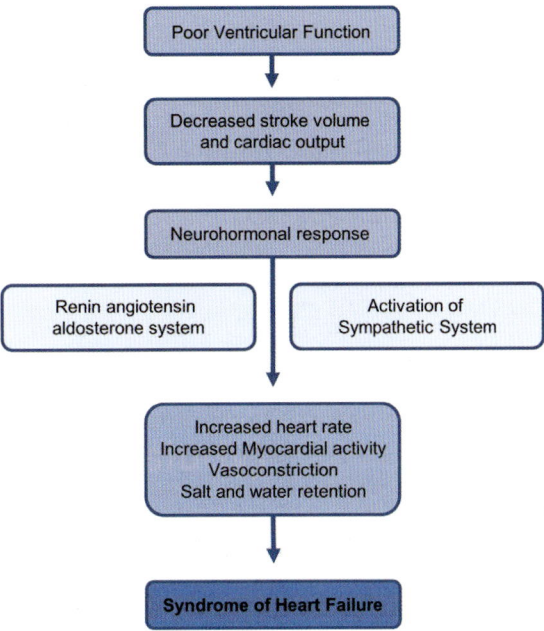

Figure 11.2: This flowchart shows the physiological impact of poor left ventricular function. In the early stages of heart failure, increased sympathetic and renin-angiotensin system activity attempts to maintain an effective cardiac output but eventually these compensatory mechanisms will fail, leading to dilated heart, increased venous pressure (distended veins), congested lungs (dyspnoea), peripheral oedema, and reduced cardiac output to other organs at the expense of maintaining brain and heart perfusion. This results in fatigue and reduced exercise tolerance.

Table 11.2: Types of heart failure

Type of heart failure	Cause	Effects
Left ventricular failure (LVF) – HFrEF	Myocardial infarction, hypertension, valve disease idiopathic	Dyspnoea, pulmonary and peripheral oedema (ankle oedema), fatigue, decreased exercise tolerance
Heart failure with preserved ejection fraction (HFpEF)	Chronic lung disease, AF, diabetes, obesity	

Drug treatment of heart failure

The aims of heart failure treatment are to improve clinical symptoms and functional capacity, enhance quality of life, reduce the incidence of hospitalisation due to acute exacerbation, and to decrease associated mortality. The overall goal of treatment for heart failure is to reduce symptoms and improve prognosis. Much of the evidence for the management of heart failure focuses on HFrEF.

Table 11.3: Summary of drugs used to treat heart failure

Examples of drugs	Action/effects
• ACE-inhibitors, such as ramipril, lisinopril, enalapril • Angiotensin II receptor antagonists (ARBs), e.g. candesartan and losartan	• Dilate blood vessels and reduce peripheral vascular resistance (PVR) and blood volume, thus reducing the heart's overall workload. • In summary, they reduce preload and afterload, which leads to improved cardiac output.
• Beta-blockers, e.g. bisoprolol, carvedilol and nebivolol	• Reduce sympathetic activity by blocking the binding of noradrenaline and adrenaline at beta 1 receptors, thereby reducing heart rate and contractility and overall heart workload. • Inhibit the increased sympathetic neurohormonal activity seen in heart failure.
• Mineralocorticoid receptor antagonists (MRAs), such as spironolactone and epleronone	• Antagonise the effect of aldosterone and can lead to reduction in fibrosis and improvement in LV function. • Furthermore, they decrease extracellular matrix turnover and myocardial collagen content and improve endothelial vasomotor dysfunction, mechanisms known to influence the progression of heart failure • Prevent formation of a protein important in Na+ and K+ exchange in kidneys. This action causes increased water and Na+ to be excreted while K+ is conserved.
• Angiotensin receptor/Neprilysin inhibitors (ARNI), sacubitril/valsartan (Entresto®)	• Inhibit RAAS, which leads to dilation of blood vessels, reduces PVR and blood volume, thus reducing the heart's overall workload. • Inhibition of neprilysin counteracts the neurohormonal activation, which also leads to vasoconstriction, sodium retention and cardiac remodelling.
• Loop diuretics, e.g. furosemide, bumetanide, torasemide • Thiazide diuretics, e.g. metolozone, bendroflumethiazide	• Cause kidneys to excrete salt and water • Reduced pulmonary and peripheral oedema • Reduces preload.

Angiotensin-converting enzyme inhibitors (ACE-inhibitors)

ACE-inhibitors have become the cornerstone of heart failure management over the last 20 to 30 years. Several randomised controlled trials (such as CONSENSUS, SOLVD and ATLAS) have demonstrated that ACE-inhibitors improve symptoms, exercise capacity and left ventricular function as well as prolonging survival in the whole spectrum of patients with left ventricular systolic dysfunction. Therefore the evidence for applying ACE-inhibitors exists for all patients with left ventricular systolic dysfunction, regardless of whether they experience dyspnoea or remain completely asymptomatic.

Patients with heart failure have increased activity from the renin-angiotensin-aldosterone system (RAAS). This leads to high levels of angiotensin II, a powerful vasoconstrictor that increases peripheral vascular resistance, thus increasing the workload of the failing heart (afterload). ACE-inhibitors inhibit the production of angiotensin II and therefore reduce the vasoconstrictor effects of angiotensin II, dilating the arterioles and reducing the heart's workload, thus increasing cardiac output. Furthermore, inhibition of this system also inhibits the formation of aldosterone and, in doing so, reduces the amount of sodium and water retained by the kidneys, thus lowering blood volume (reducing preload). See Figure 11.3, p. 204.

According to NICE (2018) guidelines, the use of ACE-inhibitors along with beta-blockers should be considered as first-line treatment for every patient who has heart failure with compromised left ventricular systolic dysfunction.

Activity 11.2
1. What is a prodrug and why are some drugs given in this form?
2. Can you identify other drugs that are given in this form?

Adverse effects of ACE-inhibitors

ACE-inhibitors are usually well tolerated but can cause severe hypotension so the patient needs to be carefully monitored and the dose of the drug titrated cautiously, especially when first prescribed. Some of the important adverse side effects associated with ACE-inhibitors are hyperkalaemia, dry coughs, angioedema (rare) and a reduction in glomerular filtration rate – hence renal function should be checked before and after increasing the dose. In people of African or Afro-Caribbean origin, who may be less responsive to ACE-inhibitors or ARBs, hydralazine in combination with nitrate should be considered after seeking specialist advice.

Angiotensin receptor blockers (ARBs)

If a patient is unable to tolerate ACE-inhibitors, an ARB should be considered as an alternative therapy. ARBs prevent angiotensin II from binding to its main receptor, the AT1 (on blood vessels), thus blocking the effect of angiotensin II. ARBs therefore have similar pharmacological effects to the ACE-inhibitors and similar adverse effects, such as hyperkalaemia, headache, dizziness, low blood pressure, diarrhoea and abnormal (metallic/salty) taste in the mouth. Candesartan and losartan are considered to be suitable for the management of patients with heart failure (CHARM and HEALS trials). ARBs tend to be used as an alternative to ACE-inhibitors because they don't usually cause a cough, although they may not be quite as effective as ACE-inhibitors. The combination of ACE-inhibitor and ARB is only recommended in exceptional cases (under specialist supervision) and is contraindicated in patients who are also undergoing mineralocorticoid receptor antagonist treatment.

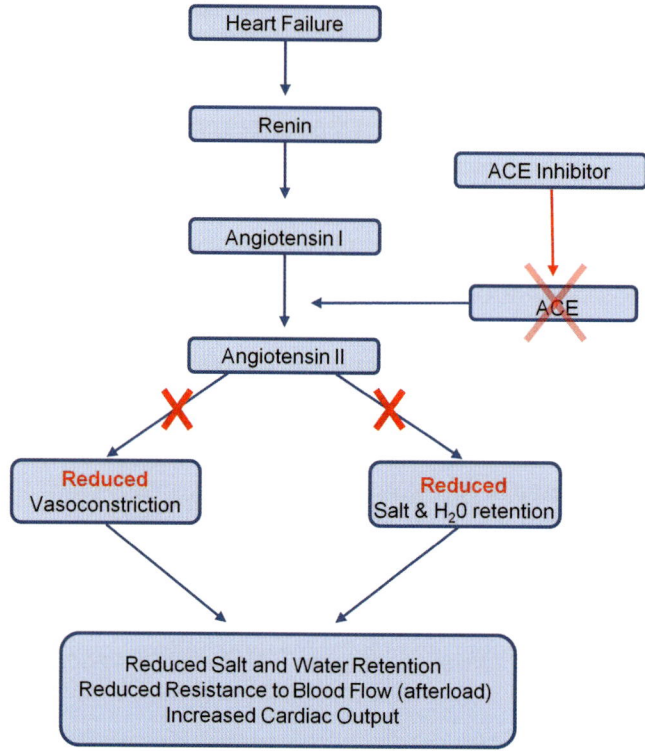

Figure 11.3: This flowchart shows the impact of ACE-inhibitors on the renin-angiotensin system in heart failure. By blocking the production of angiotensin II, they reduce the heart's workload by dilating the blood vessels as well as inhibiting the production of aldosterone, which results in reduced salt and water retention by the kidneys.

Beta-blockers

One of the earliest neurohormonal changes in heart failure is sympathetic activation. A short period of sympathetic activation improves peripheral perfusion by increasing heart rate and myocardial contractility. However, ongoing sympathetic activation adversely affects cardiac myocytes and chamber contractile function, leading to deterioration of heart function. Beta-blockers produce their effect by reducing the activity of the sympathetic nervous system on the failing heart, thus reducing the heart's workload. Large-scale clinical trials have demonstrated that beta-blockers reduce mortality and morbidity, improve left ventricular function and symptoms, and reduce hospital admission for deteriorating heart failure in patients with reduced left ventricular systolic function.

NICE (2018) has advised that beta-blockers should be started in patients who are clinically stable, immediately after diagnosis of heart failure with reduced ejection fraction. Beta-blockers and ACE inhibitors are the first-line pharmacological treatment. Beta-blockers, like ACE-inhibitors, should be started at a low dose and dosage should be increased gradually.

Absolute contraindications are relevant bradycardia, second- or third-degree heart block (without pacemaker) and bronchial asthma, and systemic hypotension. Extreme caution should be exercised as patients can sometimes experience symptoms of increasing dyspnoea on the third or fourth day following initiation or increased dose of beta-blockers due to reduced contractility. Symptoms often resolve by temporarily increasing the diuretic dose. Nevertheless, as mentioned previously, clinical trials have shown that drugs such as carvedilol and bisoprolol (in combination with ACE-inhibitors and diuretics) have reduced mortality.

Mineralocorticoid receptor antagonists (MRAs)

Mineralocorticoid receptor antagonists (MRAs), such as spironolactone, antagonise the effect of aldosterone and can lead to a reduction in fibrosis and improvement in left ventricular function. Although MRAs promote less diuresis than loop diuretics (such as furosemide), they are also considered to be diuretics as they work through the same mechanism – blocking aldosterone, inhibiting sodium and fluid reabsorption and conserving potassium. Studies such as RALES and EPHESUS have shown that MRAs reduce total and cardiovascular mortality as well as frequency of hospitalisation for worsening heart failure in patients with reduced ejection fraction when they are administered on top of ACE-inhibitors (or ARBs) and beta-blockers.

NICE (2018) have advised that patients with reduced left ventricular systolic dysfunction EF <35% who have ongoing symptoms of heart failure (despite optimal treatment with diuretics, ACE-inhibitors and beta-blockers) should be given a mineralocorticoid receptor antagonist unless this is contraindicated by the presence of renal impairment and/or elevated serum potassium concentration (K+ >5.0mmol/L).

The most important adverse effect of therapy with MRA is hyperkalaemia. Therefore, this treatment approach should be used with caution in patients with existing hyperkalaemia (K+ >5 mmol/L); and in patients with severely impaired renal function and markers, electrolytes should be checked regularly. Eplerenone can be substituted for spironolactone in patients who develop gynaecomastia.

Angiotensin receptors/neprilysin inhibitors (ARNIs)

A new drug class has recently emerged in heart failure therapy, angiotensin receptor/neprilysin inhibitors (ARNIs). This type of drug is composed of an ARB (valsartan) and sacubitril, a neutral endopeptidase (NEP) neprilysin inhibitor. Neprilysin plays a crucial role in the degradation of natriuretic peptides. The ARNI therapeutic concept is based on the established inhibition of the renin-angiotensin-aldosterone-system (RAAS) and an increase in endogenous natriuretic peptides (which are increasingly secreted in response to volume expansion and pressure overload in the failing heart) by blocking their degradation. Inhibition of neprilysin counteracts the neurohormonal activation, which would otherwise lead to vasoconstriction, sodium retention and cardiac remodelling, increasing the RAAS-blocking effects. A large multicentred randomised control trial (PARADIGM) has reported benefit from sacubitril/valsartan in comparison with enalapril. The study was terminated early because of overwhelming benefits.

The 2018 NICE guidelines recommend that patients with reduced ejection fraction (EF) <35% who have ongoing symptoms of heart failure despite optimal treatment should be given sacubitril/valsartan instead of an ACE-inhibitor or ARB unless this is contraindicated. If patients are already on an ACE-inhibitor, the ACE-inhibitor should be stopped for 36 hours before initiating sacubitril/valsartan to minimise the risk of angioedema.

Reported events of symptomatic hypotension were more common with sacubitril/valsartan in the study. Patients with very low blood pressure (systolic <100mmHg) during ACE-inhibitor treatment should therefore not be switched to ARNI. The treatment with sacubitril/valsartan should be initiated by a heart failure specialist with access to a multidisciplinary heart failure team.

Diuretics

In the majority of patients with heart failure fluid retention occurs, causing ankle oedema, pulmonary oedema or both, contributing to the symptoms of dyspnoea. Diuretic treatment relieves oedema and dyspnoea. Furosemide is a loop diuretic which is often the first-line therapy when treating clinical signs and symptoms due to fluid congestion. Loop diuretics inhibit sodium and water reabsorption in the thick ascending limb of the loop of Henle, as well as increasing urinary excretion of chloride, calcium and magnesium. Common adverse effects are often dose-related and include hypotension and electrolyte disturbances. NICE (2018) states that diuretics should be used 'routinely in patients with congestive symptoms and fluid retention in heart failure'. Bumetanide is another loop diuretic which is considered to have better oral bioavailability.

Loop diuretics can also cause metabolic disturbances such as hyperglycaemia. In older adults, diuretics are a common cause of adverse drug reactions and the ageing process enhances these adverse effects. For example, sodium depletion caused by diuretics can lead to significant reduction in blood pressure, causing hypotension, fainting, dizziness, falls and confusion. Diuretics are also involved in a number of drug interactions which can either enhance or decrease the effect of these drugs. For example, diuretics can increase retention of lithium, resulting in lithium toxicity.

Alternately, over-the-counter drugs such as NSAIDs, can reduce the effect of diuretics.

Thiazide diuretics are sometimes added on top of loop diuretics to aid diuresis, as the combination of the two drugs blocks reabsorption of sodium at different sites in the nephrons (double nephron blockade) and this action leads to greater diuretic effect. The most commonly used thiazide diuretics are metolazone and bendroflumethiazide. Combination diuretic therapy offers the potential benefit of fluid removal. However, a clinically important adverse effect is the increased risk of provoking biochemical disturbance such as hyponatraemia (low serum sodium) and hypokalaemia (low serum potassium). The dose of diuretics should therefore be as low as possible to reach and maintain euvolaemia.

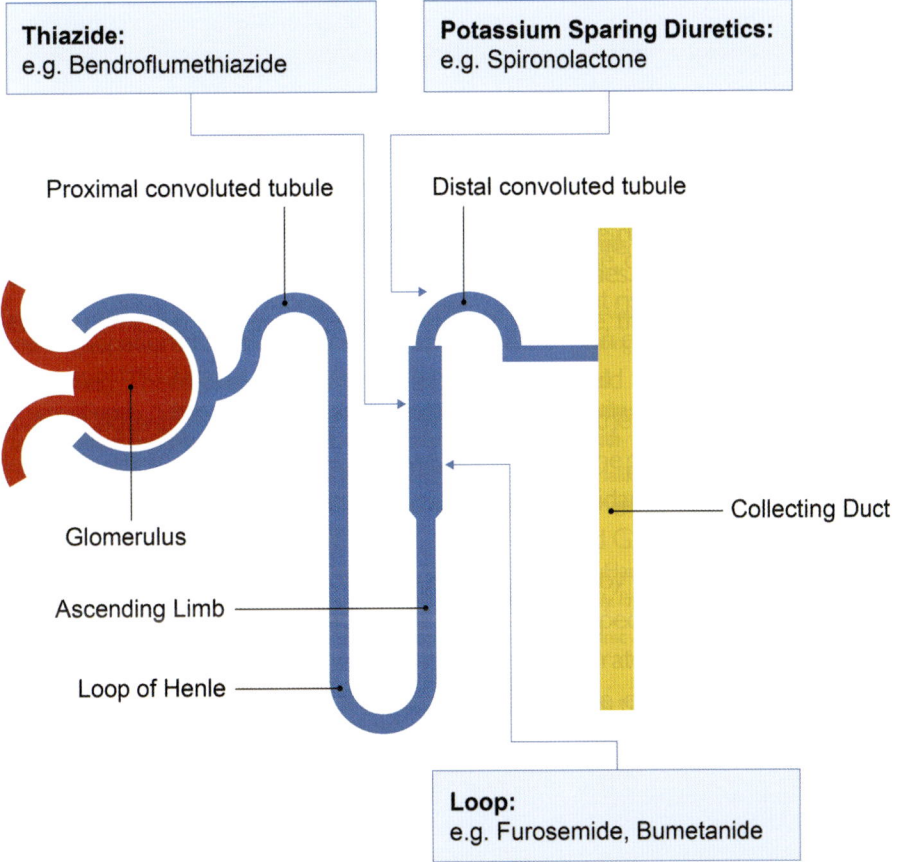

Figure 11.4: Diagram showing site of action of three groups of diuretics on the nephron. The powerful loop diuretics act on the ascending limb of the loop of Henle, where most sodium is normally reabsorbed. Thiazides act on the first part of the distal convoluting tubule. Both the loop and thiazide group cause potassium loss. Like the other two groups, the potassium-sparing group increase excretion of sodium, but with little impact on potassium loss – hence the term 'potassium sparing'. Thiazides act on the first part of the distal convoluted tubule. Both the loop and thiazide group cause potassium loss. Like the other two groups, the potassium-sparing group increase excretion of sodium, but with little impact on potassium loss – hence the term 'potassium sparing'.

Ivabradine

Ivabradine is a class of drug which targets the sinoatrial node and slows the sinus rhythm through If-channel inhibition. The SHIFT trial showed a significant decrease in heart failure hospitalisation and cardiovascular mortality in patients where ivabradine was added as an addition to an optimised heart failure medication (including beta-blockers). NICE approved its use in the treatment of chronic heart failure in 2012. Unlike beta-blockers, ivabradine does not have an adrenergic blocking effect and therefore does not affect blood pressure. Ivabradine is used with standard therapy involving ACE-inhibitors, beta-blockers and MRAs or in patients where beta-blockers are not tolerated. In Europe, the official labelling for ivabradine to treat heart failure is for patients in sinus rhythm with a heart rate >75bpm. Specialist advice should be sought before initiating ivabradine.

Hydralazine

For heart failure, hydralazine (used in combination with nitrates such as isosorbide dinitrate) is recommended in Afro-Caribbean patients with moderate to severe heart failure who do not respond well or are intolerant of ACE-inhibitors or ARBs due to renal dysfunction or hyperkalaemia. The combined arterial and venous vasodilators may cause hypotension but do not affect renal function.

When taken orally, hydralazine is well absorbed from the gastrointestinal tract. It is then rapidly broken down in the liver, which reduces its bioavailability. Hydralazine is metabolised mainly by the process of acetylation. Some individuals are slow acetylators, and in these patients a high dose can cause symptoms such as fever, malaise, muscle and joint pain, which are similar to those of systemic lupus erythematosus. On the other hand, at normal doses, slow acetylators will derive more benefits than fast acetylators. Other adverse effects of hydralazine include headaches, nausea, peripheral neuropathy, palpitations and angina in patients who have ischaemic heart disease due to reflex tachycardia.

Activity 11.3
1. Why do slow acetylators gain more benefits at normal doses than fast acetylators?
2. Why would reflex tachycardia induced by hydralazine cause angina in patients with ischaemic heart disease?

Digoxin

Digoxin is a cardiac glycoside extracted from the purple foxglove plant (*digitalis purpurea*), although today it is produced synthetically. It has been used for the treatment of heart disease since 1776, when a physician called William Withering used it to treat a woman with dropsy (peripheral oedema), whom he expected to die. Instead she made a remarkable recovery. Later it was discovered that the woman had heart failure.

Today, the role of digoxin in the management of heart failure has diminished, since trials such as the Digitalis Investigation Group (1997) demonstrated that it has no effect on all-cause mortality in patients with congestive cardiac failure. In addition, a number of studies, cited previously, have shown unequivocally that other drugs (such as ACE-inhibitors, beta-blockers and MRAs) do reduce morbidity and mortality in these patients. Nevertheless, digoxin may be beneficial if symptoms of heart failure are still present despite treatment with these drugs (NICE 2018). It is indicated in heart failure due to atrial fibrillation (AF) and it is also used in the management of arrhythmias such as supraventricular tachycardia.

Mechanism of action

Digoxin is a positive inotrope, in that it increases the force of cardiac contraction by inhibiting Na^+/K^+ ATPase pump, which leads to increased calcium in the myocardial cells. Digoxin also slows the ventricular rate through its direct effect on the action potential of the myocardial cells and indirect effects on the heart – that is, increasing vagal activity. In AF, a slower, more regular contracting heart functions more efficiently, thus increasing cardiac output.

Adverse effects

Digoxin has a very narrow therapeutic index so the risk of toxicity is high. Common adverse effects include loss of appetite, nausea, diarrhoea and vomiting, visual disturbances such as coloured halos and blurred vision; confusion, insomnia, arrhythmias such as bradycardia and couple beats. Potassium levels should be monitored because, in the presence of low and high levels, both the toxic and therapeutic effects are respectively enhanced. Practitioners should also be aware that digoxin is involved in a significant number of drug interactions (see BNF 2020 and Chapter 3).

Table 11.4: Drugs used in the management of heart failure

Drug group	Mechanism of action	Clinical effect	Examples – used in heart failure
• Angiotensin-converting enzyme inhibitors • Angiotensin receptor blockers	• ACEis inhibit the formation of angiotensin II • ARBs stop angiotensin II from binding to the ATI receptor on blood vessels	• ACEis and ARBs dilate arterioles reducing heart's workload and improving cardiac output	• ACEis, e.g. ramipril, lisinopril, enalapril • ARBs, e.g. candesartan, losartan
• Beta-adrenoceptor antagonist	• Beta-blockers block the action of the sympathetic nervous system on the heart, thus reducing heart rate and contractility	• Reduce heart's workload and prolong survival rates in patients who have heart failure that is already being treated with ACEis	• Bisoprolol, carvedilol, nebivolol
• Mineralocorticoid receptor antagonist (MRAs)	• Antagonise the effect of aldosterone	• Increase sodium and water excretion whilst conserving potassium • Reduce fibrosis and improve left ventricular function	• Spironolactone, epleronone
• Angiotensin receptor/ neprilysin inhibitor	• Inhibit RAAS and increase endogenous natriuretic peptides by blocking their degradation	• Inhibition of neprilysin leads to vasoconstriction, sodium retention and cardiac remodelling, increasing the RAAS blocking effects	• Sacubitril/valsartan (Entresto®)

• Diuretics (loop and thiazide)	• Increase the excretion of sodium and water • Each type acts on different parts of the nephron (see Figure 11.4 above)	• Reduce blood volume, pulmonary and peripheral oedema	• Loop, e.g. furosemide, bumetanide, torasemide • Thiazide, e.g bendrofluamethiazide, metolozone
• Ivabradine	• Blocks If channels in sinoatrial node	• Lowers heart rate.	• Ivabradine
• Hydralazine with nitrates in patients of African and Afro-Caribbean origin, who are less responsive to ACEis/ARBs • As an add-on to first-line therapy	• Hydralazine selectively vasodilates the smooth muscle of arterioles • Its mechanism is not fully understood but it is thought to produce this effect by blocking build-up of intracellular calcium in muscles	• Reduces heart's workload by dilating arterioles	• Hydralazine combined with a nitrate in heart failure
• Inotropes	• Increase force of contractility of myocardium • Some, such as digoxin reduce heart rate	• Improve cardiac output and reduce symptoms of HF in patients taking diuretics and ACEis • Indicated in HF due to atrial fibrillation	• Digoxin

Case studies

Throughout the course of treatment, patients with heart failure will invariably experience periods of deterioration in their condition that will require their medication to be optimised. It is therefore important that the care delivered is patient-centred and involves the family as much as possible. A great deal of time should be spent listening, understanding and responding appropriately to the patient's concerns. Alterations in medication should only be made after taking a detailed history and making a holistic assessment of the patient's needs – not solely on the presenting symptoms.

Case study: Heart failure 1

Mr Genadaire is a 56-year-old man with known severe left ventricular systolic impairment secondary to ischaemic heart disease. His GP has referred him to the cardiology clinic, with extensive peripheral oedema and diagnosed as decompensated heart failure with a NYHA score of III/IV. His past medical history also includes diabetes type 2 treated with insulin, diabetic peripheral neuropathy and a false joint in his sternum.

On examination, Mr Genadaire was generally well, with no dyspnoea, orthopnoea, chest pain, palpitations or syncope. His exercise tolerance was only limited by cramps in his legs. His vital signs were within the normal range: temperature 36.8°C, HR 76 bpm, BP sitting 110/55mmHg and standing 112/55mmHg. His weight was 85.7kg, which was a significant increase compared with his last weight of 71kg two months ago.

His current medication included bumetanide 1mg twice daily, spironolactone 25mg once daily, aspirin 75mg once daily, metformin 1g twice daily, NovoMix® 30 (biphasic insulin aspart), ramipril 5mg twice daily, simvastatin 40mg once daily, bisoprolol 3.75mg once daily and bendroflumethiazide 5mg twice weekly.

The primary aim of the heart failure team was to try to resolve the extensive oedema and optimise his heart failure treatment.

Activity 11.4 (Case study)

1. Look up the term 'decompensated heart failure'. What are the typical clinical signs and symptoms?
2. Can you suggest the type of drug and mechanism of action that will be used to reduce Mr Genadaire's peripheral oedema?

On his final visit to the clinic two months later, Mr Genadaire's peripheral oedema was resolved (weight reduced from 85.7kg on initial visit to 72.6kg) with the changes in his medication. Indeed, he reported feeling well and all other parameters were within the normal range except for his renal function which was now impaired, with creatinine levels elevated from normal levels to 244 micromol/L (60–110) and urea 35.7mg/dL (normal 6–20). Both sodium and potassium levels were within normal range. It was puzzling why his renal function should suddenly have deteriorated. On further questioning it emerged that he had returned from Africa a few days ago and suffered severe diarrhoea and vomiting which had now ceased. His current medication included bumetanide 1mg twice daily, spironolactone 25mg once daily, aspirin 75mg once daily, metformin 1g twice daily, NovoMix® 30 (biphasic insulin aspart), ramipril 5mg twice daily, simvastatin 40mg once daily, bisoprolol 3.75mg once daily and bendroflumethiazide 5mg twice weekly.

3. Which of Mr Genadaire's medications would you temporarily withdraw in order to improve his renal function and why?
4. Can you suggest a test that would give a more accurate indication of Mr Genadaire's renal function?

Case study: Heart failure 2

Mr Silveria is a 47-year-old Brazilian man who was referred to the heart failure clinic by his consultant cardiologist for titration of his heart failure treatment. He has severe biventricular failure (NYHA III-IV) secondary to mitral valve disease. His current presenting symptoms are breathlessness on minimal exertion, paroxysmal nocturnal dyspnoea and poor appetite, and he experiences dizziness with quick movements.

His past medical history includes septic arthritis with mitral endocarditis and septic emboli, mitral valve repair in 2012 and out of hospital ventricular fibrillation arrest in 2009. He has an implantable cardioverter defibrillator to manage recurrent ventricular tachycardia. Unfortunately his arrest in 2009 left him with profound short-term memory loss. His partner also stated that he often forgot to drink enough fluids. Sometimes he only drank 1–2 glasses of fluid per day whilst she was at work. Mr Silveria, however, has normal coronary arteries. His medication on the initial consultation is: lisinopril 2.5mg once daily, aspirin 75mg once daily, furosemide 40mg once daily and bisoprolol 1.25mg once daily.

On clinical examination, his observations were within the normal parameters, including a clear lung field on auscultation and no peripheral oedema. His jugular venous pressure (JVP) was not raised and his renal function and ECG were within normal limits. However, his systolic BP was relatively low, at 100/86mmHg.

In summary, his main problems were hypotension and memory loss and he was low in mood. The plan for Mr Silveria was to:

a) Increase his medication (up-titration of heart failure treatment) in order to reduce the deterioration in his current symptoms. On the first consultation, Mr Silveria's lisinopril was increased from 2.5mg to 5mg.

b) Provide support to help him address how he felt about his condition and suggest strategies to help him cope with his memory loss.

On the second consultation, Mr Silveria returned to the clinic with paroxysmal nocturnal dyspnoea. During the assessment it was discovered that he had stopped taking his furosemide but neither he nor his partner knew who had instructed him to stop it. Furosemide was recommenced.

This situation illustrates the need for good communication and clear documentation by all involved in a patient's care. The matter was investigated further, and the relevant individual was made aware of the results of their actions.

On his third visit to the clinic, Mr Silveria was generally well and more optimistic about his progress. However, his systolic BP was now 80mmHg, and although the dizziness was still present it had not worsened. No further changes were made to his medication and a follow-up appointment was made to see the consultant cardiologist. The consultant commenced Mr Silveria on spironolactone 25mg od because he was still symptomatic (hypotensive, dizziness) despite almost optimal treatment with an ACE-inhibitor and a beta-blocker.

Activity 11.5 (Case study)

1. What would be the clinical effect of increasing Mr Silveria's lisinopril? Is there anything in the clinical history that would cause concern about increasing the dose?
2. In view of Mr Silveria's hypotension and dizziness, would you consider reducing the ACE-inhibitor?
3. How would you educate Mr Silveria and his partner to manage the mild dizziness that he sometimes experiences on sudden movement?

On the fourth consultation, six months later, at the heart failure clinic, Mr Silveria was well, with clear lung fields, no peripheral oedema, and normal renal function and electrolyte levels. In addition, his vital signs were within normal range and his BP levels had improved significantly – 116/60mmHg, HR 68 sinus rhythm. In view of the improvement in his condition, especially the increase in his blood pressure, his lisinopril was increased further to 7.5mg daily.

4. What is the mechanism of action and the clinical effect of spironolactone?
5. What are the potential adverse effects of spironolactone that should be closely monitored?

Summary

Heart failure is increasing in the general population. Paradoxically, this is mainly due to improvements in the management of CHD and hypertension, which have led to increased survival rates in people with damaged heart muscle. An ageing population has also added to this trend. Survival rates for patients with heart failure are significantly reduced, but with early diagnosis and effective management the prognosis can be improved. However, the management of patients with HF is complex, in that many patients present with other health problems, both physical and psychological, which will impact on the overall management of their HF. Fortunately, guidelines, such as those drafted by NICE, have made a significant contribution in terms of guiding practitioners to deliver effective and appropriate management, and improving the overall standard and quality of care delivered nationally. Finally, although the case studies presented earlier have mainly focused on the pharmacological management, it is hoped that they have also given some insight into the complexity involved in managing patients with heart failure.

Answers to activities

Activity 11.1

Using the figures for stroke volume (SV) and heart rate (HR) given above, calculate the cardiac output.

$$CO = HR\ (75bpm) \times SV\ (70ml)$$
$$= 75bpm \times 70ml$$
$$CO = 5250ml/minute\ (5.25l/min)$$

Activity 11.2

1. What is a prodrug and why are some drugs given in this form?

A prodrug is a drug that is administered in an inactive or partially active form. When it gets inside the body, it is converted by the normal metabolic pathways to an active form. They are given in an inactive form for many reasons, often to enhance the bioavailability of the drug, especially when the oral drug is poorly absorbed in the gastrointestinal tract or to improve distribution of drug to its site of action (e.g. levodopa to provide dopamine in the central nervous system for management of Parkinson's Disease). However, often many prodrugs are not prodrugs 'by design'; they just happen to be the form in which the drug was developed or manufactured.

2. Can you identify other drugs that are given in this form?

Examples of prodrugs include: ramipril (ramiprilat), prednisone (prednisolone), levodopa (dopamine), imipramine (desipramine), diamorphine (6-acetylmorphine), codeine (morphine, norcodeine and other active metabolites).

Activity 11.3

1. Why do slow acetylators gain more benefits at normal doses than fast acetylators?

With a single dose, the fast acetylators would break down the drug faster so the drug would have less time to produce its clinical effects.

2. Why would reflex tachycardia induced by hydralazine cause angina in patients with ischaemic heart disease?

As the heart rate increases, the proportion of time it remains in diastole is reduced, meaning that the myocardium is perfused less effectively at a time when oxygen demand is increased. Reflex tachycardia is therefore likely to induce anginal symptoms in those patients with narrowed coronary arteries.

Activity 11.4 (Case study)

1. Look up the term 'decompensated heart failure'. What are the typical clinical signs and symptoms?

When the clinical signs and symptoms of someone in heart failure worsen, e.g. increasing breathlessness, paroxysmal nocturnal dyspnoea, oedema, tiredness, raised JVP.

2. Can you suggest the type of drug and mechanism of action that will be used to reduce Mr Genadaire's peripheral oedema?

Mr Genadaire's bumetanide was optimised to 5mg twice daily and his response was monitored by the team on a weekly basis. Mr Genadaire responded well to these changes. Bumetanide acts on the ascending limb of the loop of Henle in the area where a lot of sodium is reabsorbed (see Figure 11.4, p. 207). Like furosemide, bumetanide inhibits sodium pumps in this area, reducing the reabsorption of sodium and thus increasing the amount of water and salts that pass out in the renal tubules.

3. Which of Mr Genadaire's medications would you temporarily withdraw in order to improve his renal function and why?

Bendroflumethiazide, a thiazide diuretic that is known to be less effective if there is renal impairment. One of the side effects of this group is electrolyte imbalance. The BNF cautions that electrolyte level should be monitored regularly in the presence of renal impairment, and if the eGFR is less than 30mL/minute/1.73m^2 they should not be used.

4. Can you suggest a test that would be a more accurate indication of Mr Genadaire's renal function?

The eGFR (estimated glomerular filtration rate). This test assesses actual glomerular filtration rate. It is used to detect early kidney disease and monitor the condition of the kidneys. Normal values are between 90 and 120mL/min. Serum creatinine is useful to identify a trend in renal function but calculation of eGFR (or creatinine clearance) needs to be carried out to compensate for age, weight and gender.

Activity 11.5 (Case study)

1. What would be the clinical effect of increasing Mr Silveria's lisinopril? Is there anything in the clinical history that would cause concern about increasing the dose?

Lisinopril is an ACE-inhibitor and a first-line drug therapy in the management of heart failure. Lisinopril dilates arterioles, thus lowering the resistance to blood flow from the heart and so leaving less work for the heart to do (because there is less resistance to push against). The reduced retention of sodium and water thus increases cardiac output. Increasing Mr Silveria's lisinopril could reduce his blood pressure even further. Concern would be caused by the fact that he was getting dizzy spells on movement and that his BP was low.

2. In view of Mr Silveria's hypotension and dizziness, would you consider reducing the ACE-inhibitor?

Although his BP is low, Mr Silveria is not experiencing any significant symptoms, such as blackouts, falls or significant dizziness. Careful titration of his lisinopril will improve the functioning of his heart and consequently his blood pressure. The current NICE guideline (2018) states that hypotension should not be a barrier to up-titration of ACE-inhibitors, providing the patient is asymptomatic. Although he is experiencing dizziness, it is mild and he can be taught how to manage this.

3. How would you educate Mr Silveria and his partner to manage the mild dizziness that he sometimes experiences on sudden movement?

Mr Silveria and his partner need to be told how to cope with the mild dizziness that he is experiencing – for example, he should move more slowly and avoid making sudden movements, such as standing or sitting up too quickly.

4. What is the mechanism of action and the clinical effect of spironolactone?

Spironolactone is an aldosterone antagonist. It acts on the distal convoluted tubule of the nephron, competitively inhibiting aldosterone. Blocking the effects of aldosterone increases the excretion of sodium and water. Several studies have demonstrated the effectiveness of spironolactone for patients like Mr Silveria, with moderate to severe (NYHA III-IV), on optimal treatment with an ACE-inhibitor and beta-blocker. In such cases, spironolactone has been shown to reduce hospital admissions and increase survival rate.

5. What are the potential adverse effects of spironolactone that should be closely monitored?

High potassium levels, hepatic impairment, gynaecomastia. Caution: spironolactone should not be given to patients with renal impairment. Monitor renal function: urea; electrolytes (especially potassium and creatinine levels); avoid potassium-sparing diuretics and a diet that is high in potassium, e.g. salt substitutes.

References and further reading

Bristow, M.R. (1997). Mechanism of action of beta-blocking agents in heart failure. *American Journal of Cardiology*. **80**, 26–40L.

CIBIS investigators and committees (1994). A randomised trial of beta-blockade in heart failure. The Cardiac Insufficiency Bisoprolol study (CIBIS). *Circulation*. **90** (4), 1765–73.

CIBIS-II Investigators and committees (1999). The Cardiac Insufficiency Bisoprolol Study II (CIBIS II). A randomised trial. *Lancet*. **353** (9146), 9–13.

CONSENSUS Trial Study Group (1987). Effects of Enalapril on mortality in severe congestive heart failure. Results of the Cooperative North Scandinavian Enalapril Survival Study (CONSENSUS). *New England Journal of Medicine*. **316**, 1429–35.

Cowie, M.R. (2017). The heart failure epidemic: a UK perspective. *Echo Research and Practice*. **4** (1), R15–R20.

Cullington, D., Goode, K.M., Clark, A.L. & Cleland, J. (2012). Heart rate achieved or beta blocker dose in patients with chronic heart failure: which is better target? *European Journal of Heart Failure*. **14**, 737–47.

Digitalis Investigation Group (DIG) (1997). The effect of digoxin on mortality and morbidity in patients with heart failure. *New England Journal of Medicine*. **336**: 525-33. DOI: 10.1056/NEJM199702203360801. Available at: https://www.nejm.org/doi/full/10.1056/nejm199702203360801 (Accessed: 12 February 2021).

Jentzer, J.C., DeWald, T.A. & Hernandez, A.F. (2010). Combination of loop diuretics with thiazide-type diuretic in heart failure. *Journal of the American College of Cardiology*. **56** (19), 1527–34.

Joint Formulary Committee (2020). *British National Formulary*. 79th edn. BMJ Group and Pharmaceutical Press.

Kosmas, C., Silverio, D., Sourlas, A., Montan, P.D. & Guzman, E. (2018). Role of Spironolactone in the treatment of heart failure with preserved ejection fraction. *Annals of Transitional Medicine*. **6** (23), 461.

McMurry, J.J., Packer, M., Desai, A.S., Gong, J., Lefkowitz, M.P., Rizkala, A.R., Rouleau, J.L., Shi, V., Solomon, S.D., Swedberg, K. & Zile, M.R. For the PARADIGM-HF Investigators and Committee. (2014). Angiotensin-neprilysin inhibition versus enalapril in heart failure. *New England Journal of Medicine*. **371**, 993–1004.

Metra, M., Nodari, S., D'Aloia, A., Bontempi, L., Boldi, E. & Cas, L. D. (2000). A rationale for the use of B-blockers as standard treatment for heart failure. *American Heart Journal*. **139**, 511–21.

National Institute for Health and Care Excellence (NICE) (2018). Chronic Heart Failure: National clinical guidelines for diagnosis and management in primary and secondary care. London: NICE.

Packer, M., Poole-Wilson, P.A., Armstrong, P.W., Cleland, J.G., Horowitz, J.D., Massie, B.M., Rydel, L., Thygesen, K. & Urestky, R. on behalf of the ALTAS study group (1999). Comparative effects of low and high doses of the angiotensin-converting enzyme inhibitor, Lisinopril, on morbidity in chronic heart failure. *Circulation*. **100**, 2312–318.

Parker, M., Fowler, M.B., Roecker E.B., Coats, A.J., Katus, H.A., Krum, H., Mohacsi, P., Rouleau, J.L., Tendera, M., Staiger, C., Holcslaw, T.L. & Aman-Zalan, I: Carvedilol Prospective randomised cumulative survival (COPERNICUS) study group (2002). Effects of carvedilol on the morbidity of patients with severe chronic heart failure: results of the carvedilol prospective randomised cumulative survival (COPERNICUS) study. *Circulation*. **106** (17), 2194–199.

Pfeffer, M., Swedberg, K., Granger, C., Held, P., Mcmurry, J., Michelson, E., Olofsson, B., Ostergren, J., Yusuf, S. & Pocock, S. (2003). Effects of candesartan on mortality and morbidity in patients with chronic heart failure: the CHARM-Overall Programme. *Lancet*. **362** (9386), 759–66.

Pitt, B., Zanna, F., Remme, W. J., Cody, R., Castaigne, A., Perez, A., Palensky, J. & Wittes, J. (1999). The effect of spironolactone on morbidity and mortality in patients with severe heart failure. Randomised Aldactone Evaluation Study Investigators. (RALES). *New England Journal of Medicine*. **341** (10), 709–17.

Pitt, B., Remme, W., Zannad, F., Neaton, J., Martinez, F., Roniker, B., Bittman, R., Hurley, S., Kleiman, J. for the Eplerenone Post-Acute Myocardial Infarction Heart Failure Efficacy and Survival (EPHESIS) Investigators: (2003). Eplerenone, a selective aldosterone blocker, in patients with left ventricular dysfunction after myocardial infarction. *New England Journal of Medicine*. **364**, 1309–21.

Swedberg, K., Komajda, M., Bohm, M., Borer, J.S., Ford, I., Dubost-Brama, A., Lerebours, G. & Tavazzi, L. SHIFT Investigators (2010). Ivabradine and outcomes in chronic heart failure (SHIFT): a randomised placebo-controlled study. *Lancet*. **376** (9744), 875–85.

Taylor, A.L., Ziesche, S. & Yancy, C. (2004). The African-American Heart Failure Trial Investigator. Combination of isosorbide dinitrate and hydralazine in Blacks with heart failure. *New England Journal of Medicine*. **351**, 2049–57.

Testani, J.M., Brisco, M.A., Turner, J.M., Spatz, E.S., Bellumkonda, L., Parikh, C.R. & Tang, W. (2014). Loop diuretic efficiency: A metric of diuretic responsiveness with prognostic importance in acute decompensated heart failure. *Circulation: Heart Failure*. **7**, 261–70.

Tilson, L., McGowan, B. & Ryan, M. (2003). Cost effectiveness of spironolactone in patients with severe heart failure. *Irish Journal of Medical Science*. **172** (2), 70–72.

The Criteria Committee of the New York Heart Association (1994). *Nomenclature and criteria for diagnosis of the heart and great vessels*. 9th edn. Boston, Mass. Little Brown & Co.

The Digitalis Investigation Group (1997). The effect of digoxin in mortality and morbidity in patients with heart failure. *New England Journal of Medicine*. **336** (8), 525–33.

Wu, M., Chang, N., Su, C., Hsu, Y., Chen, T., Lin, Y., Hsiung, C. & Tam, K. (2014). Loop diuretic strategies in patients with acute decompensated heart failure: A meta-analysis of randomised controlled trials. *Journal of Critical Care*. **29**, 2–9.

Yusuf, S., Pitt, B., Davis, C.E., Hood, W.B. & Cohn, J.N. (1991). Effect of enalapril on survival in patients with reduced left ventricular ejection fractions and congestive heart failure (SOLVD). *New England Journal of Medicine*. **325**, 293–302.

Zannad, F., McMurry, J.J., Swedberg, K., Shi, H., Vincent, J., Pocock, S.J. & Pitt, B. EMPHASIS-HF Study Group (2011). Eplerenone in patients with systolic heart failure and mild symptoms. *New England Journal of Medicine*. **364** (1), 11–21.

12

Pharmacological case studies: Chronic obstructive pulmonary disease (COPD)

Beverley Bostock
RGN MSc MA Queen's Nurse,
Advanced Nurse Practitioner in Long Term Conditions, Committee member,
Association of Respiratory Nurse Specialists

Kola Akinlabi
BSc (Hons), MSc Advanced Cardiorespiratory (UCL);
Clinical specialist respiratory physiotherapist, North and Central London NHS Foundation Trust and University College Hospital, London.

This chapter:
- Outlines the causes and pathophysiology of COPD
- Assesses the prevalence of COPD in the UK
- Considers the latest European and UK clinical evidence and guidelines for the diagnosis and management of COPD in adults, with an emphasis on pharmacotherapy for stable COPD and exacerbations of COPD
- Shows how to apply knowledge of COPD through the use of clinical case studies.

Introduction

People with chronic obstructive pulmonary disease (COPD) classically present with symptoms which include cough, breathlessness and sputum production, all of which can impact on their day-to-day lives. Breathlessness is the hallmark of patients with chronic respiratory diseases including COPD. Breathlessness can be debilitating, especially if people with COPD continue with lifestyle habits such as smoking, are not treated with optimum pharmacological therapy and are not engaged in pulmonary rehabilitation. The National Institute for Health and Care Excellence (NICE) recommends that COPD patients should be offered smoking cessation, pulmonary rehabilitation, vaccination and optimum pharmacotherapy. This chapter will give an understanding of the prevalence, aetiologies and pathophysiology of COPD, with an emphasis on diagnosis, classification and pharmacotherapy using the Global Initiative for Chronic Obstructive Lung Disease clinical guidelines (GOLD 2019), and the NICE Chronic Obstructive Pulmonary Disease clinical guidelines (NICE 2019b). Clinical case studies will be used to show how the theories are applied in practice.

Prevalence of COPD

COPD is the cause of significant morbidity and mortality in the United Kingdom. According to the Health and Safety Executive (HSE), COPD accounted for around 30,000 deaths per year over the past decade (HSE 2019), with the vast majority being linked to cigarette smoking. The prevalence and mortality impact of COPD is difficult to estimate because COPD is an umbrella term which covers chronic bronchitis, emphysema and chronic asthma, amongst other conditions. Estimates regarding prevalence range from around 1 million cases up to 3 million, many of whom are undiagnosed (HSE 2019).

Pathophysiology of COPD

Cigarette smoking and noxious particles (such as smoke from biomass fuels) are a major cause of lung inflammation in COPD. The resulting unique pathological changes include chronic lung inflammation and systemic inflammation, which cause structural changes, repeated lung injury, and the development of secondary comorbidities. Lung inflammation, airway and structural changes increase with disease severity and persist with cigarette smoking. Lung parenchyma and airway inflammation in COPD are characterised by the increased number of CD8+ (cytotoxic cell) Tc1 lymphocytes that are only present in smokers who develop the disease. In addition, neutrophils and macrophages release inflammatory mediators and enzymes that invade the airways, causing structural changes in the lung parenchyma and pulmonary vasculature. The disease process leads to characteristic physiological abnormalities of peripheral airway narrowing, a reduced Forced Expiratory Volume in 1 second/Forced Vital Capacity (FEV1/FVC) ratio, resulting in symptoms of breathlessness, and emphysema, which cause airflow limitation and impaired gas transfer, along with cough and increased sputum production due to impaired mucociliary clearance.

Diagnosing COPD

A diagnosis of COPD should be considered in any patient over the age of 35 who has dyspnoea, chronic cough, sputum production and a history of exposure to risk factors, such as tobacco smoking, smoke from home cooking, heating fuel, occupational dust and chemicals (GOLD 2019, NICE 2019b).

Spirometry is required to confirm a diagnosis, with a ratio of FEV1 to FVC of less than 0.7 (FEV1/FVC <0.7) post bronchodilator, confirming the presence of persistent airflow obstruction and thus COPD. Although post-bronchodilator spirometry is required for the diagnosis and assessment of the severity of COPD, as seen in Table 12.1 (below), it is no longer recommended to measure the degree of reversibility. This is because measuring FEV1 before and after bronchodilator or steroids does not contribute to the diagnosis of COPD or differentiate it from an asthma diagnosis.

Table 12.1: Spirometric criteria for severity of airflow obstruction in COPD post bronchodilator

GOLD stage 1	Mild airflow obstruction	FEV1/FVC <0.7 FEV1 = 80% predicted or more (≥80%)
GOLD stage 2	Moderate airflow obstruction	FEV1/FVC <0.7 50% ≤FEV1 <80% predicted
GOLD stage 3	Severe airflow obstruction	FEV1/FVC <0.7 30% ≤FEV1 <50% predicted
GOLD stage 4	Very severe airflow obstruction	FEV1/FVC <0.7 FEV1 <30% predicted or FEV1 <50% predicted plus chronic respiratory failure

Adapted from GOLD (2019).

Comorbidities are frequently noted in COPD, as it is now recognised that COPD is a systemic disease with chronic inflammatory responses. These comorbidities include cardiovascular diseases (heart failure, pulmonary hypertension and cor pulmonale, and myocardial infarction), skeletal muscle dysfunction, metabolic syndrome, osteoporosis, depression and lung cancer. Comorbidity can occur at any stage of COPD and can affect the frequency of hospitalisation and mortality. It should therefore be routinely checked for and treated, once COPD is diagnosed.

A combination of spirometric classification and symptomatic assessment is the recommended method of assessing the impact of COPD on the individual and their risk of exacerbation. The COPD assessment test (CAT) can be used to detect the symptomatic impact of COPD. A CAT score ≥10 indicates a high level of symptoms (see Table 12.2 below). In addition to a CAT score, risk characteristics in relation to symptoms and rate of exacerbation can be used to assess the severity and the impact of COPD. Table 12.2 shows how patients' COPD GOLD stage relates to the risk characteristics, rate of exacerbation, CAT score and the modified British Medical Research Council (mMRC) Dyspnoea Scale (GOLD 2019).

Table 12.2: Classification

Patient Group	Exacerbation risk and symptoms	Spirometric classification	Exacerbations per year	CAT	mMRC
A	Low risk, fewer symptoms	GOLD 1–2	0–1	<10	0–1
B	Low risk, more symptoms	GOLD 1–2	0–1	≤10	0–1
C	High risk, fewer symptoms	GOLD 3–4	2 or more	<10	≥2
D	High risk, more symptoms	GOLD 3–4	2 or more (or 1 requiring admission)	≥10	≥2

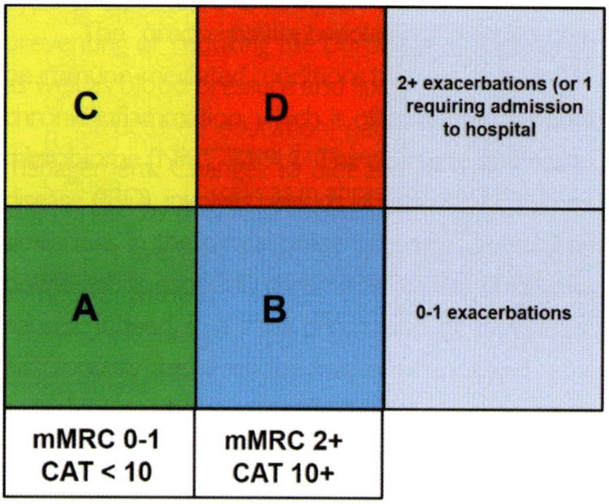

Category A: Use a bronchodilator inhaler

Category B: Use a long-acting beta2 agonist (LABA) or long-acting muscarinic antagonist (LAMA) inhaler

Category C: Use a long-acting muscarinic antagonist (LAMA) inhaler

Category D: Use a long-acting muscarinic antagonist (LAMA) inhaler OR use a dual long-acting beta2 agonist (LABA) and long-acting muscarinic antagonist (LAMA) inhaler if highly symptomatic OR use an inhaled corticosteroid (ICS)/LABA if blood eosinophils are >300cells/μL

Figure 12.1: Combined assessment of COPD, using symptoms, breathlessness, spirometric classification and risk of exacerbations with recommended initial treatment (GOLD 2019).

Drug treatments are used alongside non-pharmacological interventions, such as pulmonary rehabilitation, to improve symptoms, reduce exacerbation risk and improve exercise capacity. The two key guidelines on COPD, GOLD and NICE, offer different approaches to choosing inhaled therapies.

The NICE guidelines for COPD take a 'one size fits all approach' to classification and treatment, recommending a short-acting bronchodilator as initial therapy. In theory, this could be either a beta2 agonist (SABA) or a muscarinic antagonist (SAMA). As SABAs have a faster onset of action than SAMAs, they are more often the drug of choice (Ejiofor & Turner 2013).

For those patients who need more intensive treatment, either because they remain breathless or because they are having exacerbations, a dual bronchodilator is recommended. There are four dual bronchodilators available at the time of writing. These are:

- Vilanterol/Umeclidinium (Anoro®) in the Ellipta device
- Formoterol/Aclidinium (Duaklir®) in the Genuair device
- Glycopyrronium/Indacaterol (Ultibro®) in the Breezhaler device
- Tiotropium/Olodaterol (Spiolto®) in the Respimat device.

As with any inhaled therapy, consideration should be given to device choice as well as the drugs in each product.

For further information on inhaler device options, go to https://www.rightbreathe.com

Treatment options

Upon diagnosis of COPD, assessment of current symptoms and future risk (using CAT and GOLD stage, see Table 12.2 on p. 224 and Table 12.3 on p. 226) should be made, with a view to planning effective treatment. Goals of treatment should be to reduce symptoms, improve exercise tolerance and improve quality of life. Other goals will be to reduce risk of exacerbation, prevent faster disease progression and reduce mortality (NICE 2019b, GOLD 2019).

Recommended initial therapy (based on A, B, C, D classification)

GOLD recommends that COPD presentations are categorised and initially treated using the ABCD algorithm (see Figure 12.1) which is based on symptom scores such as the modified MRC dyspnoea scale and/or the COPD assessment test (CAT) and exacerbation risk, which can be estimated by referring to the history of exacerbations in the past year (see Figure 12.1).

Both the UPLIFT (Tashkin, Celli, et al. 2008) and POET-COPD (Vogelmeier, Hedere, et al. 2011) studies found that LAMA therapy was associated with a reduction in exacerbation risk and respiratory failure in moderate to very severe COPD. A combination of LABA/LAMA reduced healthcare utilisation in COPD patients with FEV1 <59% and history of exacerbation as shown in the SPARK study (Wedzicha et al. 2013).

If an individual does not respond adequately to this initial treatment, GOLD states that there are different factors that will influence which way to go next. These include whether the patient:

- Is predominantly breathless
- Is predominantly exacerbating
- Has raised blood eosinophils

- Has any evidence of an asthma/irreversible element.

In breathless patients, the following recommendations are made:
- Unless already being used, initiate a long-acting beta2 agonist (LABA) or a long-acting muscarinic antagonist (LAMA).
- If either of these is being used already, move up to a dual bronchodilator (LAMA/LABA).
- GOLD suggests that although inhaled corticosteroid (ICS)/LABA or triple therapy might be used in this group, eosinophil levels and exacerbation rates should inform their initiation or ongoing use. Eosinophils over 300 cells/µL suggest potential benefit, as do eosinophils over 100 cells/µL in the presence of two or more exacerbations in the past year (or one severe enough to require hospital admission).
- NICE states that in the 'breathless' group, ICS therapies should be used with caution, especially if there is a history of pneumonia, or previous use of an ICS has had no effect or it was inappropriately prescribed in the past.

In people who are exacerbating, the following recommendations are made:
- If on bronchodilator monotherapy, move to a dual bronchodilator
- Consider an ICS/LABA if eosinophils are >300cells/µL or >100cells/µL with two or more acute exacerbations of COPD (AECOPD)
- Those who are still suffering from AECOPD on either of these can be considered for a move up to triple therapy (ICS/LABA/LAMA)
- There are currently two triple therapies on the market:
    - Trimbow® (extra-fine Beclometasone with Formoterol and Glycopyrronium), and
    - Trelegy® (Fluticasone furoate with Vilanterol and Umeclidinium).

Table 12.3: Follow-up treatment (GOLD 2019)

Breathlessness is the main issue (Often category A and B)	Exacerbation is the main issue (Often category C and D)
LABA or LAMA	LABA or LAMA
Dual LABA/LAMA – consider trying different molecules/devices	Dual LABA/LAMA
Consider role of ICS/LABA: check eosinophil levels, h/o pneumonia, lack of response before prescribing/continuing	ICS/LABA – especially if eosinophil levels ≥300 cells/µL or ≥100 cells/µL + 2 AECOPD, or 1 AECOPD + hospitalisation
	Triple therapy – ICS/LABA/LAMA: check eosinophil levels, h/o pneumonia, lack of response before prescribing/continuing

NICE and GOLD both recommend caution when using ICS in people with 'pure' COPD, i.e. when there is nothing in the history or lung function to suggest that there is any reversible (i.e. asthmatic) element in their condition. To that end, NICE recommends that clinicians should be prepared to discuss the risk of side effects (such as pneumonia and diabetes) in people who take ICS for COPD. This will apply to ICS/LABAs as well as triple therapy.

Treatment options recommended for COPD by NICE (2019b) and GOLD (2019) are:

- **Influenza vaccination:** Influenza vaccination has been found to reduce serious respiratory tract infection and prevent hospitalisation and reduce morbidity in COPD. Patients are advised to have the vaccine annually (Walters, Tang, et al. 2017).
- **Pneumococcal vaccination:** The Green Book (GOV.UK 2020) recommends pneumococcal vaccine for anyone with COPD. Evidence has shown that pneumococcal vaccine can reduce the incidence of community-acquired pneumonia, especially in COPD patients over 65 years of age with FEV1 <40%.
- **Smoking cessation:** Smoking cessation, using counselling, nicotine replacement therapy, varenicline and bupropion, is said to be the most cost-effective treatment option for COPD. Despite increasing evidence to suggest that smoking cessation treatments work in people with pulmonary diseases, many individuals are still not given appropriate advice or support to quit (Jiménez-Ruiz, et al. 2015).
- **Pulmonary rehabilitation:** Pulmonary rehabilitation (PR) is an essential, evidence-based multidisciplinary option within a wider comprehensive respiratory pathway for the management of COPD and other chronic respiratory diseases (GOLD 2019). PR includes exercise training, smoking cessation, nutrition counselling and education. The principal goals of PR are to reduce symptoms, improve quality of life and increase physical and emotional participation in everyday activities. A Cochrane review found evidence that PR reduced mortality and hospital admission following exacerbation of COPD (McCarthy, Casey, et al. 2015). In all clinical trials, PR improved patients' capacity to exercise and improved activities of daily living. PR should be offered to patients diagnosed with COPD with mMRC dyspnoea scores of 3–5, who are functionally limited by breathlessness.

Influenza vaccination is associated with a 27% reduction in the risk of hospitalisation for pneumonia and a 48% reduction in the risk of death (Nichol, Nordin, et al. 2007). A systematic review of the potential benefits of the flu vaccination in people with COPD concluded that the risk/benefit profile was favourable and that people with COPD should be advised to have their annual flu jab (Bekkat-Berkani, Wilkinson, et al. 2017).

Although there is less evidence for pneumococcal polysaccharide vaccine, research has shown that it prevents pneumonia in patients aged 65 years and above and in young patients with a history of cardiac disease.

Acute exacerbations of COPD

Acute exacerbations of COPD drive progression, reduced health status and a decline in lung function. Acute exacerbations are defined as 'episodes of worsening respiratory symptoms beyond normal daily variations' and lead to change in medication (GOLD 2019).

Most acute exacerbations of COPD are caused by respiratory viral infections, especially the rhinovirus, the cause of the common cold (see Figure 12.2 below). Respiratory viruses can be detected in up to 60% of acute exacerbations of COPD. Bacteria are normally present in the lower airways in a stable state and are seldom the cause of acute exacerbation. Although viral triggers are considered a primary cause of exacerbation, viral triggers may lead to secondary bacterial load, which results in increased inflammation and worsens already chronically inflamed airways. This acute change results in bronchoconstriction, oedema and an increase in mucous production, with a resultant increase in dynamic hyperinflation and worsening dyspnoea. These are all characteristics of exacerbations in COPD. The NICE antimicrobial guidelines on acute exacerbations of COPD (AECOPD) suggest that careful consideration should be given before prescribing antibiotics for AECOPD (NICE 2018).

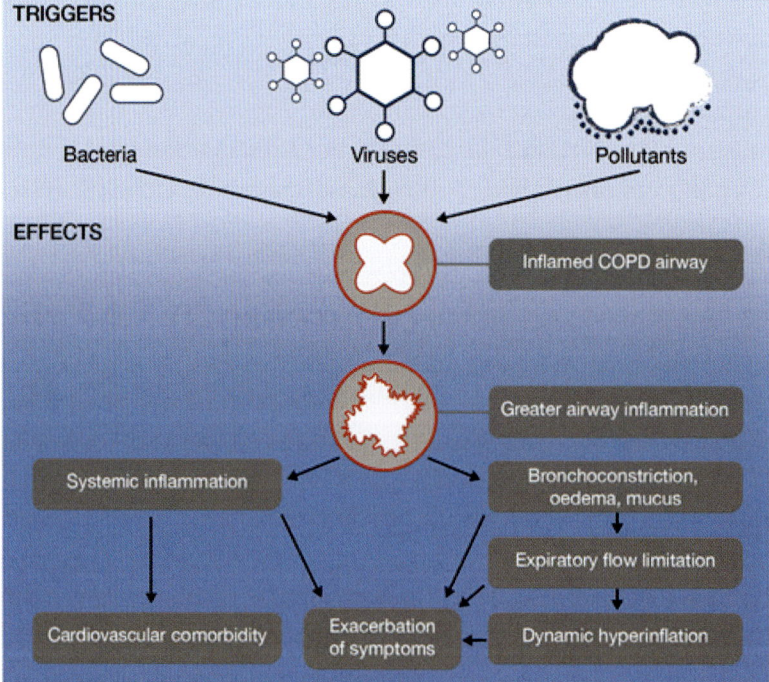

Figure 12.2: This diagram shows triggers of COPD exacerbations and their associated pathophysiological changes, which lead to increased symptoms (Wedzicha & Seemungal 2007). Reproduced with permission.

Management of acute exacerbations of COPD

The main goal of treating exacerbations of COPD is to minimise the impact of the current exacerbation and prevent development of further exacerbation. There are three classes of medication that are commonly used for exacerbations of COPD: antibiotics, corticosteroids and short-acting bronchodilators.

Antibiotics

As stated, COPD exacerbations can be either viral or due to bacteria. This is why some clinicians are cautious in their use of antibiotics. However, there is evidence to support the use of antibiotics in COPD exacerbations when patients have clinical signs of purulent sputum. Antibiotics may be given in the presence of three cardinal symptoms – increase in dyspnoea, sputum volume and sputum purulence. The recommended length of treatment is between 5 and 10 days (GOLD 2019).

Corticosteroids

The GOLD guidelines state that oral steroids can also be used to improve breathlessness, oxygen levels and lung function during exacerbations. The REDUCE study showed that a five-day course of 40mg prednisolone offered the best risk/benefit profile in terms of recovery time and earlier discharge from hospital if admitted (Leuppi, Schuetz, et al. 2013).

Although NICE previously recommended using 30mg prednisolone for upwards of 7 days, the 2019 update recommends 40mg for 7 days.

Short-acting bronchodilators

Regular short-acting bronchodilators can be used to supplement long-acting bronchodilators in acute exacerbations. Patients on long-acting beta 2 agonists (LABAs) and/or long-acting muscarinic antagonists (LAMAs) will benefit from additional short-acting beta 2 agonists (SABAs). However, short-acting muscarinic antagonists (SAMAs), should only be used in people who are not already on a LAMA.

GOLD recommends that SABAs should be used at a rate of 1 puff per hour for the first 2–3 hours then every 2–3 hours, whilst continuing to use any long-acting bronchodilators. It is important to note that hand-held devices such as pressurised metered dose inhalers (pMDIs) or dry powder inhalers (DPIs) will deliver the drugs just as effectively as (and more cost effectively than) a nebuliser, as long as the patient has adequate inspiratory flow for the device.

Case study: Breathlessness

Vicky Jeffrey is a 78-year-old woman who has recently complained of continuous breathlessness to her GP. Mrs Jeffrey has been referred by her GP for assessment and management of her continuous breathlessness. She has never smoked but previously worked in a pub and lived with a husband who was a heavy smoker and died of lung cancer. Mrs Jeffrey finds it increasingly difficult to do her daily domestic chores and can only manage 60 metres walking outdoors on a flat surface.

We know from the patient's history that she never smoked but lived with her husband who was a heavy smoker and used to work in a pub before smoking was banned in public places in the UK. From the literature, we know that COPD can occur as a result of passive smoking in non-smokers – the risk is highest with environmental tobacco exposure in multiple settings such as home and work (Hagstad, Bjerg, et al. 2014).

Past medical history revealed none of the following: asthma, heart failure, hypertension, atrial fibrillation, DVT, pulmonary embolus and no previous cardiac surgery. This information will help to rule out other causes of breathlessness.

Drug history: Atorvastatin 20mg at night, and paracetamol 500mg when needed.

The following investigations were carried out:
- Chest X-ray – showed bilateral hyperinflation
- Arterial blood gases – PH 7.37, PCO_2 4.8 kpa, PaO_2 11kpa, SaO_2 99%, HCO_3 23, BE -2
- Blood test – CRP 3mg/l, Na+ 138mmol/l, K+ 4.2mmol/l, Hb 12.5g/dL, BNP 30pg/ml, WCC 7 x 109/l, eosinophils 60 cells/μL, INR 0.9, Troponin 10
- Pulse oximetry – SpO_2 96% HR 85b/min regular
- Post-bronchodilator spirometry – result showed, FEV1/FVC ratio 45%, FEV1 40% predicted with a concave shape to the flow volume curve
- mMRC 2

Frequency of exacerbations: 2 in 12 months.

Activity 12.1 (Case study)
How would you treat Mrs Jeffrey?

Case study: COPD

A 78-year-old man, Mr David Allan, with a diagnosis of heart failure, COPD and a history of recurrent acute exacerbations with severe breathlessness has been admitted to hospital three times in the last two months, twice with acute exacerbations of COPD and once with a diagnosis of pneumonia and pulmonary oedema. In one of his admissions, Mr Allan's heart failure medication was titrated upwards to optimise his therapeutic management. He also had a follow-up chest X-ray for his pneumonia to make sure this had remained clear. However, four weeks after discharge he had another exacerbation and was treated by his GP with antibiotics and steroids and a referral back to the chest clinic due to his recurrent exacerbations. Mr Allan is currently taking a LABA via a dry powder inhaler. The GP also mentioned that Mr Allan's exacerbations were always associated with a high volume of purulent sputum and severe breathlessness, with or without wheezing.

Activity 12.2

How would you treat Mr Allan?

Case study: Smoking

Mr Andrew Clark, a 68-year-old man, has been referred by his GP, with recurrent episodes of wheezing and cough that have recently become persistent. Mr Clark is an ex-smoker with an extensive smoking history of 40 years. During the last GP visit, he was prescribed a course of antibiotics and a course of oral prednisolone for a severe productive cough with associated shortness of breath. A chest X-ray was requested but has yet to be reported. His GP reports that Mr Clark has a low BMI, severe shortness of breath when walking and oxygen saturation of 96% on air. His only regular inhaled therapy is Salbutamol 100mcg MDI with a spacer device. During a recent hospital visit, the team prescribed him Clenil® (Beclometasone) 100mcg MDI 2 puffs bd via spacer. This was switched to Fostair® (Beclometasone and Formoterol) by his GP due to his recurrent exacerbations. The GP referral records indicate that no formal respiratory diagnosis has been made.

Activity 12.3 (Case study)

What investigations and assessments are required to provide both a diagnosis and a differential diagnosis for Mr Clark? What should Mr Clark be prescribed?

Pharmacology case studies for nurse prescribers

> ### Activity 12.4 (Case study)
> Which types of smoking cessation therapy are available?

Summary

COPD is a major health and social care burden, especially in developed countries. Earlier diagnosis, vaccination, smoking cessation, pulmonary rehabilitation and optimal pharmacotherapy are required for the safe and effective management of this condition. It is important to undertake a detailed consultation that includes a history of the presenting complaint, a symptom profile and a description of lifestyle behaviours. The physical assessment must include spirometry and appropriate investigations to make a diagnosis and plan the right level of care. During assessment, care should be taken to rule out acute cardiac events and lung parenchyma damage as causes of breathlessness and worsening of the usual symptoms of COPD. A combination of mentoring, clinical experience and understanding of clinical guidelines helps to develop expertise in the practice of respiratory medicine and the management of COPD.

Answers to activities

Activity 12.1 (Case study)

How would you treat Mrs Jeffrey?

To be able to manage breathlessness, you need to find out its possible causes, as it may be due to many aetiological factors, ranging from airway narrowing due to hyper-responsiveness to noxious stimulus, airway blockage due to mucus plugging in the large airway, lung static hyperinflation exacerbated by exertional dynamic hyperinflation, fluid overload from heart failure, acute coronary syndrome, aortic stenosis, pulmonary embolus, haemo-pneumothorax, pleural effusion, pulmonary oedema, type I and type II respiratory failure, pneumonia and more. Most of these can be ruled out by history, blood tests, chest X-ray (CXR), clinical presentation and physical assessment.

Mrs Jeffrey's blood results are within the normal reference range, she has no chest pain and CXR showed no focal lesion except lung hyperinflation. Also, the patient does not have a past cardiac history and her international normalisation ratio (INR) is normal. Although Mrs Jeffrey does not have a smoking history, she has a smoke inhalation history, which suggests susceptibility to obstructive airways disease. She also has reduced exercise tolerance, which is a consequence of dynamic hyperinflation, which can be confirmed on CXR. The patient also has a spirometric result of FEVI/FVC ratio of 45% and FEVI 40% and mMRC 2. Respiratory medications are Beclometasone diprorionate 100mcg 2 puffs BD and Salbutamol 100mcg MDIs as required.

Pharmacological case studies: Chronic obstructive pulmonary disease (COPD)

The following diagnosis was made, based on the above assessment:
- CXR showed lung hyperinflation; this is usually due to poor alveoli elastic recoil as a consequence of COPD.
- Spirometry: FEV1/FVC ratio of 45% with usual concave flow-volume curve suggestive of obstructive airways disease and classification of severe, due to FEV1 40% predicted. Also to be considered is the history of smoking inhalation, the MRC 2 and the reduced exercise tolerance to 60m with 3–4 exacerbations a year.

The results above confirm Mrs Jeffrey's diagnosis of COPD, and indicate that her current therapy of salbutamol needs to be stepped up. Mrs Jeffrey fits into category D in the GOLD guidelines as she has an mMRC score of 2 and has had two exacerbations this year. As she has no history of asthma, she does not need an inhaled corticosteroid at this stage and is likely to benefit from a LAMA or a dual bronchodilator. NICE guidelines would recommend a dual bronchodilator. Mrs Jeffrey should be supported to choose the most appropriate inhaler device to deliver this treatment from the range of dual bronchodilators available. She should be reviewed to assess the impact of her new treatment on her symptoms and exercise tolerance.

To find out if Mrs Jeffrey is responding better to new medications, check the following:
- Repeat FEV1: it may be slightly improved but not significantly
- Improved exercise tolerance
- Improved breathlessness, measured with Borg scale, mMRC score and CAT score.

Activity 12.2 (Case study)

How would you treat Mr Allan?

It is important to find out if the series of exacerbations with severe breathlessness were true exacerbations of COPD or were, in fact, episodes of decompensated heart failure. You also need to establish that the patient has not had a silent myocardial infarction (MI). Evidence suggests that patients with frequent exacerbations of COPD are more at risk of cardiovascular disease, such as MI, than those with infrequent exacerbation. They may not show classic chest pain due to adaptation to chronic hypoxia. However, they may demonstrate severe breathlessness (Rothnie et al. 2014).

The following investigations were done after the physical assessment, to rule out other causes of breathlessness and to find other causes of recurrent exacerbation:
- Echocardiogram
- B-type natriuretic peptide (BNP)
- Chest X-ray (CXR)
- Computer tomography pulmonary and angiogram (CTPA)
- High resonant computer tomography (HRCT)
- Troponin and electrocardiography (ECG)
- Arterial blood gases (ABG).

The HRCT showed an area of small airways thickening, fibrosis and dilatation in the left mid lobe and both lower lobes. CXR had not changed from the previous, CTPA was normal, the patient also had normal troponin of 9mcg/L and ECG was normal. Mr Allan's BNP was also normal. However, his echocardiogram showed mild left ventricular systolic dysfunction impairment, which was in line with his previous echocardiogram. His ABG was normal, with no evidence of type I or type II respiratory failure.

Therefore, based on the above assessment, the patient was diagnosed with bronchiectasis that was probably caused by the pneumonia and recurrent exacerbation, resulting in airway damage due to chronic inflammation. It was also established, with the normal troponin and ECG, that the patient had not had an MI. There was no evidence of exacerbation of heart failure and pulmonary embolism, as BNP, echocardiogram and CTPA were normal.

The NICE antimicrobial guidance for bronchiectasis recommends that sputum samples are tested for microscopy, culture and sensitivity and that appropriate antibiotics are prescribed based on the results. Local guidelines will offer guidance which reflects local sensitivities and resistance but the guidance from NICE suggests using either amoxicillin 500mg tds for 7–14 days, or doxycycline 200mg on day one, followed by 100mg for 7–14 days or clarithromycin 500mg bd for 7–14 days (NICE 2018). Chest clearance is important in people with COPD and/or bronchiectasis. This can be achieved through the use of chest clearance devices (e.g. Aerobika® – see https://www.trudellmed.com/products/aerobika-opep-device) or through referral for chest physiotherapy.

Mr Allan must also undergo chest physiotherapy targeted at sputum clearance to avoid further infection. If the patient's sputum is too thick and difficult to clear from airways, then the use of a mucolytic agent (usually Carbocisteine 2.25g daily in divided doses or nebulised 0.9% sodium chloride 2.5ml) may be considered to reduce sputum viscosity.

The diagnosis of bronchiectasis in addition to his COPD should not prevent the patient from taking his regular inhalers, as chronic inflammation seen in COPD is part of the pathogenesis of bronchiectasis and inhalers are known to be effective. It is also important that the patient keeps a rescue pack of antibiotics at home to use, upon advice, at the start of a further acute exacerbation. His COPD is currently being treated with a LABA, but LAMAs are known to improve sputum-related symptoms, including exacerbations. Therefore, his inhaled therapy should be stepped up to a dual bronchodilator to optimise symptom control, improve exercise tolerance and reduce exacerbation risk.

Activity 12.3 (Case study)

What investigations and assessments are required to provide both a diagnosis and a differential diagnosis for Mr Clark? What should Mr Clark be prescribed?

Appropriate investigations and assessments required are:

1 Post-bronchodilator spirometry assessment
2 CXR and HRCT scan to rule out pneumonia, atelectasis and bronchiectasis
3 Blood test to rule out high CRP, WCC and troponin
4 Sputum test for colour and volume and MC&S to determine need for antibiotic therapy
5 Malnutrition University Screening Tool (MUST) score to determine need for dietetic input due to low BMI
6 Echocardiography to rule out heart failure
7 CURB 65 score (confusion, blood urea nitrogen, respiratory rate, systolic BP or diastolic BP, age = 65).

Results:

Post-bronchodilator spirometry result showed:

1 FEV1 1.23l (37% predicted), FVC 2.45l (58% predicted), FEV1/FVC ratio 50%
2 CXR showed hyperinflation of lung fields, shadowing in both middle lobes, and no area of atelectasis; CT scan showed severe emphysematous change of both middle and lower lobes; no bronchial thickening and fibrotic changes seen
3 Blood results: WCC 11.5 × 10^9/l, CRP 45mg/L, Hb 15g/dL, Na+ 138mmol/l, K+ 4.0 mmol/l
4 Sputum result revealed: *Haemophilus influenzae* sensitive to penicillin and tetracycline, no atypical bacteria
5 MUST score >2
6 Echocardiogram – normal LV function and ejection fraction of 59%
7 CURB 65 was 1, based on the data above.

Based on the post-bronchodilator spirometry result, CXR and CT scan, Mr Clark's diagnosis of severe COPD is conclusive. The CXR showed shadowing, which may be evidence of community-acquired pneumonia (CAP) and this can be confirmed by high WCC, CRP and the sputum culture result of *H. influenzae*, which is one of the usual bacteria strains of community-acquired pneumonia. As mentioned in the history, the patient has had recurrent exacerbations, recurrent wheezing, and productive cough; these could be due to the untreated pneumonia and lack of appropriate inhalers as per NICE (2019b) and GOLD (2019) guidelines.

Regarding treatment, the initial priority is to treat the pneumonia. Mr Clark may be able to receive treatment at home, as his CURB 65 score is 1. A CURB 65 score of 2 and above will require hospital admission for therapy.

According to the NICE (2019c) guidance on CAP, which was updated in 2019, the recommended treatment would be amoxicillin 500mg tds for 5 days. If the patient cannot take amoxicillin, the recommendation would be to use doxycycline 200mg on day one, followed by 4 more daily doses of 100mg (a 5-day course in total). A 5-day course of clarithromycin may also be considered (NICE 2019c). Further assessment and management should be carried out in line with NICE and local guidelines.

With respect to Mr Clark's COPD, there needs to be very careful consideration as to the advantages and disadvantages of different therapies. ICS monotherapy (i.e. without a LABA) is not licensed in COPD. However, the switch to an ICS/LABA seems to have been made without a clear rationale. A LAMA/LABA may offer key benefits in terms of symptom control and reducing the risk of future exacerbations, and a switch from his ICS/LABA to a dual bronchodilator may be a better option. However, stepping up to triple therapy (ICS/LABA/LAMA) may offer further advantages.

NICE currently states that in people with COPD who are taking an ICS/LABA, triple therapy should be offered if their day-to-day symptoms continue to adversely impact their quality of life or they have a severe exacerbation (requiring hospitalisation) or they have two or more moderate exacerbations within a year.

Furthermore, NICE says that for people with COPD who are taking a dual bronchodilator, triple therapy should be considered if:
- They have a severe exacerbation (requiring hospitalisation), or
- They have two or more moderate exacerbations within a year.

Nonetheless, the use of ICS in COPD may also increase the risk of pneumonia and, as Mr Clark has already had a confirmed diagnosis of CAP, careful consideration should be given before prescribing triple therapy.

Activity 12.4 (Case study)

Which types of smoking cessation therapy are available?

Smoking cessation interventions should be tailored to the individual, after careful discussion about the advantages and disadvantages of the different approaches: Varenicline, Nicotine Replacement Therapy, Bupropion and e-cigarettes (vaping).

Varenicline is a prescription-only medication licensed for smokers age 18+ alongside behavioural support. The most common side effects are nausea and sleep disturbance.

Nicotine replacement therapy, using patches and/or other delivery methods to replace nicotine from cigarettes, helps to reduce cravings and withdrawal symptoms.

Bupropion (Zyban®) is less commonly used than the previous two methods but can be effective for suitable smokers.

Views on vaping differ from person to person, and this includes healthcare workers. Public Health England takes the position that vaping is much safer than smoking, although the issue is not without controversy. The NHS website has a useful page on vaping, updated in 2019, which can be accessed here: https://www.nhs.uk/live-well/quit-smoking/using-e-cigarettes-to-stop-smoking/ For free further training in smoking cessation, go to https://www.ncsct.co.uk/ (NCST 2020).

References and further reading

Association of Respiratory Nurse Specialists (2020). https://arns.co.uk/ (Last accessed 15 October 2020).

Bekkat-Berkani, R., Wilkinson, T., Buchy, P., Dos Santos, G., Stefanidis, D., Devaster, J.M. & Meyer, N. (2017). Seasonal influenza vaccination in patients with COPD: a systematic literature review. *BMC Pulmonary Medicine.* **17** (1), 79. doi:10.1186/s12890-017-0420-8

British Lung Foundation (2020). https://www.blf.org.uk/ (Last accessed 15 October 2020).

Bustamante-Marin, X.M. & Ostrowski, L.E. (2017). Cilia and mucociliary clearance. *Cold Spring Harbor Perspectives in Biology.* **9** (4), a028241. doi:10.1101/cshperspect.a028241

Ejiofor, S. & Turner, A.M. (2013). Pharmacotherapies for COPD. Clinical medicine insights. *Circulatory, Respiratory and Pulmonary Medicine.* **7**, 17–34. doi:10.4137/CCRPM.S7211

Global Initiative for Obstructive Lung Disease (GOLD) (2019). *Global Strategy for the Diagnosis, Management and Prevention of Chronic Obstructive Pulmonary Disease 2020 report.* https://goldcopd.org/wp-content/uploads/2019/11/GOLD-2020-REPORT-ver1.0wms.pdf (Last accessed 15 October 2020).

GOV.UK (2020). https://www.gov.uk/government/publications/pneumococcal-the-green-book-chapter-25 (Last accessed 15 October 2020).

Hagstad, S., Bjerg, A., Ekerljung, L., Backman, H., Lindberg, A., Rönmark, E. & Lundbäck, B. (2014). Passive smoking exposure is associated with increased risk of COPD in never smokers. *Chest.* **145**, 1298–304.

Health and Safety Executive (HSE) (2019). *Work-related Chronic Obstructive Pulmonary Disease (COPD) statistics in Great Britain, 2019.* http://www.hse.gov.uk/statistics/causdis/copd.pdf (Last accessed 15 October 2020).

Jiménez-Ruiz, C.A., Andreas, S., Lewis, K.E., Tonnesen, P., van Schayck, C.P., Hajek, P., Tonstad, S., Dautzenberg, B., Fletcher, M., Masefield, S., Powell, P., Hering, T., Nardini, S., Tonia, T. and Gratziou, C. (2015). Statement on smoking cessation in COPD and other pulmonary diseases and in smokers with comorbidities who find it difficult to quit. *European Respiratory Journal.* **46**, 61–79. DOI: 10.1183/09031936.00092614

Leuppi, J.D., Schuetz, P., Bingisser, R., Bodmer, M., Briel, M., Drescher, T., Duerring, U., Henzen, C., Leibbrandt, Y., Maier, S., Miedinger, D., Müller, B., Scherr, A., Schindler, C., Stoeckli, R., Viatte, S., von Garnier, C., Tamm, M. & Rutishauser, J. (2013). Short-term vs Conventional Glucocorticoid Therapy in Acute Exacerbations of Chronic Obstructive Pulmonary Disease: The REDUCE Randomized Clinical Trial. *The Journal of the American Medical Association.* **309** (21), 2223–231. DOI: 10.1001/jama.2013.5023

McCarthy, B., Casey, D., Devane, D., Murphy, K., Murphy, E. & Lacasse, Y. (2015). Pulmonary rehabilitation for chronic obstructive pulmonary disease. Cochrane Systematic Review. https://doi.org/10.1002/14651858.CD003793.pub3 (Last accessed 15 October 2020).

National Centre for Smoking Cessation and Training (NCST) (2020). https://www.ncsct.co.uk/ (Last accessed 15 October 2020).

National Institute for Health and Care Excellence (NICE) (2018). Bronchiectasis (non-cystic fibrosis), acute exacerbation: antimicrobial prescribing. https://www.nice.org.uk/guidance/ng117/chapter/Recommendations#treatment (Last accessed 15 October 2020).

National Institute for Health and Care Excellence (NICE) (2019a). Chronic obstructive pulmonary disease (acute exacerbation): antimicrobial prescribing. https://www.nice.org.uk/guidance/ng114 (Last accessed 15 October 2020).

National Institute for Health and Care Excellence (NICE) (2019b). Chronic obstructive pulmonary disease in over 16s: diagnosis and management. https://www.nice.org.uk/guidance/ng115 (Last accessed 15 October 2020).

National Institute for Health and Care Excellence (NICE) (2019c). Pneumonia in adults: diagnosis and management. https://www.nice.org.uk/guidance/cg191 (Last accessed 15 October 2020).

NHS UK (2020). https://www.nhs.uk/live-well/quit-smoking/using-e-cigarettes-to-stop-smoking/ (Last accessed 15 October 2020).

Nichol, K.L., Nordin, J.D., Nelson, D.B., Mullooly, J.P. & Hak, E. (2007). Effectiveness of influenza vaccine in the community dwelling elderly. *New England Journal of Medicine.* **357** (14), 1373–1381.

Primary Care Respiratory Society (2020). https://www.pcrs-uk.org (Last accessed 15 October 2020).

Right Breathe (2020). https://www.rightbreathe.com (Last accessed 15 October 2020).

Rothnie, K.J., Smeeth, L., Herrett, E., Pearce, N., Hemingway, H., Timmis, A. & Quint, J.K. (2014). Explaining the mortality gap in COPD patients after myocardial infarction: Data from the UK Myocardial Ischaemia National Audit Project (MINAP). *Thorax.* **69** (2), A57–58.

Tashkin, D.P., Celli, B., Senn, S., Burkhart, D., Kesten, S., Menjoge, S., Decramer, M., for the UPLIFT Study Investigators (2008). A 4-Year trial of tiotropium in Chronic Obstructive Pulmonary Disease. *New England Journal of Medicine.* **359**, 1543–1554

Vogelmeier, C., Hedere, B., Glaab, T., Schmidt, H., Rutten-van Molken, M., Beeh, K.M., Rabe, K.F., Fabbri, L.M., for the POET-COPD Investigators (2011). Tiotropium versus salmeterol for the prevention of exacerbations of COPD. *New England Journal of Medicine.* **364**, 1993–1103

Walters, J.A., Tang, J.N., Poole, P. & Wood-Baker, R. (2017). Pneumococcal vaccines for preventing pneumonia in chronic obstructive pulmonary disease. Cochrane Database Systematic Review.1:CD001390.

Wedzicha, J.A. & Seemungal, T.A. (2007). COPD exacerbations: defining their cause and prevention. *Lancet.* **370**, 786–96.

Wedzicha, J.A., Decramer, M., Ficker, J.H., Niewoehner, D.E. & Taylor, A.F. (2013). Analysis of COPD exacerbations with dual bronchodilator QVA149 compared with glycopyrronium and tiotropium (SPARK): a randomised double-blind parallel group study. *Lancet Respiratory Medicine.* **2013** (1), 199–209.

Wedzicha, J.A., D'Urzo, A.D., Mezzi, K., Chen, H., Banerji, D. & Fogel, R. (2014). QVA149 showed significant improvements in lung function and health status and was well tolerated versus glycopyrronium and tiotropium in patients with severe COPD: The SPARK study (2014). *European Respiratory Journal.* **44** (58), 1893.

13

Pharmacological case studies: Neurological problems

Anne Preece
MSc, BSc (Hons) Nursing Studies, BSc (Hons) Clinical Nursing Studies with RN, RM ENB 148 and Specialist Practitioner Award, ENB 100,
Head Injury Clinical Nurse Specialist, University Hospitals Birmingham NHS Foundation Trust

Julie Moody
MSc, BSc (Hons), RN, DMS, PGCHE, FAETC/D32/D33,
Registered Practice Educator Lecturer, Health and Education, Middlesex University, London

This chapter:
- Gives an overview of specified neurological conditions
- Shows how to apply drug knowledge to clinical case studies
- Considers prescribing principles.

Introduction

This chapter focuses on the formulation and provision of optimum drug therapy for clients with neurological problems, and particularly on a case study involving a young client with temporal lobe epilepsy (TLE), and an elderly client with Parkinson's disease.

Epilepsy

Epilepsy is a common neurological disorder characterised by recurring seizures, and different types of epilepsy have different causes. Accurate estimates of incidence and prevalence are hard to achieve, due to difficulty in identifying all those who may have the condition. According to NICE (2019), epilepsy has been estimated to affect between 362,000 and 415,000 people in England. In addition, there are further individuals (5–30%) who have been diagnosed with epilepsy but in whom the diagnosis is incorrect. Incidence is estimated to be 50 per 100,000 per year, and the prevalence of active epilepsy in the UK is estimated to be 5–10 cases per 1000. Two-thirds of people with active epilepsy have their epilepsy controlled satisfactorily with anti-epileptic drugs (AEDs); others by surgery. Optimal management improves health outcomes and can also help to minimise other negative effects – on social, educational and employment activity.

An epileptic seizure occurs when there is a neurological dysfunction that causes abnormal neuronal activity and firing. There may be changes in motor function and control, behaviour and autonomic functions, as well as sensory changes. Faulty electrical activity that fires within the brain cells suggests an overall alteration in neurological functioning that allows seizures to occur or re-occur.

This dysfunction results from a disturbance in biochemical cellular processes, promoting hyper-excitability and hyper-synchrony, and it should be noted that a single neuron firing abnormally within a larger network of neurons can cause a seizure. Several subcortical structures and cortical structures are involved, and ion channels are specifically involved in neuronal excitation.

Temporal lobe epilepsy

In TLE, the seizure activity arises in the temporal lobe and the condition may begin with an early injury to the left or right hippocampus, causing neuron death. Such an injury may be the result of a much earlier and long forgotten childhood accident involving a bump on the head. In TLE, there may be a significant variation in quality and/or intensity of the seizure and it may be so mild as to go unnoticed; experiences vary significantly. There may be feelings of fear, pleasure or unreality or an odd smell, an abdominal sensation that rises up through the chest into the throat, an old memory or familiar feeling, or a feeling that is impossible to describe.

Epilepsy is not a single disease but a collection of heterogeneous terms, all of which are expressions of differing pathophysiology. For example, focal or partial seizures may arise locally but become diffuse, involving pathways through the whole cortex. There may, or may not, be full loss of consciousness with a variety of functional losses.

The most common seizure type in TLE is a complex partial seizure. During complex partial seizures, people with TLE tend to perform repetitive, automatic movements (called automatisms), such as lip smacking and rubbing hands together. Three-quarters of people with TLE also have simple partial seizures, and about half have tonic-clonic seizures at some time. It is worth noting that some people with TLE experience only simple partial seizures. Table 13.1 summarises the first- and second-line drug therapy suited to different types of seizure.

Table 13.1: Types of seizure and appropriate anti-epileptic drugs (AEDs)

Seizures	First-line drugs	Second line-drugs
Focal seizure, with or without secondary generalisation	Carbamazepine, lamotrigine, oxycarbazepine, sodium valproate	Clobazam, gabapentin, levetiracetam, pregabalin
Generalised seizures		
Tonic-clonic seizures	Carbamazepine, lamotrigine, sodium valproate	Clobazam, levetiracetam, oxycarbazepine, topiramate
Absence seizures	Ethosuximide, sodium valproate	Clonazepam, lamotrigine
Myoclonic seizures	Sodium valproate	Levetiracetam, clonazepam

Case study: Seizure

Sally is a 21-year-old girl who came to see you after a suspected epileptic seizure that morning, as she was trying to wake up. According to her father, Sally has had other seizures over the last two years, all of which have been related to her sleep pattern. She has never previously been medicated, due to the spasmodic nature of the seizures and her difficulty in getting a witness account. After a consultation, Sally was referred for an electroencephalogram (EEG) with sedation. During the appointment, she had another seizure, which was witnessed. Sally was noted to have a hemiparesis post-seizure, with a drooping eyelid and drooping mouth, and was also incontinent of urine. Sally was admitted and an EEG confirmed a diagnosis of temporal lobe epilepsy with generalised tonic-clonic seizures (complex). She was sent for an urgent scan, which showed an area of scar tissue in her left temporal lobe, believed to be the result of a childhood accident. There are no signs of tumour, no fever and all biochemistry is normal. After one hour, the hemiparesis resolved. Sally's boyfriend was very worried that she might have a brain tumour or could have suffered a stroke but Sally's medics confirmed that they felt this was a residual Todd's Palsy, which had corrected after full seizure recovery.

Activity 13.1 (Case study)

Reflecting on your knowledge of seizure warning signs, define Todd's Palsy.

Prescribing principles and commonly used drugs

During a seizure, excitation predominates over inhibition. Effective seizure treatment generally augments inhibitory processes or opposes excitatory processes. At the ionic level, inhibition is typically mediated by inward chloride or outward potassium currents, and excitation by inward sodium or calcium currents. Drugs can directly affect specific ion channels or indirectly influence synthesis, metabolism or function of neurotransmitters or receptors that control channel opening and closing. The most important central nervous system inhibitory neurotransmitter is gamma amino butyric acid (GABA). The most important excitatory neurotransmitter is glutamate, acting through several receptor subtypes.

Table 13.2: Common AEDs in use

Name	Action	**Contraindications** – no AEDs should be abruptly withdrawn
Sodium valproate	• Blockage of voltage-gated sodium channels and increases the levels of gamma-aminobutyric acid (GABA) – mechanism not completely understood	• Not for use in girls, women and pregnant women • Family history of severe hepatic disease, acute porphyria; avoid with hepatic impairment • Caution with renal impairment.
Lamotrigine	• Enhances the release of inhibitory GABA that attenuates neuronal electrical activity associated with paroxysms	• Caution in liver and renal impairment and pregnancy
Carbamazepine	• Sodium channel blocker that binds preferentially to voltage-gated sodium channels in their inactive conformation which prevents repetitive and sustained firing of an action potential	• AV conduction abnormalities – unless paced, bone marrow depression, acute porphyria • Caution in liver or renal impairment • Monitor plasma-carbamazepine concentration in pregnancy
Gabapentin	• Thought to inhibit the alpha 2-delta subunit of voltage-gated calcium channels – exact mechanism unclear	• Caution in renal impairment and pregnancy
Levetiracetam	• Modulation of synaptic neurotransmitter release through binding to the synaptic vesicle protein in SV2A in the brain	• Caution in liver and renal impairment and pregnancy

Topiramate	• Blocks voltage-dependent sodium and calcium channels • Also inhibits the excitatory glutamate pathways while enhancing the inhibitory effect of GABA • It also inhibits carbonic anhydrase activity	• Caution in liver and renal impairment and pregnancy
Phenytoin	• Voltage-dependent blockage of voltage-gated sodium channels; this prevents sustained high frequency repetitive firing of action potentials	• Caution in liver and renal impairment and pregnancy

Newer and more expensive AEDs are now being prescribed. Table 13.2 presents the most commonly prescribed AEDs, the drugs' mode of action and contraindications. With treatment costs likely to increase in coming years, it is essential to ensure that those AEDs with proven clinical efficacy and cost-effectiveness are identified. However, a large multicentre trial evaluating newer drugs in newly diagnosed epilepsy suggested that sodium valproate should be the drug of choice in generalised and unclassifiable epilepsies and lamotrigine in focal epilepsies. Because of these findings, it was therefore considered necessary to review the evidence regarding AEDs (NICE 2019).

Quite naturally, as newer drugs have been developed, patients' expectations have been raised. Safety is crucial, as are tolerance and lack of interactions, but crucially the efficacy of a newer AED is paramount. From this point of view, three questions are of particular clinical interest:

- How effective are new AEDs when corrected for the efficacy of placebo?
- Moreover, are new AEDs leading to seizure remission more often, compared with established agents?
- Finally, can more patients maintain seizure remission after withdrawal of new AEDs, compared with withdrawal of older agents?

The Sanad Trial (Marson, Appleton, et al. 2007) is of particular interest when looking at these questions in depth. It is noticeable that the newer drugs show comparable efficacy to the older drugs but no comparable benefit in terms of seizure remission. The Sanad II trial (2019) takes this a step further, looking at the efficacy and cost-effectiveness of the newer AEDs, as well as the quality of life of newly diagnosed patients.

Most NHS prescriptions for medicines are written using the generic drug name, and nurse prescribers will be familiar with this criterion. However, generic prescribing in epilepsy is controversial, with many specialists believing that changing the brand or specific formulation or preparation of an anti-epileptic drug means risking reduced seizure control or increased unwanted effects. Switching of anti-epileptic drugs has been identified by the MHRA as a potential harm caused to previously stabilised patients. If a patient requires a specific brand of a medication, the prescriber should either prescribe by a specific brand or write the generic name of the drug followed by the manufacturer. The dispensing pharmacist will need to be made aware so they can ensure continuity of supply. Any adverse reaction, as a consequence of switching brands, should be reported using the Yellow Card (BNF, no. 80).

In recent years, there has been a dramatic shift in drug use, with much newer drugs coming into play that claim to have fewer side effects and better results. NICE (2019) was therefore required to update its recommendations about the use of drugs to treat children, young people and adults with epilepsy.

In April 2018, important advice on the use of sodium valproate was included. This drug must not be used in girls (including those below the age of puberty), women or pregnant women, unless alternative treatments are unsuitable. Sodium valproate is also licensed to treat bipolar disorders and migraine (NICE 2019).

Activity 13.2 (Case study)

What factors would you need to consider before starting anti-epileptic treatment for Sally? How would you select a drug?

If possible, a patient should be treated with just one anti-epileptic drug, as recommended by NICE. If several drugs have been tried as monotherapy with little success, then adjunctive or combination therapy can be tried. The decision as to what drug or drugs a person takes will depend on the drug's unwanted effects as well as on its efficacy. However, such trial and error will always necessitate the intervention of the multi-disciplinary team who will need to take special care when changing from one drug to another.

All medicines have side effects so the choice should be based on the best evidence, but prescribers will also need to consider convenience of use, cost and patient preference.

Activity 13.3

AEDs can be defined as narrow-spectrum or broad-spectrum, depending on whether they are effective for treating focal onset seizures (narrow-spectrum) or both focal and generalised onset seizures (broad-spectrum).

- Give three examples of narrow-spectrum AEDs and three examples of broad-spectrum AEDs.

Nurse prescribers will understand the importance of having current information on the efficacy, adverse effects and potential interactions for any drugs they prescribe. The most common adverse effects observed with AEDs are noted in the drug's monograph. Dizziness, diplopia, blurred vision, ataxia, nausea and vomiting are associated with dose escalations, especially in patients taking carbamazepine. However, most acute side effects are reversible. AEDs have numerous side effects and some rare or very rare side effects. The nurse prescriber should fully explore the potential side effects with the patient prior to making any prescribing decisions. Interactions, caused by hepatic enzyme induction or inhibition, can be unpredictable and prescribers must diligently refer to the appropriate section in the BNF.

The incidence of rash occurs at a higher rate in patients who are concomitantly taking valproic acid. If the dose is started low and escalated slowly, the risk of rash is minimised. Patients should be instructed to watch out for a red raised rash, especially on the trunk of the body, as well as any mucosal involvement around the eyes, nose or mouth. If rash occurs, instruct the patient to contact their physician immediately for evaluation.

Activity 13.4

Based on the guidelines, how would you advise patients who asked:

1. Is it best to take this AED with food?
2. What should I do if I miss a dose of an AED?
3. How can I remember to take my medicine?

AEDs can have a narrow range within which seizures are controlled without toxicity. This concept is quantified as the therapeutic index (TI). The therapeutic range of AED serum concentrations is an attempt to translate the experimental concept of therapeutic index to the clinic. These ranges are broad generalisations, which are of limited use, and should be applied with care to individual patients. Many patients tolerate and need serum concentrations above the usual therapeutic range, while others achieve complete seizure control, or even experience adverse effects, at concentrations below it. The nurse prescriber should be mindful of the need for individualised assessment and medication review as AED dosage and side-effects can be highly idiosyncratic. Careful monitoring of plasma levels (as directed by the BNF), combined with patient need and preference and therapeutic control, will support safe prescribing.

Pharmacokinetics

Following absorption into the bloodstream, the drug is distributed throughout the body. Lipid solubility and protein binding affect the availability and distribution of the drug. Drugs can displace other drugs from albumin, and protein binding is responsible for many pharmacokinetic interactions between AEDs. An example of this is the interaction between phenytoin and valproic acid. If valproic acid is taken with phenytoin, the phenytoin is displaced from albumin-binding sites, thus resulting in more of the free drug being available and, in theory, more risk of toxicity. However, in practice, more of the free phenytoin becomes available for metabolism. While steady state levels may change, this possible interaction is therefore not necessarily clinically significant.

Most AEDs are metabolised in the liver by hydroxylation or conjugation. These metabolites are then excreted by the kidney. Some metabolites, such as the carbamazepine epoxide, are themselves active. Gabapentin undergoes no metabolism and is excreted unchanged by the kidney.

The half-life of a drug is defined as the time required for the serum concentration to decrease by 50%. The half-life determines the dosing frequency required for a drug to be maintained at a steady state in the serum. Most drugs are eliminated by the kidneys, and dosage adjustments are required in cases of renal impairment. In relation to this, nurse prescribers should refer to the instructions in the BNF/BNFc for prescribing for the elderly and for children.

Pharmacodynamic effects include both wanted and unwanted drug effects on the brain and other organs. Gabapentin, for example, has no important pharmacokinetic interactions with other AEDs. Because gabapentin and many other drugs can cause sedation and dizziness, pharmacodynamic interactions can occur. Ideally, AEDs used as combination therapy should produce an additive therapeutic effect and a sub-additive toxicity. Drug combinations with different mechanisms of action may help achieve this goal.

Case study: Seizure (continued)

Sally has suffered her first fully witnessed episode and is diagnosed with temporal lobe epilepsy, with generalised seizures and accompanying Todd's Palsy. Consider starting her on carbamazepine 200mg twice daily. Reassess accordingly and review blood tests for liver and kidney function after three months, then every six months if stable. Steady state may be reached in 1–2 weeks. However, carbamazepine is a liver enzyme auto-inducer and can therefore decrease the serum concentrations and thus the drug's therapeutic efficacy. The dosage may need to be reviewed and increased accordingly. With consideration for the therapeutic index, the patient should be advised on the signs of toxicity and the importance of regular dosages, as well as related health education such as DVLA requirements.

Parkinson's disease

In idiopathic Parkinson's disease (PD), the progressive degeneration of pigmented neurons in the substantia nigra leads to a deficiency of the neurotransmitter dopamine. The resulting neurochemical imbalance in the basal ganglia causes the characteristic signs and symptoms of the illness.

PD is evident, with cognitive and limb deficits which are both motor and non-motor and include bradykinesia, rigidity, loss of postural reflexes and tremor. It is hallmarked by dopamine deficiency, and the resulting symptoms appear most likely to be due to oscillating neuronal activity within the basal ganglia.

Case study: Parkinson's disease

John is a 68-year-old male factory worker who was referred to an outpatient clinic due to a nine-month resting tremor of his right hand, which later progressed to the contralateral leg. He has recently had a fall. Following neurological examination, he was found to have normal cognition. Myerson's sign was present. Oculomotor examination was normal. An intermittent mild resting tremor was observed in the hand, as well as mild signs of asymmetrical rigidity and bradykinesia (left > right). Gait and balance were normal, as were postural reflexes. The diagnosis of idiopathic Parkinson's disease was made. This case study looks at initiation of treatment and choices therein.

Activity 13.5 (Case study)

What is Myerson's sign?

Prescribing principles and pharmacokinetics

Drug therapy for Parkinson's disease ought to improve quality of life but cannot prevent disease progression and is not usually started until the disease becomes disabling. Dopamine agonists, levodopa or monoamine-oxidase-B (MAO-B) inhibitors can be used in the early stages. As PD progresses, more than one drug may be indicated, especially when patients develop motor complications and then require levodopa to be added into the regime. Using dopamine agonists on their own usually results in fewer motor complications but carries more risk of psychiatric upset.

The management aim is to limit degeneration, and early therapeutic intervention is vital. However, a PD diagnosis is mandatory before treatment is begun, and it is not always possible or feasible to identify pre-symptomatic PD. Sadly, the patient is unlikely to be diagnosed until they develop actual disablement, although a reported tremor which causes significant social difficulty can sometimes prompt treatment. It is also difficult to intervene early, as it may be unclear which drug will slow the progression (if any indeed do so).

Dopamine-receptor agonists

Dopamine-receptor agonists work by acting on dopamine receptors, and first treatment is often with pramipexole, ropinirole or rotigotine. The ergot-derived dopamine-receptor agonists, bromocriptine, cabergoline and pergolide, are rarely used, due to risk of fibrotic reactions.

Dopamine-receptor agonists are also used with levodopa in more advanced disease. If a dopamine-receptor agonist is added to levodopa therapy, the dose of levodopa needs to be reduced. Levodopa, the amino-acid precursor of dopamine, acts by replenishing depleted striatal dopamine. Levodopa is able to cross the blood–brain barrier and exert a therapeutic effect, while dopamine cannot. Levodopa is given with an extra-cerebral dopa-decarboxylase inhibitor, which reduces the peripheral conversion of levodopa to dopamine, thereby limiting side effects such as nausea, vomiting and cardiovascular effects. Additionally, effective brain-dopamine concentrations are achieved with lower doses of levodopa. The extra-cerebral dopa-decarboxylase inhibitors used with levodopa are benserazide (in co-beneldopa) and carbidopa (in co-careldopa).

Many patients will tolerate levodopa extremely well and it is therefore used in more severe cases. Levodopa is started gradually and then slowly increased until the lowest therapeutic dose is attained (this varies from one patient to another). When introducing levodopa therapy, nausea and vomiting may be a problem, in which case domperidone can be added.

Levodopa treatment is associated with potentially troublesome motor complications, including response fluctuations and dyskinesias. Response fluctuations are characterised by large variations in motor performance, with normal function during the 'on' period, and weakness and restricted mobility during the 'off' period. 'End-of-dose' deterioration, with progressively shorter duration of benefit, also occurs. However, one cannot overlook the fact that levodopa may greatly improve the quality of life of those with the disease, enabling improved and significant function. Modified-release preparations may help with 'end-of-dose' deterioration or nocturnal immobility and rigidity.

Levodopa is converted in the body to dopamine, and comes in tablet or capsule form. However, long-term use may cause a decline in efficacy, along with an increase in dyskinesia. Once in the body, levodopa is metabolised by enzymes reducing the amount of active medication. There are two main enzymes involved in the breakdown of levodopa: peripheral dopa-decarboxylase (DDC) and catechol-O-methyltransferase (COMT). Inhibiting these enzymes can prevent levodopa's breakdown, optimising its availability in the brain and improving symptom control.

It cannot be stressed highly enough that the prescriber should be aware of the importance of prescribing this drug so that it is tailored to the individual patient's requirements.

Table 13.3: Drugs commonly used to treat PD

Dopamine-receptor agonists	- The dopamine-receptor agonists have a direct action on dopamine receptors. Initial treatment of Parkinson's disease is often with the dopamine-receptor agonists, pramipexole, ropinirole and rotigotine. The ergot-derived dopamine-receptor agonists, bromocriptine, cabergoline and pergolide, are rarely used because of the risk of fibrotic reactions. - When used alone, dopamine-receptor agonists cause fewer motor complications in long-term treatment (compared with levodopa treatment) but the overall motor performance improves slightly less. The dopamine-receptor agonists are associated with more psychiatric side effects than levodopa. - Dopamine-receptor agonists are also used with levodopa in more advanced disease. If a dopamine-receptor agonist is added to levodopa therapy, the dose of levodopa needs to be reduced.
Apomorphine hydrochloride	- Apomorphine hydrochloride is licensed for use during 'off' episodes when inadequately controlled by co-beneldopa or co-careldopa or other dopaminergics. - Patients must be deemed capable and motivated to administer the subcutaneous drug as required.
Levodopa	- Levodopa, the amino-acid precursor of dopamine, acts by replenishing depleted striatal dopamine. It is given with an extra-cerebral dopa-decarboxylase inhibitor, which reduces the peripheral conversion of levodopa to dopamine, thereby limiting side effects such as nausea, vomiting and cardiovascular effects; additionally, effective brain-dopamine concentrations are achieved with lower doses of levodopa. - The extra-cerebral dopa-decarboxylase inhibitors used with levodopa are benserazide (in co-beneldopa) and carbidopa (in co-careldopa).
Monoamine-oxidase-B inhibitors	- Rasagiline, a monoamine-oxidase-B inhibitor, is licensed for the management of Parkinson's disease used alone or as an adjunct to levodopa for 'end-of-dose' fluctuations. - Selegiline is a monoamine-oxidase-B inhibitor used in conjunction with levodopa to reduce 'end-of-dose' deterioration in advanced Parkinson's disease. Early treatment with selegiline alone can delay the need for levodopa therapy. When combined with levodopa, selegiline should be avoided or used with great caution in postural hypotension.

(table continued overleaf)

Table 13.3 continued

Catechol-O-methyltransferase inhibitors	• Entacapone and tolcapone prevent the peripheral breakdown of levodopa, by inhibiting catechol-O-methyltransferase, allowing more levodopa to reach the brain. They are licensed for use as an adjunct to co-beneldopa or co-careldopa for patients with Parkinson's disease who experience 'end-of-dose' deterioration and cannot be stabilised on these combinations. • Due to the risk of hepatotoxicity, tolcapone should be prescribed under specialist supervision only, when other catechol-O-methyltransferase inhibitors combined with co-beneldopa or co-careldopa are ineffective.
Amantadine	• Amantadine is a weak dopamine agonist with modest anti-parkinsonian effects. Tolerance to its effects may develop, and confusion and hallucinations may occasionally occur.

Source: BNF (2020)

Activity 13.6 (Case study)

1. Which treatment options should be initiated for John (see p. 247)?
2. Which therapeutic goals would be a priority?
3. What is the best pharmacological intervention to decrease off-time?
4. What is the best pharmacological intervention to treat dyskinesias?

Summary

PD is a neurodegenerative movement disorder with a long duration and changing phenomenology that makes it challenging, even in the strict motor perspective. Different clinical problems emerge as potential therapeutic goals. Evidence-based management and application to each individual is vital to successful management (NICE 2017).

In early PD, multiple options exist, ranging from no treatment to different pharmacological agents such as levodopa, dopamine agonists and even MAO-B inhibitors. All the treatment options have drawbacks and benefits, and motor function is difficult to optimise. In further advanced stages of PD, clinical problems are often dopamine non-responsive and more difficult to manage. In these cases, the few available options lack the support of a good-quality body of evidence. Further research is therefore required.

Answers to activities

Activity 13.1 (Case study)

Reflecting on your knowledge of seizure warning signs, define Todd's Palsy.

Warning signs may include light-headedness, sweating, precipitants such as micturition, chest pain and palpitations. The person may experience a slow heart rate or low blood pressure. Déjà vu, aphasia, olfactory aura, epigastric sensation, tongue biting, post-event delirium or focal neuro-deficit may be experienced.

Todd's Palsy or Todd's paralysis (or postictal paresis/paralysis, 'after seizure') is focal weakness in a part of the body after a seizure. This weakness typically affects appendages and is localised to either the left or right side of the body. It usually subsides completely within 48 hours. Todd's paresis may also affect speech, eye position (gaze), or vision.

Activity 13.2 (Case study)

What factors would you need to consider before starting anti-epileptic treatment for Sally? How would you select a drug?

Sally's investigations would need to include full blood count, urea and electrolytes, liver function tests, electro-encephalogram, CAT scan, magnetic resonance imaging and perhaps ammonia and lactate.

The first-line choice of drug will therefore vary according to seizure type, and there are distinct advantages for monotherapy as opposed to combined therapy, such as improved life quality and compliance, reduced costs, fewer or absent interactions, reduced teratogenic effects and side effects, and better seizure control.

Consider:
- Was there a single seizure or a recurrence?
- How far apart was the recurrence?
- Were there any precipitating factors?
- Was epilepsy diagnosed on EEG?
- What are the prospects of compliance?
- What family support is available?

Other factors to consider when selecting a drug include:
- The possibility of pregnancy
- Any concomitant health needs
- The age of the patient.

Nurse prescribers should also be alert to the importance of cost-effective prescribing and ensuring that the prescribing decision is acceptable to the patient.

Activity 13.3

Give three examples of narrow-spectrum AEDs and three examples of broad-spectrum AEDs

Narrow-spectrum – phenytoin, phenobarbital, carbamazepine

Broad-spectrum – sodium valproate, lamotrigine, topiramate.

Activity 13.4

Based on the guidelines, how would you advise patients who asked:

1. Is it best to take this AED with food?

Some medicines can be taken with food or on an empty stomach. Advise patients to take the medicine the same way each day, as taking some with food may change the time it takes to be absorbed. Advise them not to take antacids or medicine for diarrhoea within 2 to 3 hours of taking phenytoin.

2. What should I do if I miss a dose of an AED?

If the patient misses or forgets a dose, instruct them to take it as soon as possible. However, if the patient has missed a dose and it is within a few hours before the next dose, advise them to take only the next scheduled dose. They must not double up or take extra medicine, unless instructed to do so by a doctor.

3. How can I remember to take my medicine?

Take medicine at the same time each day; take it at the same time as some other routine activity, such as brushing teeth, after meals, or bedtime; use a pillbox to check if they have taken a dose; use an alarm to remind them of times to take a dose; keep a written schedule or chart of when to take the medicine; review seizure first-aid techniques, seizure precautions as well as medication administration, compliance and storage issues.

Activity 13.5 (Case study)

What is Myerson's sign?

Myerson's sign is a medical condition in which a patient is unable to resist blinking when tapped on the glabella, the area above the nose and between the eyebrows. It is often referred to as the glabellar reflex. It is an early symptom of Parkinson's disease, but can also be seen in early dementia as well as other progressive neurological illness. It is named after Abraham Myerson, an American neurologist.

Activity 13.6 (Case study)

1. Which treatment options should be initiated for John (see p. 247)?

The factors that influence the decision of the clinician are related to the disease itself (rate of progression, presenting phenomenology, related physical disability), to individual characteristics of the patient (age, professional activity, expectations of benefit, fear of adverse effects) and those related to the anticipated goals of a given therapeutic intervention, namely:

- Prevention of clinical progression
- Easing of parkinsonism (mild improvement versus best benefit possible)
- Delaying motor complications.

Levodopa is most often used in combination with a dopa-decarboxylase inhibitor such as carbidopa (Sinemet®). It slows enzyme breakdown of levodopa before reaching the brain. Sinemet® can be standard or slow release and in most patients will significantly improve mobility early in the disease.

In John's case, treatment did not begin straight away; this is often the case. However it can be possible to initiate treatment with an immediate-release or a controlled-release form of levodopa, or levodopa plus entacapone, or dopamine-agonist, or MAO-B inhibitor (such as Selegiline) and an anticholinergic.

2. Which therapeutic goals would be a priority?

The occurrence of a fall is a warning of disease aggravation and increasing difficulty in effectively treating the symptoms of the disease. At this stage of the disease, manageable therapeutic goals may also include:

- Easing of parkinsonism
- Reduction in off-time
- Increase in on-time
- Reduction in the intensity and frequency of dyskinesias
- Improvement in postural instability/freezing.

The fall is significant. You should ask the patient the following questions:
- What were the symptoms just before the fall?
- When did it happen?
- Did anything trigger the fall?
- Did it happen during on- or off-time?

Ask the patient to start keeping a diary and interview the patient. Falls may be due to postural instability or orthostatic hypotension. Consider dose failure if freezing is evident. The need to decrease off-periods by optimising treatment may be the most suitable option

3. What is the best pharmacological intervention to decrease off-time?

Assuming that the reduction of off-time is a primary goal, several pharmacological options can be considered:

- Increase ropinirole
- Change to another dopamine agonist
- Increase levodopa/carbidopa
- Change the levodopa/carbidopa regime (increase frequency and not with high-protein food intake)
- Change to extended-release of dopamine agonists (consider a patch)

- Change to equivalent dose of controlled-release levodopa/carbidopa
- Add entacapone (COMT inhibitor)
- Use a combination of levodopa/carbidopa with entacapone
- Include a MAO-B inhibitor (rasagiline or selegiline).

Overall, current guidelines support the use of dopamine agonists, MAO-B inhibitors, levodopa/carbidopa and COMT inhibitors as options for the management of wearing-off. Rotigotine has been found to reduce off-time in PD patients with wearing-off symptoms, although this is not an approved indication. Most of the available data relating to the treatment of motor fluctuation deals with wearing-off phenomena or predictable on-off stages. Whatever the pharmacological option, off-time reduction ranges vary. Nevertheless, it is good practice to apply the management strategies described for wearing-off.

Apomorphine hydrochloride is a dopamine-receptor agonist used for 'off' episodes with levodopa. It is given subcutaneously, either as an infusion or injection. It can induce nausea and vomiting and will be given with domperidone. It should be initiated in a specialist clinic so that the dose can be individualised, side effects monitored, oral therapy safely prescribed and self-management initiated.

4. What is the best pharmacological intervention to treat dyskinesias?

All dopaminergic drugs have the risk of inducing or worsening dyskinesias, including the combination of levodopa with a dopamine agonist or a COMT inhibitor, or by adding an MAO-B inhibitor. An option would be to increase total levodopa dose, to increase dopamine agonist dose and to add an MAO-B inhibitor or COMT inhibitor to reduce the off-time. However, dyskinesia may increase. Amantadine 200–400mg/day may be the antidyskinetic drug of choice.

A meta-analysis individually comparing two dopamine agonists (pramipexole and ropinirole with levodopa) shows that both can cause dyskinesias. However, treating troublesome dyskinesias should not be achieved at the cost of increasing parkinsonian symptoms.

References and further reading

Braak, H., Ghebremedhin, E., Rub, U., Bratzke, H. & Del Tredici, K. (Oct 2004). Stages in the development of Parkinson's disease-related pathology. *Cell and Tissue Research.* **318** (1), 121–34.

Bradley, P., Lindsay, B., & Fleeman, N. (2016). Care Delivery and Self Management Strategies for Adults in Epilepsy. Cochrane Database of Systematic Reviews. https://doi.org/10.1002/14651858.CD006244.pub3

British National Formulary (BNF) (2020). BNF, no. 80. https://bnf.nice.org.uk/ (Last accessed 26 October 2020).

Buter, T.C., van den Hout, A., Matthews, F.E., Larsen, J.P., Brayne, C. & Aarsland, D. (2008). Dementia and survival in Parkinson disease: a 12-year population study. *Neurology.* **70** (13), 1017–22.

Chen, M.L., Shah, V., Patnaik, R., Adams, W., Hussain, A. & Conner, D. (2001). Bioavailability and bioequivalence: an FDA regulatory overview. *Pharmaceutical Research.* **18** (12), 1645–50.

Katzenschlager, R., Head, J., Schrag, A., Ben-Shlomo, Y., Evans, A. & Lees, A.J. (2008). Fourteen-year final report of the randomized PDRG-UK trial comparing three initial treatments in PD. *Neurology.* **71** (7), 474–80

Marson, A.G., Appleton, R., Baker, G.A., Chadwick, D.W., Doughty, J., Eaton, B., Gamble, C., Jacoby, A., Shackley, P., Smith, D.F., Tudur-Smith, C., Vanoli, A. & Williamson, P.R. (2007). A randomised controlled trial examining the longer-term outcomes of standard versus new antiepileptic drugs. *The SANAD trial. Health Technology Assessment Journal.* **11** (37), iii–iv, ix–x, 1–134.

Medwatch: The FDA Safety Information and Adverse Event Reporting Program (2020). https://www.fda.gov/safety/medwatch-fda-safety-information-and-adverse-event-reporting-program (Last accessed 18 October 2020).

National Institute for Health and Care Excellence (NICE) (2017). *Parkinson's disease: in Adults* (NG71). http://www.nice.org.uk/ng71 (Last accessed 18 October 2020).

National Institute for Health and Care Excellence (NICE) (2019). *The epilepsies: the diagnosis and management of the epilepsies in adults and children in primary and secondary care* (CG137). http://www.nice.org.uk/guidance/cg137 (Last accessed 18 October 2020).

Nevitt, S.J., Sudell, M., Smith, C.T. & Marsons, A.G. (2019). Topiramate versus Carbamazepine Monotherapy for Epilepsy: an Individual Participant Data Review. *Cochrane Database of Systematic Reviews.* (6) .doi.10.1002/14651858CD012065.pub3

Olanowe, C.W., Rascol, O., Hauser, R., Feigin, P.D. & Jankovic, J. (2009). A double-blind, delayed-start trial of rasagiline in Parkinson's disease. *New England Journal of Medicine.* **361** (13), 1268–78.

Sanad II (2019). http://www.sanad2.org.uk/ (Last accessed 18 October 2020).

Stowe, R., Ives, N., Clarke, C.E., Deane, K., Wheatley, K., Gray, R., Handley, K. & Furmston, A. (2010). Evaluation of the efficacy and safety of adjuvant treatment to Levodopa therapy in Parkinson's disease patients with motor complications. *Cochrane Database of Systematic Reviews.* **7** (7): CD007166. doi: 10.1002/14651858.CD007166.pub2.

14

Pharmacological case studies: Gastrointestinal disorders

Donna Scholefield
MSc, BSc (Hons), RN, PGDip HE; Cardiac Nursing (254);
Senior Lecturer, Health and Education, Middlesex University, London

Siobhan Corbett
MSc in Advanced Clinical Practice, BSc Hons, ENP, RN (Adult);
Nurse Consultant/Trauma Lead/ACP Lead in ED at Darent Valley Hospital

This chapter:
- Reviews the gastrointestinal system and structure
- Reviews a range of gastrointestinal conditions
- Develops knowledge and understanding of the major drug groups used in the management of common gastrointestinal conditions
- Discusses the pharmacokinetics and pharmacodynamics of drugs used to treat common gastrointestinal disorders
- Applies knowledge of gastrointestinal pharmacology to practice-based case studies.

Introduction

The aim of this chapter is to review the pharmacological management of some common gastrointestinal conditions, namely peptic ulcers, diarrhoea, constipation and inflammatory bowel conditions. Three case studies will be used to demonstrate the application of pharmacological knowledge to real-life scenarios.

The structure of the gastrointestinal tract and the process of acid secretion

The gastrointestinal tract (GIT) is made up of a series of hollow organs which are essentially joined via a muscular tract that extends from the mouth to the anus. The hollow organs that make up the gastrointestinal tract include the mouth, oesophagus, stomach, small intestine, caecum, colon (large intestine), rectum and anal canal. There are also a number of accessory organs (salivary glands, pancreas, liver and gall bladder) through which food does not pass. These organs produce additional enzymes or store substances that are essential to the digestion of foods. The primary function of the GIT is to digest and absorb both food and fluids in order to provide nutrients and to remove metabolic waste.

Although specific sections of the GIT are specialised for particular functions, the basic structure of this muscular tube is the same throughout, consisting essentially of layers of epithelial cells, an inner mucosal lining, circular and longitudinal muscle and an outer serosa layer made from connective tissue (see Table 14.1 and Figure 14.1 below). The control of muscular contraction, and secretion of acids and enzymes is by the autonomic nervous system (ANS), known as the enteric nervous system (submucosal and myenteric plexus), located in the gut wall, which controls the whole digestive process. However, the enteric system is also influenced by extrinsic fibres from the ANS – parasympathetic and sympathetic nerves. The parasympathetic nerves have the more dominant action on the GIT, in that they increase muscular activity (especially peristalsis) and glandular secretions.

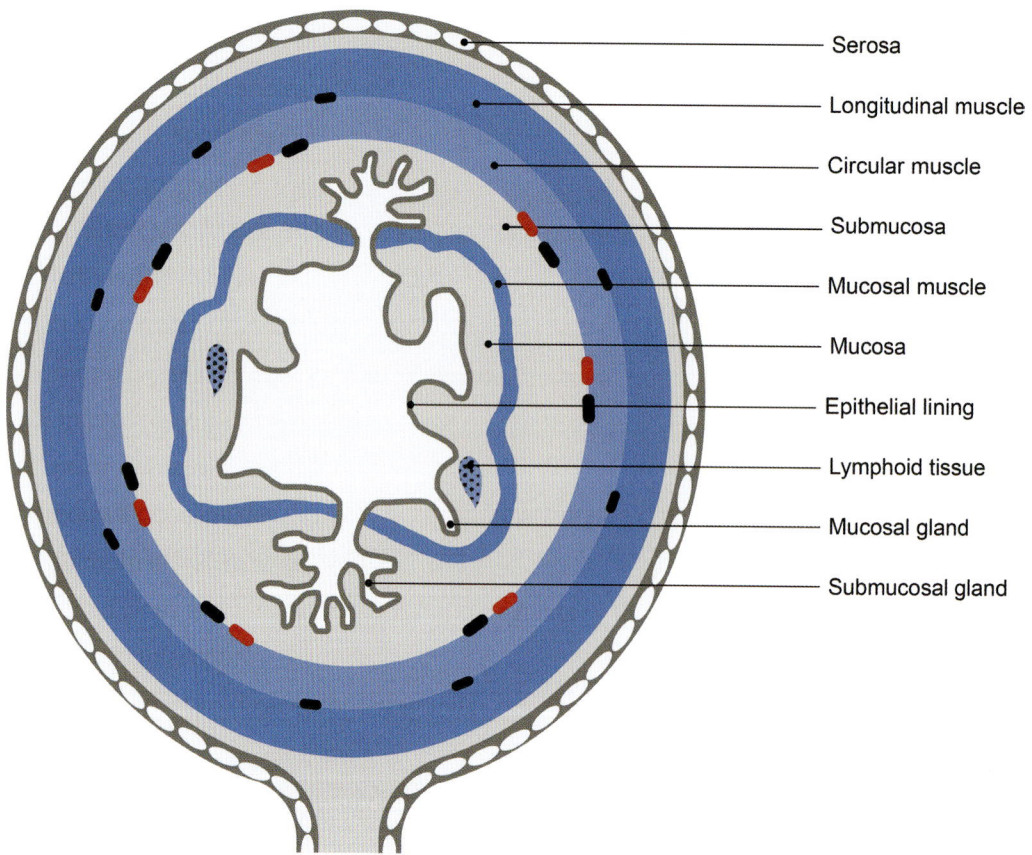

Figure 14.1: Cross-section of layers of the gut

Table 14.1: Layers of the gastrointestinal tract wall

Name	Structures	Additional
Mucosa	Epithelial cells supported by underlying connective tissue (lamina propria), containing vessels, nerves, lymphoid tissue, glands and mucosal muscle	Type of epithelium varies from simple (stomach) to stratified (mouth)
Submucosa	Connective tissue, glands, blood vessels, lymphatic vessels and enteric nervous system (nerve plexus)	Meissner plexus – supplies mucosa and submucosa
Muscularis externa; smooth muscle – most of GIT	Inner circular layer and outer longitudinal layer separated by myenteric plexus; nerve innervation controls muscle contraction, mechanical breakdown and movement of food in the gut lumen.	Skeletal muscle in mouth, pharynx, upper oesophagus, and external anal sphincter
Serosa – visceral layer of peritoneum	Fat, epithelial tissue (mesothelium)	This layer also forms the greater omentum and mesentery

Drugs acting on the gastrointestinal system

Table 14.2: The main classes of drugs acting on gastrointestinal (GI) conditions

Drug groups	Conditions
Anti-secretory drugs: • H^2 antagonists, e.g. ranitidine, cimetidine • Proton pump inhibitors, e.g. omeprazole, lansoprazole, rabeprazole and pantoprazole • Mucosal protectants, e.g. bismuth, misoprostol	Peptic ulcers, dyspepsia, gastro-oesophageal reflux, *Helicobacter pylori*; eradication with antibiotics, such as amoxicillin, clarithromycin, metronidazole
Laxatives: • Bulk, e.g. bran, methylcellulose • Osmotic, e.g. lactulose • Stimulant, e.g. senna, glycerin • Faecal softeners, e.g. docusate • Macrogols, e.g. macrogol oral powder	Constipation, prior to surgery or investigations such as colonoscopy
Anti-diarrhoeal drugs: • Anti-motility drugs, e.g. codeine phosphate, loperamide, diphenoxylate	Diarrhoea caused by viral (most often), bacterial infection

(table continued overleaf)

Table 14.2 continued

Drug groups	Conditions
Anti-inflammatory drugs: • Corticosteroids, e.g. prednisolone, budesonide • Monoclonal antibodies, e.g. infliximab, adalimumab • Immunosuppressants, e.g. azathioprine, 6-mercaptopurine • Aminosalicylates, e.g. sulfasalazine, mesalazine	Inflammatory bowel disease, Crohn's disease, ulcerative colitis
• Anti-spasmodics, e.g. hyoscine butylbromide, dicycloverine	Irritable bowel syndrome, diverticular disease
• Motility stimulants, e.g. metoclopramide and domperidone, which increase gastric emptying and speed up movement in the small intestine (see BNH/MHRA for guidance on safety of these agents in long-term use)	Functional dyspepsia, gastro-oesophageal reflux disease

Source: BNF (Joint Formulary Committee 2020a)

Drugs used to manage peptic ulcers

Ulcers are deep lesions penetrating the entire thickness of the gastrointestinal tract mucosa, the most common of which are peptic ulcers, gastric ulcers and duodenal ulcers. Gastric ulcers result from damage to the lining of the stomach, while duodenal ulcers are associated with excessive acid secretion by the stomach.

Peptic ulcers are thought to occur due to an imbalance between aggressive factors (*Helicobacter pylori*, non-steroidal anti-inflammatory drugs, gastric acid) and protective factors (mucin, bicarbonate, prostaglandins), which lead to an interruption in mucosal integrity. Under normal conditions, the linings of the stomach and duodenum are protected from the irritant action of stomach (hydrochloric) acid, and pepsin, by a barrier of mucus gel, which is about 500 micrometres thick. The mucosa also produces prostaglandins, which offer further protection by increasing blood flow and stimulating the production of mucus and bicarbonate. If this barrier is damaged, or large amounts of stomach acid are formed, the underlying tissue may become eroded, leading to the development of a peptic ulcer.

The exact prevalence of peptic ulcer disease is difficult to establish, as the definitions used vary between studies, and endoscopy is needed to make a formal diagnosis (NICE 2019a). The aetiology and causal factors for peptic ulcers have been extensively debated, with many non-organic and lifestyle considerations (including smoking, alcohol consumption and stress) featuring in the discussion. Whilst the rate of newly diagnosed peptic ulcers has remained constant, the recurrence rate seems to have fallen rapidly in the past 20–30 years, with the introduction of

Helicobacter pylori eradication therapy and widespread use of acid suppression therapy (Lanas & Chan 2017). The lifetime prevalence of peptic ulcer disease in the general population is estimated to be about 5–10% with the incidence of peptic ulcer disease about 0.1–0.3% per year but this varies with age and sex (NICE 2019a). The incidence of duodenal ulcers peaks at 45–64 years of age, and it is twice as common in men as in women. In contrast, the incidence of gastric ulcers increases with age, and the incidence is similar in men and women.

The classic presenting symptoms for peptic ulcer, particularly in duodenal ulcer, include epigastric pain, commonly arising some hours after eating, associated with dyspepsia and heartburn. The symptoms are usually relieved by eating small, frequent, non-irritating meals or taking antacids. The main risk factor predisposing to the formation of peptic ulcer disease is the presence of *Helicobacter pylori*, which is the causal agent in over 80% of cases of ulcer formation. According to the Joint Formulary Committee (2020b), the use of certain drugs is also heavily associated with peptic ulcer formation. These drugs mainly include non-steroidal anti-inflammatory drugs (NSAIDS) but also aspirin, bisphosphonates, corticosteroids, potassium supplements, selective serotonin reuptake inhibitors (SSRIs), and recreational drugs such as crack cocaine.

Complications with gastric ulcer include perforation leading to peritonitis, gastrointestinal bleeding and an increased incidence of stomach cancer. It is interesting to note that NICE (2019a) identifies upper GIT bleeding as the commonest gastrointestinal (GI) emergency managed by gastroenterologists in the UK. The underlying pathological cause is predominantly peptic ulcers, which account for up to 50% of all cases of upper GIT bleeds and an associated 5–10% fatality rate. The treatment for proven peptic ulcer disease varies depending on the cause, whether it is initial or recurrent, and whether or not there are complications. First-line treatment options tend to focus on testing and *H. pylori* eradication therapy and limiting NSAIDs usage (see below). However, it would be remiss not to also consider and advocate the use of non-pharmacological treatment, such as dietary modification and avoidance of exacerbating factors and drugs, and lifestyle modifications, particularly reducing smoking and stress levels (Joint Formulary Committee 2020a).

NSAIDs and peptic ulcer disease

As discussed previously, NSAIDs are a well-known predisposing factor for peptic ulcer disease. As NSAIDs are frequently prescribed and are known to be one of the commonest causes of serious adverse drug reactions, it is worth spending a little time exploring why this is the case in relation to the GIT.

In response to tissue injury, the prostanoid family of chemical messengers (which includes prostaglandins, prostacyclins and thromboxane) stimulate inflammation, which begins the healing process. By blocking prostaglandin synthesis, NSAIDs reduce the normal inflammatory responses (pain, swelling and vasodilation associated tissue injury). They are therefore very effective in treating inflammatory conditions ranging from minor tissue injury to conditions such as rheumatoid arthritis.

However, the problem is that NSAIDs also inhibit the cyclooxygenase (COX) enzyme responsible for prostaglandin production, thus blocking prostaglandins (especially PGE2) which protect the gastrointestinal mucosa by increasing blood flow and producing bicarbonate and mucus. By blocking these effects, NSAIDs predispose the individual to upper GIT bleeding and ulcers of the stomach and duodenum (see Figure 14.2) and also affect other systems (see Figure 14.3, p. 263). The non-selective NSAIDs block PGE2 by inhibiting both isoforms of the cyclooxygenase (COX-1) and (COX-2) enzymes (see Figure 14.2).

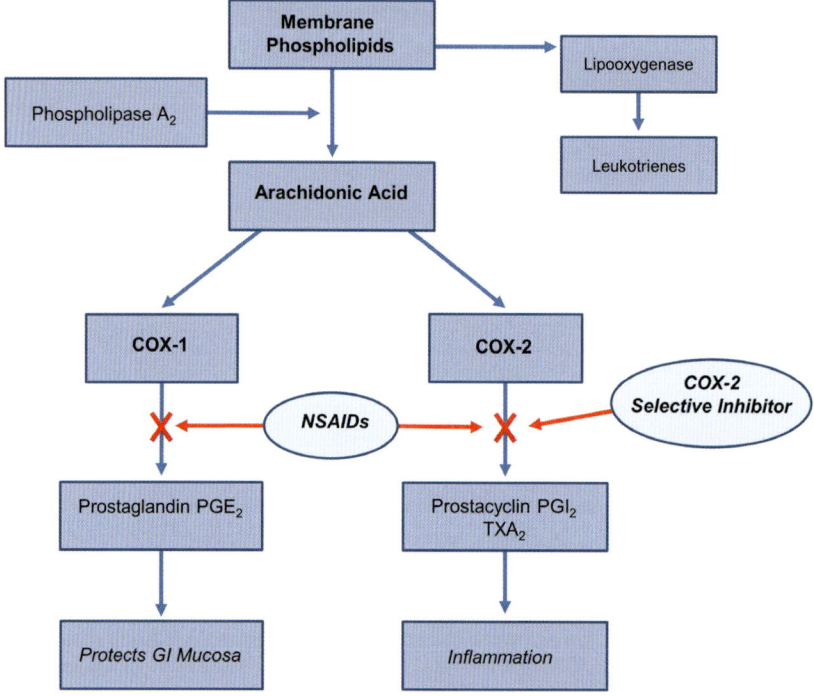

Figure 14.2: How NSAIDs cause peptic ulcers. The two isoforms of the enzyme are cyclooxygenase 1 (COX-1) and cyclooxygenase 2 (COX-2). COX-1 is responsible for producing PGE_2, which protects the gastric mucosa, and COX-2 produces PGI_2 and TXA_2, which cause pain and inflammation. The non-selective NSAIDs block both isoenzymes.

Cyclooxygenase is an enzyme involved in the formation of prostaglandins and other inflammatory mediators. COX-1 produces prostaglandins and thromboxane A2 (TXA_2), which protects the GI mucosa. COX-2 produces prostacycline (PGI_2), which mediates the inflammatory reaction. The newer selective COX-2 inhibitors, such as celecoxib, are therefore less likely to cause damage to the gastric mucosa, but they are not completely selective.

Caution: NSAIDs should be used with caution in patients with cardiovascular disease, especially with the COX-2 inhibitors, as they have been proven to cause oedema, myocardial infarction, thrombotic events, stroke and hypertension.

NSAID Side Effects:

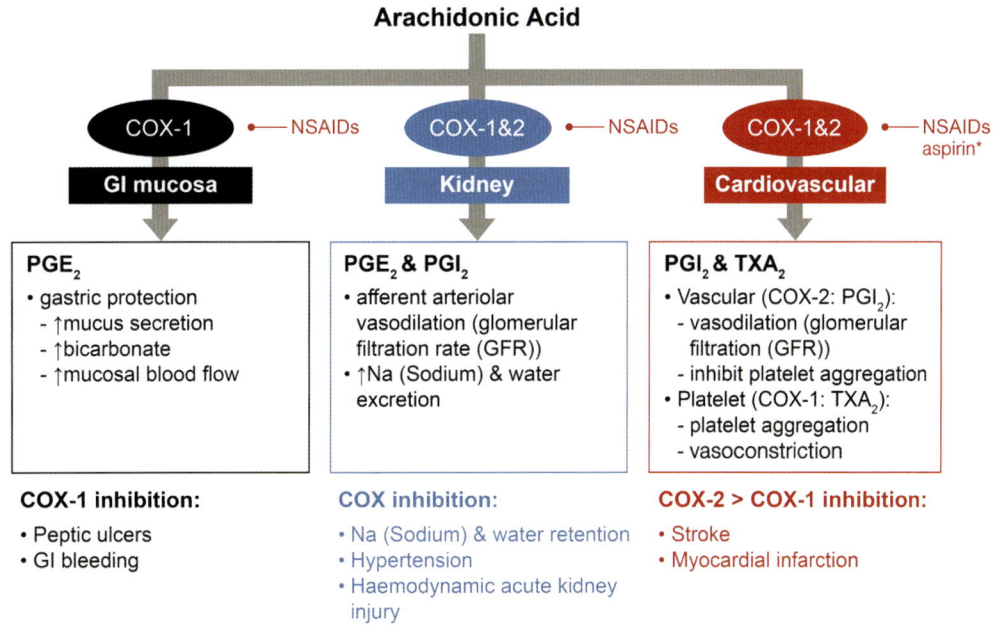

Figure 14.3 Side effects of NSAIDs

Activity 14.1

1. Draw on your knowledge of the causes of GI bleeding and list five predisposing factors.
2. Succinctly summarise the mechanism for NSAID-induced ulcers.

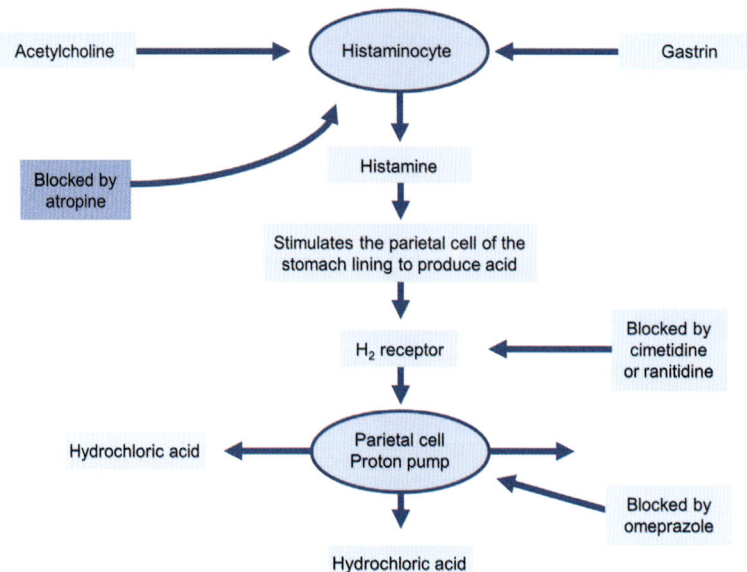

Figure 14.4: Acid production in the stomach. Adapted from Greenstein & Gould (2008), with permission from Elsevier publishers.

To gain an insight into how drugs (such as antacids, H_2 antagonists and proton pump inhibitors) produce their effects, it is important to have some understanding of gastric acid production. The H^+/K^+ATPase proton pumps in the membrane of the parietal cells in the stomach facilitate the release of hydrochloric acid (HCl) in the lumen of the stomach in exchange for potassium. The stimulation of this process is fairly complex but it is triggered by the sight and smell of food, which in turn stimulates the release of acetylcholine from the vagus nerve. Acetylcholine then interacts with muscarinic receptors on histaminocytes in the stomach, triggering the release of histamine. Food distending the stomach can also stimulate histamine release. The distension initially evokes gastrin production, which then acts on the histamine cells, releasing histamine. Histamine will in turn stimulate histamine H_2 receptors on the parietal cells to secrete hydrochloric acid (HCl) into the lumen of the stomach.

The drugs used to treat peptic ulcers aim to either neutralise secreted acid, reduce gastric acid secretion or increase mucosal resistance to acid–pepsin attack.

Antacids

These neutralise the effects of HCl by increasing the pH of the stomach, thus reducing gastric irritation. They are less effective than the H_2 antagonists (cimetidine and ranitidine) in suppressing acid secretion at night but have a similar effect on daytime secretion. They are used primarily to treat the symptoms of peptic ulcers. Frequent high doses can promote ulcer healing but such treatment is impractical, since patient adherence would be a problem, as the duration of action is short and high doses can cause alkalosis. Antacids are also indicated in dyspepsia, gastro-oesophageal reflux disease (GORD) and heartburn.

Commonly used antacids

- Magnesium hydroxide and magnesium trisilicate: These drugs are insoluble in water and have a fairly rapid action. Magnesium, however, has a laxative effect and can cause diarrhoea.
- Aluminium hydroxide: This is a slower-acting antacid that can cause constipation and interfere with phosphate absorption, leading to weakness and bone damage if taken in high doses for prolonged periods.

Caution: Antacids should be avoided or used with caution in patients with cardiac, renal or hepatic failure. In these disorders, there is reduced clearance of absorbed magnesium and aluminium. High levels of these elements can increase significantly, leading to toxicity. In addition, many antacids are high in sodium, especially sodium bicarbonate which can exacerbate tissue fluid retention and thus oedema. It is now recommended that sodium bicarbonate should not be used on its own for the treatment of dyspepsia (Joint Formulary Committee 2020a). It should be noted that the sodium content may not be immediately obvious – for example, magnesium trisilicate mixture contains 6mmol of sodium per 10ml dose.

Drug interactions

Healthcare professionals should also be aware of the fact that antacids containing magnesium, aluminium or calcium can interact with many drugs, either inactivating them or preventing their absorption from the GIT. This will reduce the efficacy and therapeutic effect of the drug.

Some antacids contain simeticone, an anti-foaming agent, to reduce flatulence or prevent hiccough in palliative care.

Case study: Use of antacids

Mr Burton is a 59-year-old part-time lecturer in Ancient History who has suffered moderate heart failure with left ventricular systolic dysfunction for the past two years. His long-term condition has been well controlled on ramipril 5mg daily, bisoprolol 7.5mg daily, aspirin 75mg daily, and metolazone 2.5mg weekly. He enjoys his job but recently (especially during assessment periods) he has found it stressful and has been experiencing bouts of heartburn, for which he takes magnesium trisilicate liquid bought over the counter.

The magnesium trisilicate is very soothing and he has been taking it regularly (up to 20ml four times daily after meals), as he thinks it's a fairly harmless substance. He has visited his GP because he has noticed that he has become breathless, with swelling of his ankles. He is also feeling constantly tired and finds himself belching frequently.

Activity 14.2 (Case study)

1. Can you suggest why Mr Burton is experiencing these symptoms since taking the antacids? How do you think the antacids may have caused these symptoms?
2. What specific advice would you offer Mr Burton?

Drugs that reduce gastric secretion

Histamine H_2 receptor antagonists (cimetidine and ranitidine) produce their effect by blocking H_2 receptors on the parietal cells, thus reducing the production of hydrochloric acid (see Figure 14.3 above). Several multicentre double-blind trials have shown that they not only significantly reduce the pain associated with peptic ulcers but also increase the healing rate, compared with placebo groups. Both drugs are absorbed rapidly when taken orally. Ranitidine may also be given intramuscularly or intravenously. These drugs undergo little metabolism in the liver and are excreted mainly by the kidneys. The half-life of ranitidine is approximately 3 hours but it is prolonged in the elderly and patients with renal impairment so the dose should be adjusted to account for this effect. Cimetidine has been shown to (albeit rarely) cause gynaecomastia.

Cimetidine is known to impede drug metabolism by binding to hepatic cytochrome P450 enzymes, increasing blood levels of drugs such as theophylline, phenytoin, warfarin and benzodiazepines. However, other H_2 receptor antagonists, such as ranitidine, famotidine and nizatidine, do not inhibit P450 hepatic enzymes, and are now used more frequently than cimetidine because of this.

Proton pump inhibitors

Proton pump inhibitors (PPIs), omeprazole and lansoprazole, reduce gastric acid secretion more effectively than the H_2 antagonists, by inhibiting the proton pump (H^+/K^+ATPase) on the parietal cell that pumps out H^+ ions into the stomach lumen. These are indicated, preferably over a short-term period, for peptic ulcers, dyspepsia, gastro-oesophageal reflux disease and conditions causing excessive acid production such as Zollinger-Ellison syndrome (ZES). They are also used effectively in combination with antibiotics to eradicate *Helicobacter pylori* (*H. pylori*).

There is an increasing clinical use of prolonged and lifetime treatment with PPIs and this is leading to a growing risk of developing adverse effects. Recent studies (such as Kumar, Ashwlayan & Verma 2019) have shown some inappropriate prescribing in both primary and emergency settings, with an increased rate of PPI prescribing related to chronic treatments, unlicensed indications and therapeutic substitutions. PPIs are also available over the counter, without any medical consultation.

Despite this, PPIs are a generally safe group of drugs and they have been successfully linked to a significant reduction in the need for surgery. However, they do have some common side effects, such as headaches, nausea, diarrhoea, abdominal discomfort and dizziness, which disappear when the user stops taking the drug. Recent studies have demonstrated a correlation between the PPIs and an increased risk of *Clostridium difficile* disease. Furthermore, prolonged use of these drugs is also associated with a reduction in bone density and thus a propensity to fractures.

Most PPIs are administered orally, though omeprazole and pantoprazole can also be administered intravenously. All PPIs are administered orally as enteric-coated preparations because they are degraded at low pH. They are prodrugs, which are converted to active sulfenamide or sulfenic acid that inhibit gastric secretion. Absorption is in the small intestine and they have good bioavailability, with a short half-life of about an hour, and they are rapidly metabolised in the liver.

Antibiotics

Helicobacter pylori (H. pylori) is a spiral shaped Gram-negative rod bacterium, found deep in the mucosa layer of the gut and able to survive over a wide pH spectrum. It causes excessive production of hydrochloric acid, which in turn damages the mucosa, leading to ulcers and gastritis. Due to *H. pylori's* ability to survive in pH extremes, no single therapy can eradicate it effectively and drug combination therapy is usually needed. In this case, antibiotics such as clarithromycin, amoxicillin and metronidazole are normally used in clinical management, and the precise choice of antibiotic may depend on the patient's recent antibiotic exposure.

Combined therapy with proton pump inhibitors has been successful in eradicating the bacteria through multiple actions – direct antimicrobial action against *H. pylori*, increased intra-gastric pH becoming more sensitive to antibiotics, increased antibiotic stability and efficacy, and reduced gastric emptying and mucous viscosity. Refer to the BNF (Joint Formulary Committee 2020a) for examples of combination therapy.

Drugs used to manage constipation – laxatives

Constipation is a prevalent symptom in which the individual passes hard and sometimes painful stools or goes to the toilet less often than is usual for them. It is a somewhat subjective term and, as a result, the definition is variable. Indeed, more recently it has been defined by including a range of symptoms such as abdominal pain, straining, passing hard stools, and bloating that should be present 25% of the time. Perhaps the most succinct yet comprehensive definition is the one formulated by the Joint Formulary Committee (2020c): 'Defaecation that is unsatisfactory because of infrequent stools, difficult stool passage, or seemingly incomplete defaecation'. Although the symptom of constipation can be found in anyone, it is often associated with the elderly but is commonly found in other groups such as pregnant women.

There are many possible causes of constipation. These may include certain clinical conditions (e.g. hypothyroidism or hypercalcaemia), genetic disposition, intestinal motility and absorption, pharmacological factors (e.g. use of opiates), or lifestyle issues including insufficient dietary fibre, exercise or fluid. With such a long and variable list of causative factors, caution should be used when applying therapeutic treatment based on only one cause. Dietary advice should be considered as a first and general treatment option for constipation; and osmotic and stimulant laxatives should be used as the first-line pharmacological treatment (Forootan, Bagheri & Darvishi 2018).

Although laxatives are commonly used, especially amongst certain groups of patients like the elderly, their use is often unwarranted. If used inappropriately, they can cause more serious problems, including worsening serious abdominal conditions such as appendicitis. They can also induce chronic constipation, diarrhoea, dehydration and electrolyte imbalance so they should not be prescribed indiscriminately. Before constipation is diagnosed, any serious underlying causes (such as acute appendicitis) should be excluded by taking a careful history, followed by a clinical examination as directed by the history (Chodhury 2006, Ford & Talley 2012).

How constipation develops

Throughout the lower gastrointestinal tract, waves of muscular contraction and relaxation, known as peristalsis, push undigested food along. The last stage of digestion occurs in the large intestine where very strong periodic (three or four times a day) peristalsis, known as mass peristalsis, pushes the faecal material along the colon to the rectum, stimulating the urge to defaecate. By the time the faeces reach the rectum, they are of a solid consistency due to water absorption along the large intestine. Absorption of water is controlled by the autonomic nervous system (sympathetic and parasympathetic). If too much water is absorbed, constipation will occur. If too little water is absorbed, diarrhoea results.

Peristaltic movements in the colon occur at a much slower rate than in other parts of the GIT so the transit time is slower. Factors that alter motility in the large intestine, either directly or indirectly, will therefore affect the transit time, as both the absorption and secretion rate are proportional to transit time. If, for example, peristaltic movement and transit time become too short (because of bacterial infection), diarrhoea results. Conversely, if the transit time is too slow (because of factors such as drugs, disease, diet or immobility), constipation will occur.

Intestinal motility is mainly controlled by the parasympathetic nervous system so drugs that block the activity of the parasympathetic nerve (such as anticholinergic drugs like hyoscine) will reduce motility and cause constipation. The opioid drugs delay the movement of faeces through the large intestine by other mechanisms, such as increasing smooth muscle time and reducing forward peristalsis as well as the urge to defaecate. This delay, as mentioned earlier, will cause more absorption of water and electrolytes from the colon, leading to constipation.

Table 14.3: Commonly prescribed laxatives used to manage constipation

Types	Effects	Side effects/adverse effects
Bulk laxatives, e.g. bran, ispaghula	They increase bowel content, stimulate peristalsis and soften stools. Many contain methylcellulose or ispaghula husk	• Flatulence and abdominal bloating • Rarely obstruction of the gut, especially if not enough fluid is ingested – hence care needed when prescribing for the elderly
Stool softeners, e.g. docusate sodium, liquid paraffin	Moistens and softens the faeces	• Liquid paraffin can disturb the absorption of vitamins A, K and D • Can also cause anal seepage and is no longer recommended
Stimulant laxatives, e.g. senna (active ingredient sennosides) and bisacodyl	Increase peristalsis by stimulating the parasympathetic nerves in the wall of the colon and rectum increasing muscular contraction	• Can cause abdominal cramp • Reduces the activity of the bowels over time • Do not administer in pregnancy
Osmotic laxatives, e.g. lactulose	Makes bowel content more fluid. Laxatives retain fluid in the bowels by osmosis. Thus less fluid is absorbed into the circulation. They are broken down to lactic acid, which exerts an osmotic effect.	• Can cause abdominal pain and bloating. • May take 2–3 days to produce its effects but this depends on adequate fluid intake • Unsuitable for quick relief of constipation

Case study: Constipation and pharmacological management of peptic ulcer

Mrs Green is a 78-year-old lady who has attended your clinic with a presenting history of not having had a bowel movement for four days. She states that she is 'always regular every day'.

Mrs Green lives in a residential home and suffered a sprained ankle two weeks ago, for which she has been taking co-codamol, which has been effective in managing the pain. She admits that the injury has restricted her movements and she has been unable to 'get about' as she usually does. She also reveals that she has been experiencing heartburn on a regular basis, especially after a spicy meal or after a glass of whisky, which she sometimes takes to help her to relax since the injury

She has been taking an antacid for the last few days, which initially helped but she is still experiencing the indigestion.

Mrs Green has a past medical history of hypertension and persistent atrial fibrillation (AF), for which she takes digoxin 125micrograms od, aspirin 75mg od and ramipril 5mg od. On examination, she appears well. Her AF and blood pressure are well controlled, with BP 138/80mmHg, HR 72bpm, and ECG showing an irregularly irregular rhythm.

Laxatives are prescribed for Mrs Green. Consideration is given to withdrawing the co-codamol but Mrs Green states that she is still experiencing pain and that it is effective. She is also prescribed omeprazole to address the dyspepsia. A follow-up appointment is made for four weeks hence.

Activity 14.3 (Case study)

1. Constipation commonly occurs in the elderly. Can you list common causes for constipation and suggest reasons why Mrs Green has become constipated?
2. What type of laxatives would you prescribe for Mrs Green? How will they be administered? And can you briefly outline their mechanism of action?
3. What advice would you offer about taking antacids?
4. What lifestyle advice would you discuss with Mrs Green?

Case study (continued)

On her second visit to the clinic, Mrs Green is generally well. She states that her ankle is back to normal and she stopped taking the co-codamol weeks ago. She is also over the moon that her bowels are now back to being 'regular'. However, although the omeprazole initially worked, she is still experiencing pain at night, especially a few hours after eating. Mrs Green is referred to a gastroenterologist, to exclude the presence of *Helicobacter pylori*. The presence of this bacterium is confirmed and she is started on triple therapy treatment of amoxicillin, omeprazole and metronidazole for seven days to eradicate the bacteria.

Activity 14.4 (Case study)

1. Explain the mechanism of action of the triple therapy that has been prescribed for Mrs Green.

2. What advice would you give Mrs Green about taking the medication?
3. Can you identify four pharmacokinetic factors that could cause adverse drug reactions in the elderly? Refer back to Chapters 1 and 3.

Drugs used to manage diarrhoea

The World Health Organisation (WHO 2013) defines diarrhoea as 'passage of three or more loose or liquid stools per day'. Acute diarrhoea is usually infective and is mainly caused by bacterial, viral and parasitic organisms. In the UK, infective diarrhoea generally resolves fairly quickly without the need for pharmacological intervention.

Nevertheless, it is important to mention that diarrhoea contributes significantly to mortality and morbidity rates worldwide, especially in developing countries, where it is the second-biggest cause of death in children under five years (WHO 2013). In many of these cases, death is usually due to dehydration and electrolyte imbalance. The main approach in the management of diarrhoea of any cause is therefore through the use of oral rehydration therapy. In such circumstances, anti-diarrhoeal drugs should be used cautiously, as flushing out the infective agents is beneficial, provided patients are managed appropriately to prevent dehydration and electrolyte loss.

The previous section described the role of laxatives in facilitating bowel movements and this was predominantly achieved by increasing the motility of the gut. The anti-diarrhoea drugs have the opposite effect. They reduce the motility or peristaltic action of the GIT by acting on the circular and longitudinal muscles in the small and large intestine. Many of these drugs, such as codeine and loperamide, are opioid based. Codeine and morphine interact with mu (μ) receptors in the mesenteric plexus of the GIT and this in turn increases the inward movement of potassium into the nerve cells. The consequent effect is to prevent the release of acetylcholine from the plexus into the gut wall, thus reducing gut motility. Acetylcholine, as discussed earlier, is released by the parasympathetic nerve, which is the main nerve responsible for gastric motility.

Loperamide (Imodium®) co-phenotrope (diphenoxylate with atropine sulphate as Lomotil®) and codeine are used in the treatment of acute diarrhoea. They are fairly well absorbed orally, distributed in the plasma, broken down in the liver and excreted mainly in the faeces. Side effects are few but they include constipation, abdominal distension, dizziness, dyspepsia and nausea. Loperamide is a commonly used opioid drug that acts locally. As it does not easily cross the blood–brain barrier, the potential for dependency is significantly reduced. Some authorities suggest that antimotility drugs should be avoided in pregnancy. In the case of loperamide, the manufacturers specifically state that it should not be used in pregnancy, as opioids are known to suppress breathing and cause withdrawal symptoms in the neonate if given close to labour. Atropine-containing products may also suppress lactation.

Antibiotics are used in diarrhoea caused by specific infective agents, such as cholera, *campylobacter* enteritis, *shigellosis*, *salmonellosis* and *bacillary dysentery*. When travelling, antibiotics such as ciprofloxacin are sometimes used prophylactically to prevent diarrhoea but this should be done with caution and only for a short period of time.

> ### Activity 14.5
> What general measures would you recommend for the treatment of acute diarrhoea?

Drugs used to manage inflammatory bowel disease

Crohn's disease and ulcerative colitis are two common chronic inflammatory conditions of the gastrointestinal system (GBD 2019). Indeed, ulcerative colitis is thought to be the most common type of inflammatory bowel disease in the UK. Ulcerative colitis mainly affects the colon, whilst Crohn's disease – although generally confined to the terminal ileum – can also spread to other parts of the whole of the GIT.

The precise pathophysiology of the two conditions is not known but they are considered to be immune-mediated conditions that lead to damage to the protective epithelial layer of the GIT and chronic inflammation, which is often caused by environmental factors such as alterations in the gut microbiome (NICE 2019b). The course of both conditions, collectively known as inflammatory bowel disease (IBD), involves periods of relapse and remission. Symptoms are variable and there are many similarities in the clinical presentations of both disorders. These can include recurrent pain, altered bowel habits especially chronic diarrhoea which may contain fresh unaltered blood, weight loss and nausea. Indeed, in a small proportion of individuals it is often difficult to determine the difference histologically between the two conditions and according to NICE (2019b) the term 'inflammatory bowel disease type-unclassified' (IBDU) is then assigned.

Management of these conditions has undergone a recent major review, with new guidelines on emerging therapies (Lamb, Nicholas, et al. 2019, NICE 2019a & 2019b), consisting of pharmacological treatments, nutritional and lifestyle changes, psychological therapies and surgical intervention, to address complications associated with the diseases.

Studies (Mikocka-Walus, Pittet, et al. 2016 and Frolkis, Vallerand, Shaheen, et al. 2019) have shown that individuals with depression have significantly greater risk of developing inflammatory bowel disease; and drugs used to treat depression, such as tri-cyclic anti-depressants (TCAs) and selective serotonin reuptake inhibitors (SSRIs), have been shown to protect against both Crohn's disease and ulcerative colitis. However, treatment therapies not previously recommended include low-dose TCAs and SSRIs (see Chapter 17) and antispasmodics.

Studies (Frolkis, Vallerand, Shaheen, et al. 2019) involving TCAs and SSRIs showed an effect on gut transit times, and central and peripheral pain sites as well as anti-inflammatory and analgesic properties. Meanwhile antispasmodics are thought to block anticholinergic or calcium channel action which in turn relaxes smooth muscle in the gut. However, using antidepressants to treat inflammatory bowel disease (IBD) could be seen as a healthcare professional dismissing IBD as a psychological disease. It therefore requires considerable patient education regarding the benefits and actions of antidepressants to ensure adherence.

In the UK, some of the drugs used to manage these chronic inflammatory disorders are outlined in Table 14.4 (below)

Table 14.4: Commonly prescribed drugs used to manage inflammatory bowel disease

Types	Effects	Indications	Side effects/adverse effects
Corticosteroids, e.g. prednisolone, budesonide	Reduce the inflammatory process	• Main drugs in severe acute attacks • Short-term use • Local application if IBD localised to rectum/recto-sigmoid region • Diffuse disease • Can be used in combination with aminosalicyclic acid	• Many adverse effects, including suppression of the adrenal glands, fluid retention, hypertension, hypokalaemia, metabolic effects, infections • Budesonide gives less adrenal suppression
Amino salicylates, e.g. sulfasalazine, mesalazine	The active ingredient is 5-aminosalicylic acid; these drugs are anti-inflammatory; their mechanism of action is not fully understood	• Mild disease to reduce symptoms and prevent relapse • Local application in mild to moderate disease • Local for diffuse disease – proctitis or distal colitis • Can be used in combination with steroids	• Nausea, blood disorders, rashes, male infertility • Mesalazine has fewer adverse effects; it acts locally in the gut
Immunosuppressants	• Reduce immune system mediated inflammation	• Severe Crohn's disease and ulcerative colitis disease that is not responsive to conventional treatment	• Patients prone to infection and blood disorders

(table continued overleaf)

Table 14.4 continued

Types	Effects	Indications	Side effects/adverse effects
Biologics, e.g. infliximab, adalimumab	Monoclonal antibodies that inhibit tumour necrosis factor alpha, suppressing the inflammatory process	• Severe Crohn's and ulcerative colitis disease that is not responsive to conventional treatment • More effective in healing anal fistulae caused by Crohn's	• Patients may experience shortness of breath, nausea, chest pain and immune reactions during the treatment • Information about adverse reactions is still being gathered

Corticosteroids

Corticosteroids are used locally in mild to moderate and diffuse disease if the inflammation is localised or systemic. The Joint Formulary Committee (2020d) suggests that the aminosalicylates should be used initially, especially in mild disease, as they are more effective. However, if the patient does not respond, a corticosteroid (such as prednisolone or budesonide) may be added. Budesonide is an oral slow-release preparation and causes less adrenal suppression than prednisolone and is licensed for use in Crohn's disease (ileum and ascending colon). If symptoms are severe or unresponsive to oral therapy, hospital admission with intravenous drug and nutritional therapy is indicated. Intravenous corticosteroids (such as hydrocortisone or methylprednisolone) are the suggested choices.

Other immunosuppressant drugs

Severe unresponsive conditions can be treated with immunosuppressant drugs such as azathioprine and methotrexate or newer monoclonal antibodies such as infliximab.

Infliximab as stated earlier (see Table 14.4) blocks tumour necrosis factor alpha, which is an important cytokine released from activated macrophages that stimulates the inflammatory process in Crohn's disease. Indeed, NICE (2019b) and the Joint Formulary Committee (2020d) recommend both infliximab or adalimumab for severe Crohn's disease that is refractory to conventional treatment. Both drugs are licensed for use in Crohn's and ulcerative colitis. Infliximab is given intravenously and the patient is usually admitted to hospital as a day case, as they need to be observed for infusion-related reactions.

Acute pain management

Abdominal pain is a common reason for a visit to primary care or the Accident and Emergency department (A & E), as it is often a symptom of severe or life-threatening disorders such as cancer, acute intestinal obstruction and acute appendicitis. Misdiagnosis of abdominal pain may occur and, in some countries, is the subject of a large number of litigation cases brought against practitioners (Kachalia, Gandhi & Puopolo 2007). In some patients a diagnosis is not always attained, hence the term non-specific abdominal pain (NSAP). NSAP makes up 13–40% of all surgical admission with abdominal pain and is generally defined as acute abdominal pain of less than seven days' duration where no diagnosis is reached after both examination and extensive investigations (Sanders, Iman & Hurlstone 2006). The ultimate causes of NSAP can include gynaecological conditions, irritable bowel syndrome (IBS), gastroenteritis and abdominal wall pain.

An accurate history taken from the patient is generally the cornerstone of an accurate diagnosis. To facilitate a comprehensive assessment, the pain assessment method known by the acronym PQRST is used to prompt and obtain a holistic pain history from the patient. PQRST stands for positional, palliating, and provoking factors such as, quality, region, radiation referral, severity and temporal factors (such as time, mode of onset, progression and previous episodes). Once a history and pain assessment has been completed, it may not be possible to undertake a physical assessment until pain control has been achieved.

The World Health Organisation (WHO) pain ladder (1986) is a widely used and widely advocated step-wise approach to analgesia administration, starting with simple analgesics, followed by weak opioids and then strong opioids. The administration of opioid analgesics does not obscure the diagnosis or interfere with the treatment of the patient and does not affect diagnostic accuracy in patients with acute abdominal pain. For pre-existing abdominal conditions where a flare-up is considered, such as gallstones and pancreatitis, the patient may already identify successful analgesic therapies which do not follow the WHO (1986) approach. It is worth taking a patient-centric approach to pain management, including the consideration of existing therapies as well as the clinical consequences of polypharmacy.

Case study: Gastrointestinal conditions affecting drug absorption

Lavinia Adjei is 50 years old. She has suffered from hypertension and type 2 diabetes for the past four years. For these long-term conditions, she takes aspirin 75mg daily, enalapril 20mg daily, simvastatin 20mg every night and metformin 500mg three times a day. She was also diagnosed with Crohn's disease when she was 20 years old. This illness is usually well managed by diet alone and she has been in remission for the last 10 years. Investigations at that time confirmed distal iliac disease. Lavinia goes to the gym on a regular basis, does not drink alcohol but does smoke between 5 and 10 cigarettes per day, depending on her level of anxiety. Due to her recent promotion to a senior position in her company and the increased level of stress, her smoking has increased. She has also suffered a relapse of her Crohn's, with an average of 10 bowel movements each day, persistent bloody diarrhoea, abdominal cramps and weight loss.

She also noticed that when she carried out her usual home monitoring of her blood pressure and diabetes, both were out of control. On examination by her GP, Lavinia was anxious, pale with slight tenderness in her right iliac fossa. Rectal examination revealed no abnormalities. The GP discussed the use of prednisolone to manage Lavinia's clinical symptoms but she explained that during the last flare-up of her condition 10 years ago, she was unable to tolerate them as she constantly felt agitated and restless and her blood pressure and diabetes were not well controlled. In the light of her intolerance of conventional steroids, the GP prescribed another drug.

Activity 14.6 (Case study)

1. Why do you think Lavinia's diabetes and blood pressure, which were normally well controlled, should have become unstable at about the same time as her flare-up?
2. What alternative drug was prescribed for Lavinia instead of prednisolone?

Case study (continued)

The new drug worked well, and even after the dose was tapered down Lavinia's condition improved and remained stable. Lavinia asked her GP about her treatment options in order to remain in remission. This was discussed with Lavinia, as well as relevant lifestyle advice.

Activity 14.7 (Case study)

1. Outline the type of advice Lavinia should receive in order to help her make a decision about her plan of care.
2. Suggest two maintenance drugs that could be prescribed to help Lavinia remain in remission, and briefly outline their mechanism of action.
3. Briefly identify an important lifestyle change that Lavinia should try to address as soon as possible.

Summary

Gastrointestinal disorders, such as peptic ulcers, constipation, diarrhoea and inflammatory bowel conditions, are just a few of the most common conditions that the healthcare professional will come across either acutely or chronically.

It is hoped that this chapter has given some insight into the pharmacological principles that are necessary to prescribe safely for these conditions.

Answers to activities

Activity 14.1

1. Draw on your knowledge of the causes of GI bleeding and list five predisposing factors.

- Bacterial infection: A significant cause of peptic ulcer is the presence of *Helicobacter pylori* (*H. pylori*) in the stomach. The bacteria stimulate an increase in gastric acid production, which leads to ulcer formation.
- NSAIDs: These drugs block the action of cyclooxygenase (COX-1), which is important for the production of prostaglandins such as PGE2. PGE2 protects the mucosa from the damaging effects of gastric acid. Celecoxib is a selective COX-2 inhibitor and does not inhibit the production of gastroprotective PGs such as PGE2. It is therefore associated with a lower risk of peptic ulcer formation than non-COX-2 selective NSAIDs. All COX-2s are associated with cardiovascular risk.
- Smoking: The risk of peptic ulcer formation increases in the presence of *H. pylori*.
- Alcohol: The risk of peptic ulcer formation increases in the presence of *H. pylori*.
- Gastric tumour: Zollinger Ellison syndrome is a rare tumour that causes a significant increase in the production of gastrin, which results in hypersecretion of gastric acid.

Other factors that could increase the clinical signs and symptoms include spicy meals, stress, coffee, caffeine and eating habits.

2. Succinctly summarise the mechanism for NSAID-induced ulcers.

The non-selective NSAIDs cause peptic ulcers by blocking the synthesis of the protective gastrointestinal mucosal PGE2s. This is because they block both COX-1 and COX-2 enzymes, the former being the one that produces these protective prostaglandins. Remember, it is important to determine the role of prostaglandin in other parts of the body in order to understand the other adverse effects of the NSAIDs.

Activity 14.2

1. Can you suggest why Mr Burton is experiencing these symptoms since taking the antacids? How do you think the antacids may have caused these symptoms?

One likely cause is that the antacids have interfered with the absorption of Mr Burton's cardiac drugs, especially the angiotensin-converting inhibitor (ramipril). The most probable cause is the sodium content of the magnesium trisilicate (20ml qds = 48mmol sodium), which contributed to Mr Burton's oedema.

2. What specific advice would you offer Mr Burton?

The manufacturers of quinapril, trandolapril and moexipril caution that antacids may reduce the bioavailability of some ACEis but there is no evidence of this in practice. However, the manufacturers of fosinopril do suggest separating it from the administration of antacids by at least 2 hours.

If a patient's drug treatment fails or there is a suspected adverse effect, healthcare professionals should always exclude obvious causes such as other medications taken by the patient. Antacids interact with many important drugs, leading to treatment failure in these individuals. You should therefore ask the patient if they are taking an OTC drug such as an antacid.

In addition, individuals should always seek advice from the pharmacist before taking any OTC drugs, no matter how innocuous they may seem. Antacids are a major cause of adverse drug reactions and interactions.

For patients taking ramipril, the antacids should be taken after food if ramipril is taken before food.

Activity 14.3

1. Constipation commonly occurs in the elderly. Can you list common causes for constipation and suggest reasons why Mrs Green has become constipated?

Mrs Green's constipation may be due to immobility caused by the injury, a low fibre diet, the ageing process. Other general causes include: drugs, e.g. opiates, antidepressants; inadequate fluid intake, overuse of laxatives, disorders that affect bowel movements, e.g. hypocalcaemia, myxoedema, bowel lesions. Comprehensive history and abdominal examination are needed to exclude more serious causes.

2. What type of laxatives would you prescribe for Mrs Green? How will they be administered and can you briefly outline their mechanism of action?

Suggested options:
- Stimulants – good for short-term, quick relief
- Lactulose – takes 2–3 days for onset of action so undesirable
- Bulk formers – poor choice in the elderly; insufficient fluid intake.

She was prescribed senna tablets × 2 at night and a glycerin suppository on the following day was prescribed for her constipation. Senna increases motility of the gut wall by stimulating the nerve plexus. Glycerin suppositories stimulate nerve receptors in the gut wall.

3. What advice would you offer about taking antacids?

Avoid taking antacids, as these could interact with her current medication (digoxin) and reduce its effect. Antacids are known to reduce absorption. The high sodium content of these drugs could also exacerbate Mrs Green's hypertension. If antacids *are* taken, the patient's prescribed drug should be taken before a meal and the antacids after the meal. The healthcare professional should always exclude other causes, such as interactions with antacids or non-adherence, before increasing prescribed drug dosage.

4. What lifestyle advice would you discuss with Mrs Green?
Dietary advice should include small frequent meals, reducing spicy foods and alcohol intake, ways of improving mobility and increasing the amount of exercise. She should also seek advice from a healthcare professional before taking OTC drugs such NSAIDs and antacids.

Activity 14.4

1. Explain the mechanism of action of the triple therapy that was prescribed for Mrs Green.
Amoxicillin destroys the bacterial cell wall, while metronidazole inhibits bacterial nucleic acid synthesis. A combination of antibiotics is more effective in destroying the bacteria and also reduces the risk of resistance developing. Omeprazole is a proton pump inhibitor (PPI), which reduces acid formation. The combination effectively eradicates the *H. pylori* infection.

2. What advice would you give Mrs Green about taking the medication?
Advise her to complete the course of treatment and avoid taking alcohol with metronidazole, as it can produce unpleasant reactions like flushing, nausea, vomiting and tachycardia. The treatment is successful in most people (80%) but a few may require a second course. Some patients experience diarrhoea and stomach cramps during the course of the treatment. Mrs Green should inform her GP if this occurs. She may also need a PPI for a short time.

3. Can you identify four pharmacokinetic factors that could cause adverse drug reactions in older people? Refer back to Chapters 1 and 3.
Factors contributing to adverse drug reactions in the elderly include reduced first-pass hepatic metabolism, half-life of drugs prolonged, drug interactions and a loss in protein-binding sites.

Activity 14.5

What general measures would you recommend for the treatment of acute diarrhoea?
Drink as much as possible and continue to drink. Have a range of fluids, including water and soups, but avoid having drinks containing too much sugar and dairy products. Rehydration drinks are available from the chemist but are usually used for the elderly, the frail, infants and children, or people with other underlying disorders. Try to eat small, easily digestible meals. Continue to drink even if appetite is poor. If symptoms continue for more than 2 days or there are any signs of dehydration (such as confusion, dizziness, muscle cramps, or passing only a small amount of urine), consult your GP.

Activity 14.6 (Case study)

1. Why do you think Lavinia's diabetes and blood pressure, which were normally well controlled, should have become unstable at about the same time as her flare-up?
The explanation in this case is impaired absorption of enalapril and metformin, due to the damaged surface area of the small intestine caused by her Crohn's disease.

2. What alternative drug was prescribed for Lavinia instead of prednisolone?

The alternative drug was budesonide. Budesonide is a corticosteroid that suppresses the inflammatory process in Crohn's disease. It is not as effective as prednisolone but it does have fewer side effects. As Lavinia experienced a number of adverse effects when she was taking prednisolone, budesonide is an appropriate choice.

Activity 14.7 (Case study)

1. Outline the type of advice Lavinia should receive in order to help her make a decision about her plan of care.

She should be given verbal information about the types of drugs used to maintain remission and their side effects. This should be supported by written information. Whether she uses drugs or not, there is a risk that the inflammatory flare-ups could worsen. A plan of care should be put in place regardless of the decision Lavinia makes. This should include frequency of follow-up appointments, how to recognise important symptoms of deterioration (e.g. weight loss, diarrhoea, abdominal pain) and how to access help at an early stage, contact details of support groups such as Crohn's and Colitis UK and a specialist irritable bowel syndrome (IBS) nurse. Lavinia's decision should also be respected, valued and documented.

2. Suggest two maintenance drugs that could be prescribed to help Lavinia remain in remission and briefly outline their mechanism of action.

Azathioprine or mercaptopurine can be used as maintenance medication (NICE 2019b). Both drugs are immunosuppressants. Azathioprine inhibits DNA synthesis in proliferating cells (T & B) of the immune system. Azathioprine is a prodrug, which is converted to mercaptopurine in the gut wall, liver and red blood cells. Adverse reactions include suppression of the bone marrow, which can lead to anaemia, and increases the patient's susceptibility to infections. Blood counts are monitored regularly.

3. Briefly identify an important lifestyle change that Lavinia should try to address as soon as possible.

Smoking cessation should be discussed with Lavinia. Emphasise that research has shown that there is less chance of a Crohn's relapse if she stops smoking, as conversely smoking appears to be beneficial in ulcerative colitis. Nutritional advice should be a high-fibre/low-residue diet.

References and further reading

Chodhury, S. (2006). Exploring the science of laxatives: mechanism and mode of action. *Nurse Prescribing.* **4** (3), 107–12.

Dial, S., Alrasadi, K. & Manoukian, C. (2002). Risk of Clostridium difficile diarrhoea among hospital inpatients prescribed proton pump inhibitors: cohort and case-control studies. *Canadian Medical Association Journal.* **171**, 33–38.

Ford, A.C., & Talley, N.J. (2012). Laxatives for chronic constipation in adults. *British Medical Journal.* **345**, e6168.

Forootan, M., Bagheri, N. & Darvishi, M. (2018). Chronic constipation. A review of literature. *Medicine.* **97**, 20.

Frolkis, A.D., Vallerand, I.A., Shaheen, A.-A., et al. (2019). Depression increases the risk of inflammatory bowel disease, which may be mitigated by the use of antidepressants in the treatment of depression. *Gut.* **68**, 1606–12.

Global Burden of Disease (GBD) (2019). The global, regional, and national burden of inflammatory bowel disease in 195 countries and territories, 1990–2017: a systematic analysis for the Global Burden of Disease Study 2017. *Lancet: Gastroenterology and Hepatology.* **5**, 17–30. https://www.thelancet.com/action/showPdf?pii=S2468-1253%2819%2930333-4 (Last accessed 22 October 2020).

Gotfried, J. (2020). Chronic Abdominal Pain and Recurring Abdominal. MSD Manual. https://www.msdmanuals.com/home/digestive-disorders/symptoms-of-digestive-disorders/chronic-abdominal-pain-and-recurring-abdominal-pain (Last accessed 22 October 2020).

Greenstein, B. & Gould, D. (2008). *Trounce's Clinical Pharmacology for Nurses.* London: Churchill Livingstone, Elsevier.

Joint Formulary Committee (2020a). *British National Formulary.* https://bnf.nice.org.uk/treatment-summary/antacids.html (Last accessed 22 October 2020).

Joint Formulary Committee (2020b). *British National Formulary.* https://bnf.nice.org.uk/treatment-summary/peptic-ulcer-disease.html (Last accessed 22 October 2020).

Joint Formulary Committee (2020c). *British National Formulary.* https://bnf.nice.org.uk/treatment-summary/constipation.html (Last accessed 22 October 2020).

Joint Formulary Committee (2020d). *British National Formulary.* https://bnf.nice.org.uk/treatment-summary/crohns-disease.html (Last accessed 22 October).

Kachalia, A., Gandhi, T.K. & Puopolo, A.L. (2007). Missed and delayed diagnoses in the emergency department: a study of closed malpractice claims from 4 liability insurers. *Annals of Emergency Medicine.* **49** (2), 196–205.

Kumar, A., Ashwlayan, V. & Verma M. (2019). Diagnostic approach and pharmacological treatment regimen of Peptic Ulcer Disease. *Pharmacy and Pharmaceutical Research Open Access Journal.* **1** (1) 1–11.

Lamb, C.A., Nicholas, A., Kennedy, R.T., Hendy, P.A., Smith, P.J., Limdi, J.K., et al. (2019). *British Society of Gastroenterology consensus guidelines on the management of inflammatory bowel disease in adults.* doi:10.1136/gutjnl-2019-318484 https://www.ncbi.nlm.nih.gov/pubmed/31562236 (Last accessed 22 October 2020).

Lanas, A. & Chan, F.K.L. (2017). Peptic ulcer disease. *Lancet.* **390** (10094), 613–24. doi: 10.1016/S0140-6736(16)32404-7.

Mikocka-Walus, A., Pittet, V., Rossel, J.B. & von Kanel, R. (2016). Symptoms of depression and anxiety are independently associated with clinical recurrence of inflammatory bowel disease. *Clinical Gastroenterology and Hepatology.* **14**, 829–35.

National Institute for Health and Care Excellence (NICE) (2013). Acute upper intestinal bleeding. (QS38). http://www.nice.org.uk/guidance/QS38 (Last accessed 22 October 2020).

National Institute for Health and Care Excellence (NICE) (2019a). Gastro-oesophageal reflux disease and dyspepsia in adults: investigation and management (CG 184). https://www.nice.org.uk/guidance/cg184/ifp/chapter/Peptic-ulcer. (Last accessed 22 October 2020).

National Institute for Health and Care Excellence (NICE) (2019b). Crohn's disease: management (NG129), https://www.nice.org.uk/guidance/ng129/resources/crohns-disease-management-pdf-66141667282885 (Last accessed 22 October 2020).

National Institute for Health and Care Excellence (NICE) CKS (2020), Ulcerative colitis: Summary. https://cks.nice.org.uk/ulcerative-colitis#!topicSummary (Last accessed 22 October 2020).

Neal, M.J. (2012). *Medical Pharmacology at a Glance.* 7th edn. London: Wiley Blackwell.

Rang, H.P., Dale, M.M., Ritter, J.M., Flower, R.J. & Henderson, G. (2012). *Pharmacology.* Edinburgh: Churchill Livingstone, Elsevier.

Sanders, D.S., Iman, A.F. & Hurlstone, D.P. (2006). A new insight into Non-Specific Abdominal Pain. *Annals of the Royal College of Surgeons of England.* **88** (2), 92–94. doi: 10.1308/003588406X85751

Tortora, G.J. & Derrickson, B.H. (2016). *Principles of Anatomy and Physiology.* 15th edn. US: John Wiley & Sons.

Wongrakpanich, S., Wongrakpanich, A., Melhado, K. & Rangaswami, J. (2018). A comprehensive review of Non-steroidal Anti-Inflammatory Drug use in the elderly. *Aging and Disease.* **9** (1), 143–50.

World Health Organisation (WHO) (1986). *Cancer Pain Relief.* Geneva, Switzerland: World Health Press.

World Health Organisation (WHO) (2013). Diarrhoeal disease [online] Fact sheet No 3330. http://www.who.int/mediacentre/factsheets/fs330/en/ (Last accessed 22 October 2020).

15

Pharmacological case studies: Urinary incontinence in adults

Alison Harris MSc, BSc (Hons), RN, DipDN, PGCertHE, Registered Practice Educator, Community Practitioner Nurse Prescriber. Senior Lecturer, Health & Education, Middlesex University, London

This chapter:

- Outlines the common causes of urinary incontinence
- Describes the holistic assessment required before making a prescribing decision
- Discusses the drugs available to treat urinary incontinence, their pharmacological actions and adverse effects
- Develops and applies knowledge of drugs used in the treatment of urinary incontinence

Introduction

Urinary incontinence is the complaint of involuntary leakage of urine (International Continence Society 2020). It needs no definition beyond this except that which the individual gives as to how it affects their daily activities, ability to cope and well-being. Studies on the general population have demonstrated that urinary incontinence has a profound impact on the quality of an individual's life (Kwon, Kim, et al. 2010). In the UK, 14 million men, women and young people are estimated to suffer with bladder-related problems of differing severity (Buckley & Lapitan 2009). The prevalence of urinary incontinence increases with age, and the figure increases further for those over the age of 70 and those in nursing homes (Milsom & Gyhagen 2019). This chapter will explore the pharmacological treatments available for some of the most common types of urinary incontinence: stress urinary incontinence, urgency urinary incontinence and the overactive bladder, and mixed urinary incontinence.

Overview of approach to management

The clinician's aim in managing urinary incontinence is to maximise the potential for a return to effective bladder control and continence. In conditions where the renal tract is susceptible to damage, the aim is to protect the kidneys (Pannek, Stöhrer, et al. 2012). For maximum efficacy, drug therapy is usually used alongside non-pharmacological modalities, such as bladder retraining or pelvic floor exercises. This approach also promotes patient empowerment and increases the likelihood of possible future withdrawal of the drug. Pharmacological treatment should be started at the lowest dose and titrated, with regular review, either until care goals are met or until adverse effects become intolerable.

Before prescribing, the clinician should review the whole picture. The Royal Pharmaceutical Society (RPS) Competency Framework for all Prescribers (2016) explicitly states that the prescriber is responsible for their prescribing decision. That decision must follow a well-conducted assessment and therefore, as stipulated by the RPS Framework, only those clinicians with a clear understanding of the causes and management options for urinary incontinence should be prescribing for this group. Prescribers have a responsibility to ensure that they reach a shared decision with the patient or carer prior to any treatment (RPS 2016). Shared decision-making also upholds the principle of informed consent and safeguards the patient's preferences and cultural values in any decisions made about their treatment. This includes being made aware of the associated side effects and any prescribing data. Putting patients at the centre of the prescribing decision means establishing the effect incontinence has on their life, and getting a clear idea of their expectations of treatment, as well as their health beliefs.

Some conditions that contribute to urinary incontinence, including urinary tract infection, diabetes and Parkinson's disease, require a complex and integrated plan of care. Nurse prescribers should be alert to the importance of a well-conducted assessment, which may include a symptom profile and a measure of any residual urine, and the possibility that a prescription may not always be the necessary clinical outcome. A multi-agency approach to care, as laid down in the RPS Prescribing Competency Framework (RPS 2016), is essential to providing ethical, effective, safe, patient-centred, holistic care.

Activity 15.1

Reflect on the individuals you have cared for with continence difficulties and list the causes of urinary incontinence.

Continence physiology

The maintenance of continence can be thought of in two phases: the storage phase and the voiding phase. In order to store urine, the healthy adult bladder is able to hold approximately 300–400ml (Lukacz, Sampselle, et al. 2011). The autonomic (sympathetic and parasympathetic) and the somatic nervous systems control the storage and voiding functions of the bladder.

The detrusor muscle is a layer of the urinary bladder that is made up of smooth muscle. As the bladder distends, the excitatory effect on the parasympathetic nerves results in a contraction of the bladder. This is only one part of the mechanism. For voiding to take place, the involuntary controlled internal sphincter and the somatic and voluntary controlled external sphincter must simultaneously relax and open. In some neurological diseases, such as multiple sclerosis, this coordinated action does not occur. In such cases, individuals can experience urgency and urinary retention as the bladder contracts but simultaneous contraction of the urethral sphincter prevents micturition. Conversely, incontinence can result from an involuntary relaxation of the urethral sphincter. This uncoordinated response is known as bladder-sphincter dyssynergia.

The storage of urine requires a suppression of bladder contractions and inactivity of the sphincters. Any damage to the innervation of the bladder and its supporting structures can cause urinary incontinence (see Figure 15.1).

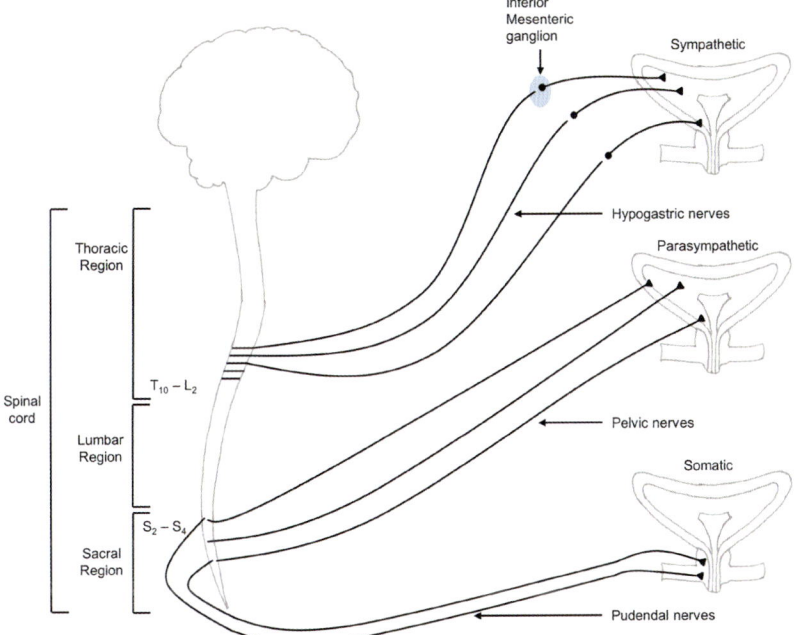

Figure 15.1: The innervation of the lower urinary tract

Neurotransmitters

Acetylcholine (ACh) is one of several neurotransmitters that have an effect on the bladder. ACh acts on muscarinic receptors, which are located on the detrusor smooth muscle, leading to a synchronised and sustained contraction of the bladder. Acetylcholine that binds to muscarinic receptors found in the bladder presents the greatest opportunity for pharmacological treatment specifically in the overactive bladder, as anticholinergic drugs (also called antimuscarinics) that interfere with the receptor binding can supress bladder contractility, and reduce urgency and urge urinary incontinence.

Muscarinic receptors are located throughout the body. By studying where in the body the antimuscarinic drugs take their effect, the nurse prescriber can understand why many of the side effects of drugs with anticholinergic properties occur. Examples of unwanted side-effects resulting from anticholinergic medication include: dry mouth, blurred vision, constipation, dry eyes, urinary retention, tachycardia and confusion.

> ## Activity 15.2
> 1. Outline, in some detail, the role of the neurotransmitter acetylcholine in producing a bladder contraction.
> 2. Consider how interference with the neurotransmitter may affect bladder control.

Types of urinary incontinence

Stress urinary incontinence

In people who have damage to the urethral sphincter (for example, after childbirth or post-prostatectomy), the sphincter cannot remain sufficiently contracted under provocation such as coughing or exercising. Stress urinary incontinence (SUI) occurs when, in the absence of a detrusor contraction, the pressure inside the bladder exceeds the urethral closing pressure, and the individual experiences an involuntary loss of urine. Characteristically, urine loss is small and continence is restored after the exertion has stopped.

According to Opara and Czerwinska-Opara (2014), SUI affects 20–25% of the European female population over the age of 20. However, differing definitions and diagnosis of SUI, as well as differing sampling strategies, give rise to discrepancies in prevalence (Bedretdinova, Fritel, et al. 2016).

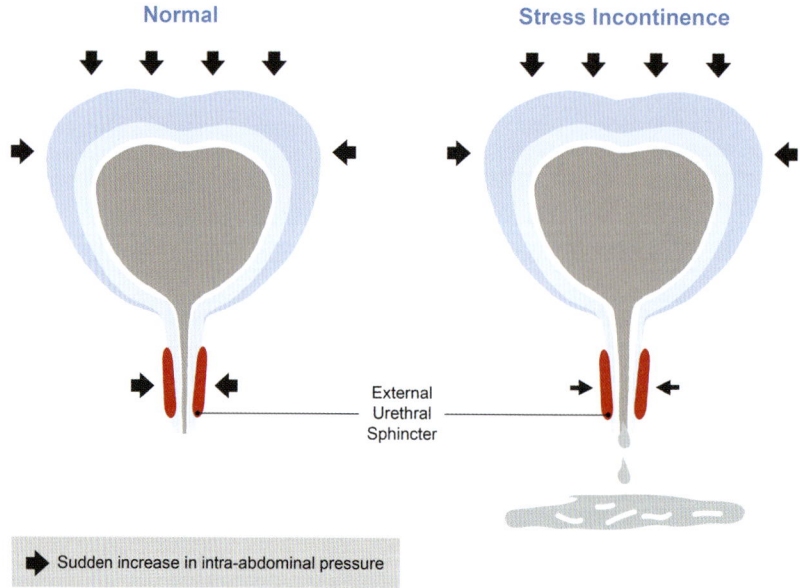

Figure 15.2: Stress urinary incontinence.

Urgency urinary incontinence and the overactive bladder

The overactive bladder (OAB) is known to predominate in the elderly but it can affect all ages (Buckley & Lapitan 2009; Irwin, Milsom, et al. 2006). The overactive bladder gives rise to involuntary bladder contractions that can result in an urgent desire to void. If the individual is unable to either inhibit the urge or to reach the toilet in time, an episode of urge urinary incontinence (UUI) may result. Some sufferers report complete emptying of the bladder.

In the frail elderly, most notably where there is impaired mobility or dexterity, urgency can have a catastrophic impact on their ability to be continent. Urgency has been independently associated with an increased risk of falls and fractures in older women (Brown 2000).

Individuals experiencing increased daytime frequency, nocturia (voiding one or more times at night) and urgency, with or without incontinence, and in the absence of a urine infection, should be considered for treatment.

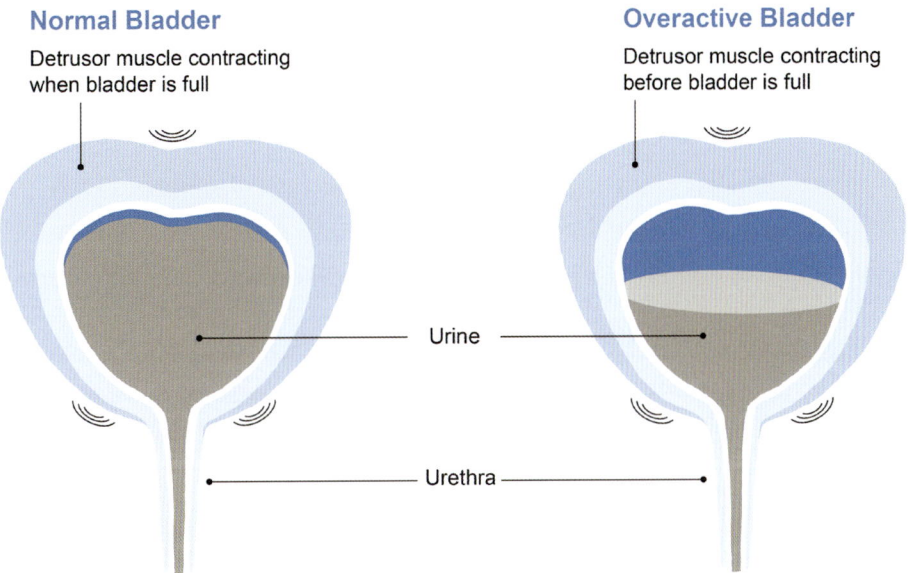

Figure 15.3: Urge urinary incontinence.

Mixed urinary incontinence

Patients with symptoms of involuntary leakage associated with urgency and exertion, effort, coughing or sneezing are said to have mixed incontinence. In such cases, management and treatment should be aimed at those symptoms that the individual identifies as being most troublesome (NICE 2019).

Assessing incontinence

Prior to instigating pharmacological treatments, nurse prescribers need to perform a structured consultation with their client. Past medical and surgical history and current drug regimens (including over-the-counter, internet-purchased and complementary remedies) must be recorded; any allergies and previous adverse drug events must also be noted (RPS 2016).

A holistic continence assessment in women should include checking the perineum for atrophic vaginitis and prolapse. If competent, a cough test to demonstrate stress urinary incontinence can be performed, as well as urinalysis to eliminate the possibility of a urinary tract infection (UTI) and assessment for post-void residual urine. A pelvic floor muscle assessment should be performed or be requested by the competent assessor. In men the assessment is guided by the urological symptoms. If there are symptoms of an outflow obstruction, or if the man is concerned about prostate cancer, he should be referred to a specialist where the physical examination will include a digital rectal examination (NICE 2015).

Furthermore, a thorough and close questioning approach to bowel habits, an assessment of fluid intake (both type and quantity) and the impact of the incontinence on the individual will facilitate a thorough assessment. Obesity is a risk factor for incontinence. Anyone with a BMI greater than 30 should be advised of this and encouraged to lose weight (NICE 2019; Subak, Wing, et al. 2009).

A urinary symptom profile will elucidate the frequency of micturition, nocturia, number of incontinent episodes and the amount of urinary loss. For any cause urinary incontinence, individuals should be directed to keep a bladder diary for a minimum of three days to aid diagnosis and to evaluate therapy (NICE 2019, NICE 2015).

UTIs are a common cause of sudden onset urinary incontinence. UTI should therefore be the first consideration when anyone reports a recent history of urinary incontinence. Presenting symptoms can be similar to those of an overactive bladder and the person may also report dysuria, haematuria, lower abdominal and loin pain and be febrile. The detection of leucocytes with nitrites on dipstick, in the symptomatic patient, is confirmation of a UTI and prescribers are directed to collecting a mid-stream urine sample and prescribing an appropriate course of antibiotics pending microscopy and culture results (NICE 2018, NICE 2019, Gray & Malone-Lee 1995).

Microscopic haematuria, and either dysuria or a raised white cell count on blood test in patients aged over 60, and any findings of macroscopic haematuria, should be referred to specialist services. Microscopic haematuria in the over-45s (where it is unexplainable, persistent or where UTIs are recurring) should also be referred (NICE 2017). Other abnormalities in the presenting history, including severe prolapse (protruding below the introitus), previous history of pelvic cancer, bladder pain, post-void residual urine greater than 100ml and neurological dysfunction, require urgent referral to a specialist (NICE 2019, ICS 2020). In men, post-void residual urine should be assessed and the patient referred to a specialist if an enlarged prostate is suspected (NICE 2015).

Any abnormalities should be addressed and followed by a review of lower urinary tract symptoms. Multi-professional team working is important in facilitating clinical care pathways, including referral to specialist services and key clinical investigations. The International Continence Society has produced a glossary of terminology to standardise definitions and care pathways (ICS 2020) and these are further supported by NICE guidance (NICE 2018, NICE 2019). Nurse prescribers should refer to these guidelines to ensure prescribing is evidence based.

Pharmacological management of stress urinary incontinence

This section, based on information in the online BNF (Joint Formulary Committee 2020), discusses the major classes of drugs used to treat urinary incontinence. It is assumed that nurse prescribers will be referring to the monograph in the BNF when making clinical decisions pertaining to drugs used in urinary incontinence. Cautions and contraindications for drugs listed are readily available in the online BNF.

Care protocols advise as to the benefit of trying non-pharmacological as well as pharmacological therapies prior to any surgical intervention for the treatment of stress urinary incontinence (SUI). Supervised pelvic floor exercises, following digital assessment of the strength and duration of a pelvic floor contraction, are a first-line therapy for SUI and should be trialled for a minimum of three months prior to beginning pharmacological therapy (NICE 2018, NICE 2019). Men who have failed to respond to conservative methods may require a referral to specialist services (NICE 2018).

Duloxetine

Duloxetine is primarily used for the treatment of major depressive disorders and it is the only pharmacological preparation available in the UK for the treatment of SUI in women. The efficacy of duloxetine in SUI is based on inhibiting the re-uptake of the neurotransmitters serotonin and norepinephrine. It is suggested that this leads to an increased concentration of the neurotransmitter, enhanced stimulation of the receptors and a marked increase in the tone of the 'guarding' reflex of the external urethral sphincter. This guarding reflex prevents voiding that is initiated by coughing and sneezing. Duloxetine has also been found to have some effect on increasing bladder capacity (Jost & Marsalek 2005).

Studies on duloxetine in women with SUI have reported up to a 50% reduction in incontinence episodes (Mariappan, Alhasso, *et al.* 2007). However, duloxetine prescribed for SUI has also been found to have a high discontinuation rate due to patients experiencing adverse effects (Maund, Schow, *et al.* 2017). Duloxetine is not recommended as first-line therapy for SUI and is to be offered as second-line therapy only to women who prefer to avoid or are not suitable for surgery (NICE 2019). All women need to be counselled about the potential side effects, with nausea and sexual dysfunction being the most common. In line with the RPS Framework, nurse prescribers must ensure that they prescribe medications only within their scope of practice and they must counsel women about the potential side effects (RPS 2016, NICE 2019).

There is evidence that a combination of pelvic floor exercises with duloxetine is more efficacious than duloxetine alone (57% reduction in incontinence episodes with combination therapy, compared with 35% reduction with pelvic floor exercises alone) (Ghoniem, Van Leeuwen, et al. 2005).

Oestrogen

Atrophic vaginitis does not in itself cause urinary incontinence; and oestrogen hormone replacement therapy is no longer a recommended treatment for SUI (NICE 2019).

Pharmacological management of overactive bladder (OAB) symptoms

Antimuscarinic drugs

The first line of treatment for individuals presenting with symptoms of OAB is a programme of behavioural interventions, for up to 12 weeks, including modification of high or low fluid intake, caffeine reduction, weight reduction if appropriate and supervised bladder retraining (NICE 2019).

Bladder retraining involves over-riding the sensation to void, thus enhancing the ability to inhibit micturition and to increase bladder capacity. Antimuscarinics (sometimes called anticholinergics) have been the mainstay of OAB drug treatment for many years. Current preparations have been found to be similarly efficacious, when used as monotherapies, with varying degrees of adverse effects (Hsu, Chandler, et al. 2019; Chapple, Khullar, et al. 2008). These drugs reduce symptoms of urgency and urge urinary incontinence, decrease detrusor overactivity, reduce frequency and increase bladder capacity.

Antimuscarinic drugs can also reduce bladder contractility by blocking the muscarinic receptors on the smooth-muscle membranes of the detrusor muscle. When administered in higher doses, antimuscarinics can diminish detrusor contractility and sometimes cause urinary retention. However, urgency and frequency are recognised as sensory symptoms of OAB. Antimuscarinics have an effect on these sensory symptoms and research has studied the role of the afferent (sensory) innervation of the bladder lining, the urothelium, and the mode of action of antimuscarinics on the urothelium (Smith & Wein 2010, Andersson 2004). The bladder urothelium releases acetylcholine and, in turn, the neurotransmitter adenosine triphosphate or ATP (a coenzyme used as an energy carrier in all cells), both in response to increasing bladder distention. ATP acts on purinergic receptors (membrane receptors that mediate relaxation of smooth muscle as a response to the release of ATP) on afferent nerve terminals, providing a link with acetylcholine and helping to establish a sensory mechanism of action for antimuscarinic drugs.

When assessing for the pharmacological agent of choice, the nurse prescriber will be guided by the history-taking and symptom profile and by local and national guidelines. NICE guidelines (2019) recommend that the first choice of anticholinergics for OAB should be the drug with the lowest acquisition cost. If first-line treatment does not work, offer another drug with a low acquisition cost. Transdermal medication can be offered to individuals who are unable to tolerate oral medication (NICE 2019). For maximum efficacy, anticholinergics should be taken in conjunction with bladder retraining and fluid modification (NICE 2019; Burgio, Locher & Goode 2000).

The annual cost of antimuscarinics can be reduced by ensuring the lowest-cost drug is prescribed and the effectiveness and tolerability of the drug is regularly reviewed (NHS PrescQIp, 2014).

Nurse prescribers will be aware of the concomitant effect of taking other drugs with anticholinergic or antimuscarinic properties, and manufacturers will recommend that time intervals are allowed when changing antimuscarinics. With antimuscarinics, patients should be informed that the drug may take four weeks to have any therapeutic benefit and be made aware of the common side effects – dry mouth, constipation and headaches. Antimuscarinic drugs can cause adverse cardiac events such as tachycardia (Shaukat, Habib, *et al.* 2014). While these side effects may be merely bothersome in the younger and healthier population, they can be serious in those with underlying heart complaints. The BNF therefore advises that all antimuscarinic drugs should be used with caution in older adults and in adults with cardiac disease, including those with acute myocardial infarction, arrhythmias, autonomic neuropathy, cardiac insufficiency, cardiac surgery and congestive heart failure.

Adherence to drugs used to treat OAB has been shown to be poor, due to the side effects. A study from a UK general practice found that less than 25% of patients continued on their prescribed medication (Wagg, Foley, *et al.* 2017). Therapeutic failure can be averted by regularly reviewing both the condition and the prescribed treatment. In drugs with known debilitating and unpleasant side effects, the prescription should be reviewed at regular intervals, and the prescriber should be prepared to discontinue or alter the treatment. This approach further supports the nurse prescriber in delivering care that is acceptable to the patient and is cost-effective.

Activity 15.3

1. Drawing on your knowledge of pharmacodynamics (see Chapter 2), what is meant by an antagonist drug?
2. Explain why the action of an antagonist drug is not permanent.

Oxybutynin hydrochloride

Oxybutynin is a competitive antagonist for M1, M2 and M3 muscarinic receptors. When oxybutynin binds to the muscarinic receptors, it prevents their activation and has a relaxant effect on the smooth muscle of the bladder. However, it also produces a range of side effects and for some patients these adverse events make the drug intolerable. Oxybutynin is available in immediate-release (IR) and modified-release (MR) forms.

The most commonly reported side effect from this group of drugs is a dry mouth (M1 and M3 receptors), constipation (M2 and M3 receptors), headache and dry eyes (M3 and M5 receptors). Immediate-release oxybutynin 7.5–15mg a day (as well as propiverine extended-release 20mg a day and solifenacin 10mg a day) are significantly associated with a risk of withdrawal from treatment due to side effects (Madhuvrata, Cody, et al. 2012; Chapple, Khullar, et al. 2008). Starting patients on a low dose and titrating after 2–4 weeks can aid adherence.

Oxybutynin crosses the blood–brain barrier with resulting cognitive adverse events, specifically in children and the frail elderly; and the BNF advises caution (Andersson 2004). Consideration should be given to the frail elderly, where cerebrovascular disease may alter the permeability of the blood–brain barrier or where alterations in the elimination of the drugs may cause accumulation and toxicity. Immediate-release oxybutynin is therefore not to be prescribed for older women who may be at risk of a sudden deterioration in their physical or mental health (NICE 2019). The nurse prescriber, following their NMC-approved programme of study, will be alert to the need for a holistic assessment, including mental health, a comprehensive reassessment before repeat prescribing and the pharmacological differences required when prescribing for these special groups.

As well as being available in immediate-release and modified-release forms, oxybutynin is also licensed as a transdermal. The nurse prescriber should scrutinise each patient for idiosyncratic and expected side effects and therapeutic response. Consideration of the mode of action, the duration of action and the potential side effects, as well as the cost and likely adherence to treatment, will all inform the prescribing decision.

Activity 15.4

With reference to your knowledge of pharmacokinetics, what advantages might the transdermal patch of oxybutynin have over the oral form in promoting patient adherence? (See Chapter 2.)

Activity 15.5

1. Some of the antimuscarinics can cross the blood–brain barrier. What are the properties of a drug that would make them more likely to cross the blood–brain barrier?
2. What symptoms could be reported as adverse side effects in a drug that was able to cross the blood–brain barrier?
3. Why might some anticholinergic drugs produce unwanted side effects?

Tolterodine tartrate

Tolterodine has no specific selectivity for muscarinic receptors but is claimed to have selectivity for the bladder over the salivary glands. Tolterodine is rapidly absorbed and has a half-life of 2–3 hours. It also undergoes first-pass metabolism and its metabolite is very similar (in its pharmacokinetic action) to the parent compound and contributes significantly to the drug's therapeutic action. Tolterodine is not very lipophilic so it cannot cross the blood–brain barrier. Adverse effects on the central nervous system (CNS) are therefore unlikely (Andersson 2004).

Tolterodine is available as IR or MR. A daily 4mg dose of the MR preparation has been found to be the most effective (Chapple, Khullar, et al. 2008). Tolterodine has been shown to have similar outcomes to oxybutynin and solifenacin for incontinence due to OAB. However, tolterodine has a significantly higher incidence of a dry mouth than mirabegron but a lower incidence of a dry mouth than oxybutynin (Hsu, Chandler, et al. 2019). In clinical practice, studies showing comparable data between antimuscarinic drugs enable the prescriber to offer patients an informed choice.

Fesoterodine fumarate

Fesoterodine is rapidly metabolised to 5-hydroxymethyltolterodine (5-HMT), the same primary active metabolite of tolterodine. While the two drugs have similar antimuscarinic activity, fesoterodine has fewer cognitive side-effects (Smith & Wein 2010). Both drugs have lipophilic properties that could enhance their ability to penetrate the blood–brain barrier. However, fesoterodine appears to have less CNS penetration due to its larger molecular size. Like tolterodine, this compound is a non-subtype-selective muscarinic receptor antagonist (Smith & Wein 2010).

Fesoterodine is comparable to solifenacin in reducing OAB symptoms (urgency, frequency and nocturia) but more people discontinue fesoterodine (compared to solifenacin), due to its adverse side effects. When compared with tolterodine, there is some evidence that patients, who have achieved continence, favour fesoterodine. However, side effects of a dry mouth and constipation again appear to be higher (Hsu, Chandler, et al. 2019).

Trospium chloride

Trospium chloride, like tolterodine, has no selectivity for any of the muscarinic receptors. Its bioavailability is low. Like tolterodine, it does not cross the blood–brain barrier and seems to have no negative cognitive effects. It is not metabolised and is renally excreted in unchanged form (Andersson 2004). In a systematic review, trospium has been found to be comparably efficacious with darifenacin in reducing OAB symptoms, and both drugs had a similar side effect of constipation (Manjunatha, Purushotama, et al. 2015).

> ### Activity 15.6
> 1. Some of the antimuscarinic agents are metabolised by the cytochrome P450 enzyme. Drawing on your knowledge of these important metabolising enzymes, explain the effect of the cytochrome P450 enzyme (see Chapter 1).
> 2. List some of the drugs or foods that could interfere with the metabolism of the antimuscarinic agents.

Propiverine hydrochloride

Propiverine combines antimuscarinic action and inhibition of calcium influx in the smooth muscle of the urinary bladder, causing reduced bladder contractility and an increase in bladder capacity.

It is almost completely absorbed from the gastrointestinal tract, and plasma concentrations are largely unaffected by food. It undergoes extensive first-pass metabolism and the resulting metabolites are thought to contribute to the efficacy of the drug (eMC Summary of Product Characteristics).

Prescribers are reminded always to assess for allergies to foods as well as medicines, as individuals with an allergy to the colouring agent cochineal should be advised to avoid this drug.

Darifenacin

Darifenacin was developed to deliver greater selectivity of the M3 receptors that are responsible for contractions of the detrusor. Darifenacin is primarily metabolised by the cytochrome P450 enzymes, CYP2D6 and CYP3A4. A low starting dose is recommended, as well as careful observation when doses are titrated up. Darifenacin undergoes a high first-pass metabolism and bioavailability is low (eMC Summary of Product Characteristics).

Solifenacin succinate

Solifenacin has some competitive selectivity for M3 receptors. It is well absorbed from the gastrointestinal tract and undergoes hepatic first-pass metabolism involving the cytochrome P450 group of enzymes.

Combination therapy, involving solifenacin and mirabegron, have resulted in significant improvements in OAB symptoms and specifically with the number of urgency episodes. This is a significant finding, as prescribers should be considering symptom relief that enhances quality of life (Gratzke, Van Maanen, et al. 2018). Solifenacin, given as single therapy, compares favourably with mirabegron in reducing the frequency of micturition (Hsu, Chandler, et al. 2019).

Mirabegron

Some individuals find they have a sub-optimal response to antimuscarinic drugs and/or they find the side effects intolerable. This can limit the clinician's prescribing options. A different class of drug, mirabegron, has proven beneficial in treating OAB symptoms. Mirabegron stimulates the β³-adrenoceptors, which are found in the urothelium, leading to a relaxation of the bladder, and subsequent improved compliance and filling, and delayed micturition (Nitti, Khullar, et al. 2013).

Mirabegron has also been found to reduce the number of incontinent episodes and the frequency of micturition, as well as the predominant side effect of a dry mouth, when compared to tolterodine (Khullar, Amarenco, et al. 2013).

Mirabegron may be prescribed in combination with an antimuscarinic. Improvements in the patient's symptoms of urgency and frequency have been observed when mirabegron has been combined with solifenacin (Gratzke, van Maanen, et al. 2018).

Oestrogen

Oestrogen deficiency may be a factor in urinary incontinence. Systemic oestrogens are contraindicated in the treatment of urinary incontinence, with the risk of serious adverse effects (including carcinoma) and some suggestion that it may worsen incontinence. However, there is some evidence that intravaginal oestrogens are indicated for short-term use in post-menopausal women who present with vaginal atrophy. They have been found to improve the vaginal epithelium and reduce frequency, nocturia and urgency (Cody, Jacobs, et al. 2012). The nurse prescriber may therefore offer intravaginal oestrogens to treat symptoms of the overactive bladder (urgency, frequency and nocturia) in postmenopausal women with vaginal atrophy (NICE 2019).

Drugs that can cause or exacerbate bladder dysfunction

Drugs can affect continence status by acting directly on the lower urinary tract, by increasing urinary output, by inducing constipation and by impairing cognition, which may lead to functional type incontinence.

Table 15.1: Types of drugs that can cause or exacerbate bladder dysfunction

Drug type	Side effects/potential effects on continence status	Effects on continence status
Acetylcholinesterase inhibitors, e.g. donepezil hydrochloride	• Increase bladder overactivity	• Urgency and urge incontinence
Antihistamines, e.g. cetirizine hydrochloride	• Antimuscarinic action • Sedation	• Urinary retention • Urinary function
Antipsychotics, e.g. olanzapine	• Reduce bladder contractions • Constipation • Confusion	• Urinary retention • Urinary function
Benzodiazepines, e.g. diazepam	• Sedation	• Urinary function

(table continued overleaf)

Table 15.1 continued

Drug type	Side effects/potential effects on continence status	Effects on continence status
Beta-adrenergic antagonists, e.g. propranolol	• Contraction of urethral sphincter	• Urinary retention
Diuretics, e.g. furosemide	• Increase diuresis	• Exacerbation of urgency, frequency, nocturia
Opioid analgesics, e.g. morphine	• Constipation • Reduce bladder contractions • Confusion	• Urinary retention • Urinary function
Selective alpha blockers, e.g. prazosin	• Relax bladder outlet	• Stress urinary incontinence
Selective serotonin re-uptake inhibitors (SSRIs), e.g. citalopram	• Antimuscarinic properties, with reduced contractility of the bladder	• Urinary retention
Tri-cyclic antidepressants, e.g. amitriptyline	• Antimuscarinic action • Sedation	• Urinary retention • Urinary function
Caffeine and alcohol	• Increase diuresis • Increase bladder overactivity	• Exacerbation of urgency, frequency and nocturia

Case study: Mixed urinary incontinence

Mrs Lorraine Parks is 62 years old, married and works as a secondary school teacher. She presents for help after an episode of severe (self-evaluated) urinary incontinence while out for dinner with her husband, their 30-year-old son and his wife. This was a devastating and humiliating occurrence.

Presenting symptoms are severe urgency (a sudden, compelling desire to pass urine which is difficult to defer), urgency urinary incontinence (1–2 times per week) and urinary leakage on coughing. On closer questioning, she has a diurnal frequency of 10–15 voids a day (on average we may expect a daytime frequency of 7 voids) and nocturia, getting up usually twice in the night to void (once a night is acceptable). Other symptoms include a strong desire to void, and sometimes incontinence, just as she nears home, 'the key in the door syndrome'.

Menopause occurred at 52 years, and the urgency and urgency urinary incontinence became notable around this time. Lorraine has three children, who were all vaginal deliveries. She reports that slight stress urinary incontinence initially occurred after her first delivery.

She has no other past medical history. She takes no prescription drugs, does not buy any herbal or over-the-counter remedies, denies taking any recreational drugs and reports no allergies.

She weighs 65kg, is a non-smoker and drinks one to two glasses of wine most evenings. She reports regular bowel movements. Urinalysis is negative. A post-void bladder scan reveals no residual urine.

The nurse prescriber ascertains that the most bothersome symptom for Lorraine is the urgency urinary incontinence.

Activity 15.7 (Case study)

Bearing in mind Lorraine's identification of the most bothersome urinary incontinence symptom, what would be your choice of first-line management for her?

Activity 15.8

Oxybutynin is an antimuscarinic. With reference to their pharmacological properties, describe how antimuscarinics can lead to the side effects of dry mouth and constipation.

Case study (continued)

At Lorraine's 12-week follow-up appointment, she has reduced her frequency to 8–12 times a day, with behavioural interventions, but the urgency and urge incontinence persist. Recently an incontinent episode resulted in total bladder emptying. At this point, Lorraine could be offered the choice of continuing with behavioural modalities or starting medication. Lorraine has expressed a preference for medication.

Activity 15.9 (Case study)

In view of Lorraine's expressed wish to try pharmacological treatment for the urgency and urge incontinence, what will your prescribing decision be?

Summary

Within almost every domain of healthcare, within every speciality, someone is likely to present with urinary incontinence. Prescribers treating someone for urinary incontinence may find that they are prescribing for an underlying condition (such as obesity, constipation or a UTI), for a long-standing complaint of incontinence or for short-term relief until behavioural methods prove effective (as in primary nocturnal enuresis).

The pharmacological management of urinary incontinence significantly benefits individuals who suffer from this common and distressing condition. There are a range of agents for treating OAB available to the prescriber, such as mirabegron, solifenacin and darifenacin. They offer the patients choice and a more flexible dosing regimen and enhanced titration. Nurse prescribers must adhere to the RPS Competency Framework (2016), ensuring that patients are given access to non-pharmacological interventions and are fully involved in any prescribing decisions, including information on any common side effects.

Answers to activities

Activity 15.1

Reflect on the individuals you have cared for with continence difficulties and list the causes of urinary incontinence.

Urinary incontinence has been standardised, based on patient's symptoms, by the International Continence Society (2020) as follows:

- Urgency urinary incontinence is the complaint of involuntary loss of urine associated with urgency. Causes: overactive bladder, neurological condition, UTI.
- Stress urinary incontinence is the complaint of involuntary loss of urine on effort or physical exertion, including sporting activities, or on sneezing or coughing. Causes: childbirth, multiple and traumatic vaginal deliveries, instrumentation (e.g. repeated cystoscopy), total prostatectomy, obesity, straining (including a chronic cough).
- Mixed urinary incontinence is the complaint of both stress and urgency urinary incontinence, i.e. involuntary loss of urine associated with urgency and also with effort or physical exertion (including sporting activities) or on sneezing or coughing.

Causes not discussed in this chapter:

- Nocturnal enuresis is the complaint of involuntary voiding that occurs at night during the main sleep period (i.e. bedwetting). Causes: OAB, lack of waking in response to sensation of a full bladder, insufficient production of vasopressin responsible for concentrating urine at night, increased diuresis (as may be seen after diuretics or on raising oedematous legs when in bed).
- Post-micturition incontinence is the complaint of a further involuntary passage of urine following the completion of voiding. Cause: A weakness of the pelvic floor muscles; may be associated with erectile dysfunction (Yang & Lee 2019).

- Overflow incontinence is the complaint of urinary incontinence in the symptomatic presence of an excessively (over-)full bladder (no cause identified). Possible underlying causes: any obstruction of the urethra including an enlarged prostate, urethral stricture, vaginal prolapse, chronic constipation, tumour. Reduced contractility of the bladder caused by denervation of the bladder, as may be found in diabetes or some neurological conditions (ICS 2020).

Activity 15.2

1. Outline, in some detail, the role of the neurotransmitter acetylcholine in producing a bladder contraction.

During the bladder filling and storage phase, there is a release of acetylcholine (ACh). When released from the cholinergic nerve terminals, ACh binds to the muscarinic receptors in the detrusor to produce an effect. There are five muscarinic receptors found in the bladder (M1 to M5). It is believed that M2 is involved in bladder relaxation and it is the M3 receptor that is mainly responsible for the bladder contraction.

2. Consider how interference with the neurotransmitter may affect bladder control.

It is understood that the release of ACh may increase in overactive bladder syndrome and current antimuscarinic drugs thus have a role to play in treating the condition. By blocking the action of the neurotransmitter ACh, the bladder will be less contractile. Symptoms of overactivity, including frequency, urgency and nocturia, will therefore be reduced.

Activity 15.3

1. Drawing on your knowledge of pharmacodynamics (see Chapter 2), what is meant by an antagonist drug?

Antagonist drugs that competitively bind to receptors prevent agonists thus binding and so hinder the action of that receptor.

2. Explain why the action of an antagonist drug is not permanent.

The duration of action of an antagonist depends on the antagonist-receptor complex, and the action of an antagonist may or may not be reversible. Strong competition from an agonist, either one that is naturally occurring or a drug, may remove the antagonist from the receptor.

Activity 15.4

With reference to your knowledge of pharmacokinetics, what advantages might the transdermal patch of oxybutynin have over the oral form in promoting patient adherence? (See Chapter 2.)

The oral form of oxybutynin undergoes significant first-pass metabolism and it is its active metabolite that exerts the greatest effect. It has a plasma half-life of 2 hours. This can vary significantly between individuals. The transdermal patch avoids first-pass metabolism and needs reapplying just twice weekly, delivering continuous therapeutic levels of the active drug. Transdermal delivery of oxybutynin has been found to significantly decrease the number of incontinence episodes and to significantly increase the average voided volume.

Activity 15.5

1. Some of the antimuscarinics can cross the blood–brain barrier. What are the properties of a drug that would make them more likely to cross the blood–brain barrier?

Lipophilic drugs are more likely to cross the blood–brain barrier. Lipophilic drugs are fat soluble (as opposed to hydrophilic drugs, which are water soluble). Lipophilic drugs can more readily diffuse across cell membranes.

2. What symptoms could be reported as adverse side effects in a drug that was able to cross the blood–brain barrier?

Adverse side effects of an antimuscarinic drug that was able to cross the blood–brain barrier might include somnolence, sedation and confusion.

3. Why might some anti-cholinergic drugs produce unwanted side effects?

There are five types of muscarinic receptors located throughout the body. For example, acetylcholine, acting as a neurotransmitter in the heart, causes the rate and intensity of the heartbeat to decrease. Oxybutynin is frequently prescribed to treat urinary urge incontinence. Oxybutynin is a muscarinic receptor antagonist, inhibiting the binding of the acetylcholine and preventing it exerting its effect of initiating a bladder contraction. Thus, while the therapeutic calming effect of oxybutynin (an antimuscarinic drug), on the overactive bladder is a desirable outcome, the drug's wider distribution may allow it to become attached to the predominant M2 receptors in the heart, causing an unwanted and adverse reaction of palpitations.

Activity 15.6

1. Some of the antimuscarinic agents are metabolised by the cytochrome P450 enzymes. Drawing on your knowledge of these important metabolising enzymes, explain the effect of the cytochrome P450 enzymes (see Chapter 1).

Metabolism inactivates drugs or breaks them down into their active metabolites. The cytochrome P450 enzymes are part of a large group of enzymes involved in the metabolism of drugs. Two enzymes from this group, CYP3A4 and CYP2D6, are responsible for metabolising most drugs. Genetic variability in these enzymes can influence an individual's response to certain drugs, causing varying adverse events or treatment failure. Drugs can act to induce or inhibit the enzyme. Drugs that induce the enzyme will increase metabolism. Those that inhibit the enzyme will reduce metabolism. Dose, and the ability of a drug to bind to the enzyme, will determine the extent of the effect. Propiverine is a weak inhibitor of cytochrome P450, and mild interactions would be expected with other drugs metabolised by the enzymes with minimal increases in drug concentrations.

2. List some of the drugs or foods that could interfere with the metabolism of the antimuscarinic agents.

Darifenacin is primarily metabolised by the cytochrome P450 enzymes, CYP3A4 and CYP2D6. Therefore inhibitors of these enzymes may potentiate the antimuscarinic effect – for example, paroxetine, grapefruit juice and erythromycin. Solifenacin is metabolised by CYP3A4 and simultaneous administration of a potent CYP3A4 inhibitor (such as ketoconazole) is known to significantly increase the potency of solifenacin. Nurse prescribers should be alert to the need to reduce the dose of solifenacin when it is given with potent inhibitors such as ritonavir or itraconazole

Activity 15.7 (Case study)

Bearing in mind Lorraine's identification of the most bothersome urinary incontinence symptom, what would be your choice of first-line management for her?

Lorraine could be started on a 12-week course of non-invasive modalities, including keeping a bladder diary (for a minimum of three days), bladder retraining (holding on past the first desire to void) and caffeine reduction.

Activity 15.8

Oxybutynin is an antimuscarinic. With reference to their pharmacological properties, describe how antimuscarinics can lead to the side effects of dry mouth and constipation.

Oxybutynin is a competitive antagonist for M1, M2 and M3 muscarinic receptors. Antagonist drugs that competitively bind to receptors thus prevent agonists binding and so hinder the action of that receptor. However, muscarinic receptors are located throughout the body, including the salivary gland and the gastrointestinal tract. The most commonly reported side effect of this group of drugs is a dry mouth (M1 and M3 receptors) and constipation (M2 and M3 receptors).

Activity 15.9 (Case study)

In view of Lorraine's expressed wish to try pharmacological treatment for the urgency and urge incontinence, what will your prescribing decision be?

Lorraine could be started on a 12-week course of a first-line antimuscarinic – one with the lowest cost, such as oxybutynin IR, 5mg twice daily. If tolerated, this can be increased to 5mg 3 times daily, after 4 weeks, and to a maximum of 5mg 4 times daily if effective and side effects are tolerated. She should be advised to contact the prescriber if she experiences any adverse and intolerable side effects. Continuing bladder retraining will augment the effect of the antimuscarinic.

References and further reading

Andersson, K.E. (2004). Antimuscarinics for treatment of overactive bladder. *The Lancet Neurology*. **3**, 46–53.

Bedretdinova, D., Fritel, X., Panjo, H. & Ringa, V. (2016). Prevalence of female urinary Incontinence in the general population according to different definitions and study designs. *European Urology*. **69** (2), 256–64.

Brown, J.S. (2000). Urinary incontinence: Does it increase risk for falls and fractures? *Journal of the American Geriatric Society*. **48** (7), 721–25.

Buckley, B.S. & Lapitan, M.C.M. (2009). Prevalence of urinary and faecal incontinence and nocturnal enuresis and attitudes to treatment and help seeking amongst a community-based representative sample of adults in the United Kingdom. *International Journal of Clinical Practice*. **63** (4), 568–73.

Burgio, K.l., Locher, J.L. & Goode, P.S. (2000). Combined behavioural and drug therapy for urge incontinence in older women. *Journal of the American Geriatric Society*. **48**, 370–74.

Chapple, C.R., Khullar, V., Gabriel, Z., Muston, D., Bitoun, C.E. & Weinstein, D. (2008). The effects of antimuscarinic treatments in overactive bladder: an update of a systematic review and meta-analysis. *European Urology*. **54**, 543–62.

Cody, J.D., Jacobs, M.L., Richardson, K., Moehrer, B. & Hextall, A. (2012). Oestrogen therapy for urinary incontinence in post-menopausal women. Cochrane database, Systematic Review. Oct 17.

eMC, electronic Medicines Compendium, Summary of Product Characteristics. https://www.medicines.org.uk/emc (Last accessed 27 October 2020).

Ghoniem, G.M., Van Leeuwen, J.S., Elser, D.M., Freeman, R.M., Zhao, Y.D., Yalcin, I. & Bump, R.C. (2005). A randomized controlled trial of duloxetine alone, pelvic floor muscle training alone, combined treatment, and no active treatment in women with stress urinary incontinence. *Journal of Urology*. **173**, 1453–54.

Gratzke, C., van Maanen, R., Chapple, C., Abrams, P., Herschorn, S., Robinson, D., Ridder, A., Stoelzel, M., Paireddy, A., Yoon, S.J., Al-Shukri, S., Rechberger, T. & Mueller, E.R. (2018). Long-term safety and efficacy of mirabegron and solifenacin in combination compared with monotherapy in patients with overactive bladder: a randomised, multicentre phase 3 study (SYNERGY II). *European Urology*. **74** (4), 501–509. Doi: 10.1016/j.eururo.2018.05.005.

Gray, R.P. & Malone-Lee, J. (1995). Review: Urinary tract infection in elderly people – Time to review management. *Age and Ageing*. **24**, 341–45.

Hsu, F., Chandler, E.W., Selph, S.S., Blazina, I., Holmes, R.S. & McDonagh M.S. (2019). Updating the evidence on drugs to treat overactive bladder: a systematic review. *International Urogynecology Journal*. **30**, 1603–17. doi: 10.1007/s00192-019-04022-8

International Continence Society (ICS) (2020). ICS Glossary of Terminology. https://www.ics.org/glossary (Last accessed 27 October 2020).

Irwin, D.E., Milsom, I., Reilly, K., Hunskaar, S., Kopp, Z., Herschorn, S., Coyne, K.S., Kelleher, C.J., Hampel, C., Artibani, W. & Abrams, P. (2006). Population-based survey of urinary incontinence, overactive bladder and other lower urinary tract symptoms in five countries: results of the EPIC study. *European Urology*. **50** (6), 1306–14.

Joint Formulary Committee (2020). British National Formulary Online. https://bnf.nice.org.uk/treatment-summary/urinary-incontinence-and-pelvic-organ-prolapse-in-women.html (Last accessed 27 October 2020).

Jost, W.H. & Marsalek, P. (2005). Duloxetine in the treatment of stress urinary incontinence. *Therapeutics and Clinical Risk Management*. **1** (4), 259–64.

Khullar, V., Amarenco, G., Angulo, J.C., Cambronero, J., Høye, K., Milsom, I., Radziszewski, P., Rechberger, T., Boerrigter, P., Drogendijk, T., Wooning, M. & Chapple, C. (2013). Efficacy and tolerability of mirabegron, a b3-adrenoceptor agonist, in patients with overactive bladder: Results from a Randomised European–Australian Phase 3 Trial. *European Urology*. **63**, 283–95.

Kwon, B.E., Kim, G.Y., Son, Y.J., Roh, Y.S. & You, M.A. (2010). Quality of life of women with urinary incontinence: A systematic literature review. *International Urology Journal*. **14** (3), 133–138. doi: 10.5213/inj.2010.14.3.133

Lukacz, E.S., Sampselle, C., Gray, M., MacDiarmid, S., Rosenberg, M., Ellsworth, P. & Palmer, M.H. (2011). A healthy bladder: a consensus statement. *International Journal of Clinical Practice*. **65** (10), 1026–1036. doi:10.111/j.1742-1241.2011.02763.x

Manjunatha, R., Purushotama, H., Hanumantharaju, B.K. & Anusha, S.J. (2015). A prospective, comparative study of the occurrence and severity of constipation with darifenacin and trospium in overactive bladder. *Journal of Clinical and Diagnostic Research*. **9** (3), FC055-9. doi:10.7860/JCDR/2015/11884.5677.

Mariappan, P., Alhasso, A., Ballantyne, Z., Grant, A. & N'Dow, J. (2007). Duloxetine, a serotonin and noradrenaline reuptake inhibitor (SNRI) for the treatment of stress urinary incontinence: A systematic review. *European Urology*. **51**, 67–74.

Maund, E., Schow Guski, L. & Gøtzsche, P.C. (2017). Considering benefits and harms of duloxetine for stress urinary incontinence: a meta-analysis of clinical study reports. *Canadian Medical Association Journal*. **189** (5), E194-E203

Milsom, I. & Gyhagen, M. (2019). The prevalence of urinary incontinence. *Climacteric*. **22** (3), 217–22. https://doi.org/10.1080/136971 37.2018.1543263 (Last accessed 27 October 2020).

Monz, B., Chartier-Kastler, E., Hampel, C., Samsioe, G., Hunskaar, S., Espuna-Pons, M., Wagg, A., Quail, D., Castrol, R. & Chinn, C. (2007). Patient characteristics associated with quality of life in European women seeking treatment for urinary incontinence: results from PURE. *European Urology*. **51** (4), 1073–81.

Madhuvrata, P., Cody, J.D., Ellis, G., Herbison, G.P. & Hay-Smith, E.J.C. (2012). Which anticholinergic drug for overactive bladder symptoms in adults? *Cochrane Systematic Review – Intervention*. 18 January. https://doi.org/10.1002/14651858.CD005429.pub2 (Last accessed 27 October 2020).

National Institute for Health and Care Excellence (NICE) (2015). Lower urinary tract symptoms in men: management. https://www.nice.org.uk/guidance/cg97 (Last accessed 27 October 2020).

National Institute for Health and Care Excellence (NICE) (2017). Suspected cancer: recognition and referral. https://www.nice.org.uk/guidance/ng12/ (Last accessed 27 October 2020).

National Institute for Health and Care Excellence (NICE) (2018). Urinary tract infection (lower); antimicrobial prescribing. https://www.nice.org.uk/guidance/ng109/ (Last accessed 27 October 2020).

National Institute for Health and Care Excellence (NICE) (2019). Urinary incontinence and pelvic organ prolapse in women: management. https://www.nice.org.uk/guidance/ng123/ (Last accessed 27 October 2020).

NHS England (2018). Excellence in Continence Care: Practical guidance for commissioners, and leaders in health and social care. https://www.england.nhs.uk/wp-content/uploads/2018/07/excellence-in-continence-care.pdf (Last accessed 27 October 2020).

NHS PrescQIPP (2014). Drugs for urinary frequency, enuresis and incontinence. Bulletin 58. https://www.prescqipp.info/media/1719/b58-urinary-incontinence-20.pdf (Last accessed 27 October 2020).

Nitti, V.W., Khullar, V., Kerrebroeck, P., Herschorn, S., Cambronero, J., Angulo, J.C., Blauwet, M.B., Dorrepaal, C., Siddiqui, E. & Martin, N.E. (2013). Mirabegron for the treatment of overactive bladder: a prespecified pooled efficacy analysis and pooled safety analysis of three randomised, double-blind, placebo-controlled, phase III studies. *International Journal of Clinical Practice*. **67** (7), 619–32.

Opara, J. & Czerwińska-Opara, W.E. (2014). The prevalence of stress urinary incontinence in women studying nursing and related quality of life. *Menopause Review*. **13** (1), 32–35.

Pannek, J., Stöhrer, M., Blok, B., Castro-Diaz, D., Del Popolo, G., Kramer, G., Radziszewski, P., Reitz, A. & Wyndaele, J.J. (2012). Guidelines on neurogenic lower urinary tract dysfunction. *European Association of Urology*. https://uroweb.org/wp-content/uploads/20_Neurogenic-LUTD_LR.pdf (Last accessed 27 October 2020).

Royal Pharmaceutical Society (RPS) (2016). A Competency Framework for all Prescribers. https://www.rpharms.com/resources/frameworks/prescribers-competency-framework (Last accessed 27 October 2020).

Shaukat, A., Habib, A., Lane, K.A., Shen, C., Khan, S., Hellman, Y.M., Boustani, M. & Malik, A.S. (2014). Anticholinergic medications: An additional contributor to cognitive impairment in the heart failure population? *Drugs and Aging*. **31** (10), 749–54. Doi: 10.1007/s440266-014-0204-2.

Shaw, C., Gupta, R.S., Bushnell, D.M., Assassa, R.P., Abrams, P., Wagg, A., Mayne, C., Hardwick, C. & Martin, M. (2006). The extent and severity of urinary incontinence amongst women in UK GP waiting rooms. *Family Practice*. **23**, 497–506.

Smith, A.L. & Wein, A.J. (2010). Recent advances in the development of antimuscarinic agents for overactive bladder. *Trends in Pharmacological Sciences*. **31** (10), 470–75.

Subak, L.L., Wing, R., Smith West, D., Franklin, F. & Vittinghoff, E. (2009). Weight loss to treat urinary incontinence in overweight and obese women. *New England Journal of Medicine*. **360** (5), 481–90.

Wagg, A.S., Foley, S., Peters, J., Nazir, J., Kool-Houweling, L. & Scrine, L. (2017). Persistence and adherence with mirabegron vs antimuscarinics in overactive bladder: retrospective analysis of a UK general practice prescription database. *International Journal of Clinical Practice*. **71** (10). doi: 10.1111/ijcp.12996.

Yang, D.Y. & Lee, W.K. (2019). A current perspective on post-micturition dribble in males. *Investigative and Clinical Urology*. **60** (3), 142–47.

16

Pharmacological case studies: Diabetes

Alison Harris
MSc, BSc (Hons), RN, DipDN, PGCertHE, Registered Practice Educator,
Community Practitioner Nurse Prescriber.
Senior Lecturer, Health & Education, Middlesex University, London

This chapter:

- Explains how to diagnose and classify diabetes
- Recognises that anti-diabetic agents, alongside diet and exercise, are vital to the management of hyperglycaemia in type 2 diabetes in order to reduce the burden of complications
- Considers the pharmacology of oral and injectable anti-diabetic agents available for prescribing in type 2 diabetes
- Applies knowledge of anti-diabetic agents to practice-based case studies.

Introduction

Diabetes, with its associated health complications and links with obesity and lifestyle, has now become a public health issue. The World Health Organisation (WHO) estimated worldwide prevalence, in 2014, to be 422 million (WHO 2019), with 80% of the cases found in low- and middle-income countries (International Diabetes Federation 2019). In the United Kingdom, there are 3.8 million known cases and if the incidence continues to rise, this figure will reach 5 million by 2025 (Diabetes UK 2018). The increasing prevalence of younger age groups with type 2 diabetes is a cause for concern.

Nurse prescribers will be involved in managing people with diabetes, either prescribing directly to control blood glucose or as part of a wider treatment plan to manage and control complications as outlined below. This chapter looks at all the oral and injectable anti-diabetic agents available to nurse prescribers for the management of hyperglycaemia in type 2 diabetes, for use as monotherapy, dual or triple combination.

Insulin production and resistance

Energy use is continuous but our intake of energy (in the form of food) is intermittent. Excess fuel taken in with a meal must be stored for subsequent use in between meals. The liver is the main organ responsible for ensuring that circulating blood glucose levels are maintained at 4–7mmol/l. Glucose is laid down in the liver as glycogen; when blood sugars drop to below 4mmol/l, glycogen is converted to glucose (glycogenolysis). Glycogenolysis is hormonally regulated by insulin and its counter-regulatory enzyme, glucagon, which is produced in the alpha cells of the Islets of Langerhans and unaffected in diabetes. In a 'fight or flight' response, or in a period of fasting, non-carbohydrates (including amino acids) are converted to glucose, chiefly in the liver and to a much lesser extent in the kidneys and intestine, through a process called gluconeogenesis. This process will become important when considering the mode of action of some anti-diabetic drugs.

Insulin is a hormone (produced in the beta cells of the pancreas) that acts as a transporter, carrying glucose into the cells of the body, where the glucose is converted into energy. Glucose is the main stimulator of insulin release from the beta cells, and glucose levels below 4mmol/l do not induce insulin release. Once released, insulin binds to the receptors found on the cell membranes in skeletal muscle, adipose tissue and the liver.

In type 2 diabetes, receptors on the cell membranes initially become less sensitive to the effects of insulin (insulin resistance), resulting in high circulating levels of insulin (hyperinsulinaemia), which are harmful. Obesity and insufficient exercise contribute to a lack of sensitivity to insulin. As the disease progresses, so beta cells decline and insulin synthesis is reduced. The resulting hyperglycaemia and hyperinsulinaemia give rise to a range of complications.

Diagnosis and classification of diabetes

The term 'diabetes' describes a group of metabolic disorders characterised and identified by the presence of hyperglycaemia in the absence of treatment. The aetio-pathology for all types of diabetes (see Table 16.1) includes defects in insulin secretion, insulin action, or both. Furthermore, due to the role that insulin plays, disturbances are seen in the regulation of carbohydrate, fat and protein metabolism. All forms of diabetes are characterised by the dysfunction or the destruction of the pancreatic beta cells. Genetic and environmental factors play a role in the progressive loss of the beta cells (WHO 2019, American Diabetes Association 2019).

The World Health Organisation (WHO), and the American Diabetes Association (ADA), while not consensual, are at the forefront of deciding on the terminology to be used in the classification and diagnosis of diabetes. The WHO reclassified the types of diabetes in 2019, primarily because of the growing body of research that now considers that there is a blurring between the two distinct groups: type 1 diabetes (T1D) and type 2 diabetes (T2D). There are now a significant number of adults presenting with T1D (previously thought to affect only the under-25s), and there has been a marked growth in the numbers of children with T2D (previously thought to affect mostly the over-45s and obese individuals). Furthermore, science has advanced to identify sub-groups of diabetes and therefore the nomenclature has changed.

Table 16.1 brings together the terminology agreed by NICE and Diabetes UK and incorporates the newer classification from the WHO and the ADA. The nurse prescriber caring for individuals with diabetes will need to adopt the classification and diagnostic criteria that are accepted in their practice setting.

Table 16.1: Types of diabetes

Types of diabetes (NICE 2019)	**Brief description**
Type 1 diabetes	• Beta cell destruction (mostly immune-mediated) and absolute insulin deficiency; onset most common in childhood and early adulthood. • Two or more islet auto-antibodies are predictors for developing T1D
Type 2 diabetes	• Most common type; various degrees of beta cell dysfunction and insulin resistance; commonly associated with being overweight and obese
Changes in terminology in classifying diabetes (WHO 2019, ADA 2019)	
Diabetes during pregnancy	• Hyperglycaemia that presents in pregnancy; may have been present pre-conception and should be managed as T2D (T1D is rarely detected during antenatal check) • Managed as gestational diabetes if the hyperglycaemia is at the low end of the diagnostic threshold for diabetes detected during pregnancy (hyperglycaemia is managed with insulin during pregnancy until normoglycaemia returns after delivery and women will then require lifelong screening)
Slowly evolving, immune-mediated diabetes of adults	• Similar to slowly evolving T1D in adults but more often has features of the metabolic syndrome, a single GAD auto-antibody* and retains greater beta cell function • Other characteristics are: individual is older than 35 years at diagnosis; and insulin therapy is not required in the first 6–12 months after diagnosis

(table continued overleaf)

Table 16.1 continued

Changes in terminology in classifying diabetes (WHO 2019, ADA 2019)	Brief description
Slowly evolving, immune-mediated diabetes of adults	• In the UK, the category of latent auto-immune diabetes in adults (LADA) is still used (Diabetes UK 2020) • The ADA and the WHO recognise that this is a slowly evolving form of type 1 diabetes and have therefore abandoned the term LADA
Ketosis-prone type 2 diabetes	• Presents with ketosis and insulin deficiency but after treatment with insulin the beta cells recover, there is remission and further insulin is not required • Characteristically there are further episodes of ketosis. • There is no evidence of auto-immunity or genetic markers
Monogenic diabetes	• Monogenic diabetes was previously called maturity-onset diabetes of the young (MODY) and this term is still in use in the UK (Diabetes UK 2020) • It is caused by a single inherited mutated gene • This is a rare form of the condition that requires specialist diagnosis and treatment
Neonatal diabetes	• Seen in children diagnosed with diabetes in the first 6 months of life • They should have immediate genetic testing
Other classified types of diabetes; all requiring specialist management	• Cystic fibrosis-related diabetes; OGGT testing required; treat with insulin
	• Some drugs or chemicals are known to impair insulin secretion or action or to destroy beta cells (e.g. glucocorticoids, HIV treatment)
	• Unclassified diabetes is a temporary diagnosis when the presenting condition does not fit into any category

*In type 1 diabetes, a number of auto-antibodies are thought to circulate, including those which target glutamic acid decarboxylase (GAD). A GAD test is a blood test that measures whether the body is producing a type of antibody that destroys its own GAD cells.

Most patients are classified as having type 1 or type 2 diabetes. Type 1 diabetes mellitus (T1D) is an autoimmune disorder characterised by loss of the insulin-producing pancreatic beta cells in genetically predisposed individuals, ultimately resulting in insulin deficiency and hyperglycaemia. T1D is most common among children and young adults, and its incidence is rising across the world. A common characteristic of T1D is the presence of multiple auto-antibodies and, in the pre-symptomatic phase, individuals may, if tested, have raised fasting plasma glucose (Insel, Dunne, *et al.* 2015). Progression varies according to age of onset and number and types of auto-antibodies. As blood glucose rises, those newly diagnosed with T1D, will present with diabetic ketoacidosis. This form of diabetes accounts for 5–10% of the total diabetes population (ADA 2019).

Type 2 diabetes (T2D) is the most prevalent form and accounts for 90–95% of all diabetes. T2D is defined as a relative insulin deficiency with insulin resistance (ADA 2019). Risk factors for T2D include ageing, a sedentary lifestyle and obesity, ethnicity (South Asian, Middle Eastern or African-Caribbean), hypertension and a history of gestational diabetes. There is a genetic predisposition or family history in a first-degree relative with T2D, more so than for T1D (ADA 2019).

Type 2 diabetes can go undetected for many years, as blood glucose slowly and insidiously rises and the complications of hyperglycaemia may already be manifest at diagnosis (ADA 2019). Treatment includes diet, lifestyle modifications and anti-diabetic medication and, as diabetes is a progressive disorder, eventually insulin may be required.

Gestational diabetes is a further classification applied to women who did not clearly have diabetes prior to conception and who are assessed as having developed diabetes for the first time during pregnancy. Gestational diabetes is a risk factor for developing type 2 diabetes later in life.

In addition to a diagnosis of diabetes, there is a recognised phase of glucose regulation impairment, determined by people with a glycated haemoglobin (HbA1c) of 39–47mmol/mol (5.7–6.4%). A category of impaired glucose tolerance (IGT) is given when an oral glucose tolerance test (OGTT) is in the range of 7.8–11mmol/l. A diagnosis of impaired fasting glycaemia (IFG) follows a fasting glucose of 5.6–6.9mmol/l. These impaired glucose values can be explained to patients as 'putting them at a high-risk of developing diabetes' (ADA 2019). Patients should also be made aware that IGT and IFG are risk factors for cardiovascular disease and therefore need to be managed by the nurse prescriber and the wider team, and through behavioural changes that the individual must be encouraged to make.

Earlier studies have demonstrated that for individuals with impaired glucose regulation, tight glycaemic control (with diet alone or with the addition of metformin) can reduce the risk of progression to type 2 diabetes by up to 58% (Tuomilehto, Lindström, *et al.* 2001; Diabetes Prevention Program Research Group 2002). Furthermore, the 'legacy effect', of tight glycaemic control very early after diagnosis, has a lasting effect on the micro- and macro-vascular complications of diabetes (Laiteerapong, Ham, *et al.* 2019; Lindström, Peltonen, *et al.* 2013). The fruition of these diabetes prevention and reduction of complications studies is now being seen in prevention programmes and screening tools across the globe with the NHS Diabetes Prevention Programme, which identifies those at high risk and refers them to behavioural change programmes (NHS England 2020).

A diagnosis of diabetes should be made in the presence of a recognisable symptom or symptoms (such as polyuria, polydipsia, blurred vision and unexplained weight loss) and if plasma glucose levels are raised (as set out in Table 16.2). If the individual does not present with any recognisable symptoms, but has risk factors such as obesity or a familial history of diabetes, then two blood tests are required, on separate days, preferably using the same test (WHO 2019). Recently, the American Diabetes Association has recommended screening for pre-diabetes or T2D in women who are overweight or obese and/or who have one or more risk factors for diabetes and are planning a pregnancy (ADA 2019).

The nurse prescriber needs to work collaboratively to empower their patients who may have risk factors for developing diabetes in the future, but whose current blood glucose values do not show that they have hyperglycaemia.

Furthermore, early diagnosis and effective treatment can reduce the many complications of diabetes. Diabetes can potentially stigmatise people in such areas as employment and travel. Support and self-help strategies are necessary to promote well-being and good diabetic control.

The most commonly used test for the management of diabetes is the glycated haemoglobin, or HbA1c, test. This test indicates the amount of glucose carried by the haemoglobin and can therefore indicate the blood glucose levels for the previous two to three months. In some diseases that reduce red cell lifespan (for example, sickle cell disease or thalassaemia), the HbA1c test may be invalid. Fructosamine estimation, plasma glucose profiles or total glycated haemoglobin estimation can then be used (NICE 2019). HbA1c results, sometimes combined with self-monitoring of blood glucose, will inform prescribing decisions.

Table 16.2: Methods and criteria for diagnosing diabetes mellitus (WHO 2019)

Random venous plasma glucose	> 11.1mmol/l
Fasting plasma glucose	> 7.0mmol/l (whole blood > 6.1mmol/l)
Oral glucose tolerance test (OGGT), 2-hour post 75mg oral glucose	> 11.1mmol/l
HbA1c	> 48mmol/mol (6.5%)

Complications of diabetes

Undiagnosed or poorly managed diabetes mellitus is characterised by a triage of symptoms associated with rising blood sugars, of polydipsia, polyuria and, notably in T1D, weight loss. Other commonly reported symptoms of unmanaged hyperglycaemia may include recurring infections, non-healing of wounds, blurred vision and lethargy.

Left untreated, hyperglycaemia will eventually lead to a life-threatening ketoacidosis or hyperglycaemic hyperosmolar state (severe hyperglycaemia without ketones present). The treatment of diabetes is aimed at reducing circulating glucose levels and preventing or reducing the complications of diabetes.

The long-term complications of diabetes can be divided into microvascular and macrovascular. While not the focus of this chapter, the pharmacological management of blood glucose, blood pressure, dyslipidaemia and weight control are all very important in reducing the burden of diabetes. (See Chapters 9 and 10 for discussion of the pharmacological management of lipids and hypertension.)

Microvascular complications are closely related to hyperglycaemia. The most common microvascular complication is retinopathy, with potential loss of vision. The United Kingdom Prospective Diabetes Study (UKPDS) was a highly influential study of micro- and macro-complications in type 2 diabetes. This study found that a 1% reduction in glycated haemoglobin (HbA1c) equates to a 31% reduction in retinopathy (Kohner, Aldington et al. 1998). The UKPDS also found that a 10mmHg reduction in systolic blood pressure led to significant improved outcomes in retinal diabetic disease. The legacy effect of good glycaemic and blood pressure control early in the disease has been demonstrated and, when prescribing for this group, nurses should be alert to the evidence for establishing tight control early in the diagnosis (Laiteerapong, Ham, et al. 2019, ACCORD study 2008).

Diabetic nephropathy can be tracked in the diabetic population, from microalbuminuria to macroalbuminuria and on to renal failure. Furthermore, there is clear evidence of an increased risk of cardiovascular death with progressive diabetic nephropathy (Adler, Stevens, et al. 2003; Sasso, Chiodini et al. 2012). While diabetic nephropathy is the leading cause of end-stage renal failure, there is a greater likelihood that the individual with macroalbuminuria will succumb to a cardiovascular event. Both glycaemic and blood pressure control are important in preventing diabetic nephropathy.

Diabetes and hyperglycaemia can, over time and with advancing age and duration of diabetes, cause neuropathies. Nerve endings throughout the body can be affected, leading to a range of symptoms, including pain in legs and feet, diabetic ulcers, non-healing wounds leading to amputation, urinary and sexual dysfunction and difficulties in controlling blood pressure.

Individuals with diabetes may have dyslipidaemia, even with relatively good glycaemic control, as the usual role of insulin in regulating lipids is diminished. Raised triglyceride levels and reduced quantities of the vascular protective high-density lipoproteins are seen. There is a high incidence of arteriosclerosis seen in those with diabetes, with peripheral vascular, cardiovascular and cerebrovascular disease resulting from the extensive arterial plaques laid down. The vascular plaques are more unstable and prone to breaking free and thrombolytic cerebral vascular accident and myocardial infarction are associated with diabetes (Vergès 2015). Hypertension is a complication, as well as a risk factor, for diabetes and the nurse prescriber will be managing complex drug regimens in these groups of patients.

Prescribing for blood glucose, blood pressure and lipid control are the cornerstones of pharmacological management in type 2 diabetes (NICE 2019).

The management of type 2 diabetes

Current diabetes treatment is aimed at maintaining target blood glucose, blood pressure and lipid levels. Individual targets are determined, in conjunction with the individual's preferences, based on age, the duration of diabetes, any comorbidities, diabetes-related complications, and the number of hypoglycaemia events as well as any hypoglycaemia unawareness.

NICE sets a general HbA1c target of 6.5% (48mmol/mol) when diabetes is managed by a single drug that does not cause hypoglycaemia, e.g. metformin, and diet and lifestyle alone. When an individual is prescribed a drug that can cause hypoglycaemia, e.g. a sulfonylurea, or they are on two or more anti-diabetic drugs, the aim is for an HbA1c of 7.0% (53mmol/mol). However, the HbA1c may be higher, depending on the individual's target, their general health, the number of oral anti-diabetic drugs they are taking and their risk of hypoglycaemia. Individuals who are frail, have complex health problems or have a reduced life expectancy may benefit from having their target HbA1c relaxed (NICE 2019).

Alongside the move towards individualised target blood glucose levels, a better understanding amongst healthcare practitioners of the aetio-pathology of diabetes will allow for advances in adjusted treatments, including pharmacological therapies (WHO 2019).

It has been recognised in clinical practice that some ethnic groups respond better to specific anti-diabetic drugs. Pharmacogenomics (the study of how genes affect a person's response to drugs) is evident in the genetically induced response to sulfonylureas exhibited by some people. It is hoped that future advancements in pharmacogenomics will support individualised treatments and improved diabetes outcomes (WHO 2019; Semiz, Dujic & Causevic 2013).

Exercise has been shown to reduce insulin resistance and have a beneficial effect on many of the known complications. Current advice is that pharmacological treatment should only be started if the individual has not responded to a three-month alteration in their diet and lifestyle (NICE 2019). However, while diabetes management must always put lifestyle at the heart of the treatment plan, there is some debate about whether any potential delay to reducing hyperglycaemia may compromise the legacy effect (Laiteerapong, Ham, et al. 2019).

Nurse prescribers caring for individuals with diabetes should be alert to the progressive nature of the disease. Over time, insulin secretion is likely to decline and resistance to the effects of the insulin may worsen. Progression of the condition is largely unpredictable, as are the complications. The majority of individuals with diabetes will move from monotherapy to dual or triple therapy as time passes, and a proportion will require insulin. The chief consideration for nurse prescribers is to evaluate the effectiveness of drug therapy over time and to ensure that those in their care have access to a minimum of an annual review. Furthermore, the nurse prescriber, in observing the standards set out by the Royal Pharmaceutical Society's Competency Framework must reach a shared decision, with their patient or service user, on any prescribed or de-prescribed treatment (RPS 2016).

The DIRECT study (Lean, Leslie, et al. 2018) has found that a primary-care-based weight loss programme (particularly a loss of ≥10Kg) can lead to a remission in T2D (remission is classified as maintaining HbA1c below 48mmol/mol / 6.5% after at least 2 months without anti-diabetic medication). While many anti-diabetic agents have beneficial properties that go beyond glycaemic control (see below), weight loss in those with T2D is also associated with less reliance on anti-diabetic agents, a reduction in serious adverse events, such as cancers and cerebrovascular accidents, and a reduction in blood pressure and cholesterol as well as an improvement in quality of life. Weight loss also resulted in a reduction in the amount of fat in the liver and pancreas, allowing insulin production to resume (Lean, Leslie, et al. 2018). Diabetes UK and Health Education England are taking this intensive low-calorie programme forward, potentially offering hope that T2D can be put into remission (Diabetes UK 2018).

Case study: Type 2 diabetes

Fatimah Aswad is a 55-year-old married woman of Middle Eastern origin. She lives with her husband. Her two daughters are married and live nearby. Her mother (deceased) had type 2 diabetes. Her father is well. She has a body mass index of 32. She seldom smokes and does not drink alcohol. She denies taking any recreational drugs. She buys St John's Wort over the counter, as she feels anxious and depressed at times. She has no allergies. Her past medical history reveals that she has had two caesarean sections.

She presents with oral thrush, a second occurrence in three weeks. On questioning, she reports thirst, lethargy and some deterioration in her vision. Her blood pressure is 152/89.

Activity 16.1 (Case study)

1. Consider Mrs Aswad's risk factors for a possible diagnosis of type 2 diabetes.
2. Outline the tests that Mrs Aswad needs to have, in order to confirm a diagnosis of type 2 diabetes.
3. Draw on your knowledge of the complications of type 2 diabetes and consider what mutually agreed goals you could set, to minimise progression of any diabetes-related complications.

Anti-diabetic medication

Currently there is a range of medications whose modes of action differ. NICE guidelines direct prescribers as to which drugs should be first-line and second-line therapy, which drugs can be used as monotherapy, and which drugs can be used in combination and according to what clinical parameters (NICE 2019). Nurse prescribers should ensure that they are familiar with the recognised national guidance, as well as with local formularies and care pathways. In addition, the American Diabetes Association have published a consensus report on the management of hyperglycaemia in type 2 diabetes that offers more detailed and up-to-date standards for evidence-based practice in the UK (ADA 2019).

Anti-diabetic medication should only be prescribed after an assessment that takes account of the patient's preferences as to how they wish their condition to be managed, their agreed target HbA1c, their comorbidities and any polypharmacy. Behavioural and lifestyle modifications must be appropriately instigated either before medication is prescribed or as an important part of the overall patient-specific management plan. Individuals with diabetes should receive education at the time of diagnosis and this should be reinforced at every healthcare intervention. Anti-diabetic medication should always be prescribed at the lowest therapeutic dose, and regular blood tests taken to ensure that target glycaemic control is maintained. Prescribing to control blood glucose requires a balance between maintaining agreed HbA1c targets and avoiding hypoglycaemia (ADA 2019).

Metformin hydrochloride

Standard-release metformin is the first-line pharmacological treatment for an individual newly diagnosed with type 2 diabetes. It must be prescribed in combination with diet and lifestyle changes (NICE 2019). It can be used as monotherapy or with other anti-diabetic drugs, or with insulin. Its chief mode of action is the suppression of glucose production by the liver (gluconeogenesis and glycogenolysis). Metformin also increases insulin sensitivity and enhances peripheral glucose uptake. Metformin can only act in the presence of endogenous insulin; as such, it cannot exert a therapeutic effect when there are no functioning beta cells. Metformin is recognised as preventing cardiovascular complications (Scheen & Paquot 2013). Furthermore, metformin does not produce weight gain and is increasingly appropriate for obesity-related type 2 diabetes.

Metformin can be started at a low dose (500mg) and stepped up over several weeks, to reduce the possible unpleasant gastrointestinal side effects. There is a discrepancy between the BNF and the product literature regarding the starting dose and the maximum dose; it is usually prescribed to a maximum dose of 2g a day. Modified-release (MR) metformin can be used if gastrointestinal disturbances are not resolved. Metformin use is associated with vitamin B12 deficiency and worsening of symptoms of neuropathy (ADA 2019).

Metformin should be prescribed cautiously for those who have renal disease, especially older people who are likely to have a degree of renal decline. The nurse prescriber needs to follow the advice for titrating the medication in accordance with the BNF. Nurse prescribers should work in a multi-professional manner to ensure that renal function is regularly monitored and the correct dosage is prescribed.

Metformin is excreted by the kidneys so the individual's renal function should be determined before prescribing. In addition, all individuals should be monitored at least annually and those with renal impairment monitored more closely. Lactic acidosis is a rare but life-threatening adverse event that can occur due to metformin accumulation, primarily in those with significant renal failure. Caution is advised with anyone with an estimated glomerular filtration rate (eGFR) below 30ml/minute/1.73m^2 and metformin has to be stopped in those with any sudden deterioration in renal function or a recent myocardial infarction (NICE 2019). This instruction may be modified as more evidence becomes available regarding the risks and benefits of metformin (ADA 2019, Scheen & Paquot 2013).

Sodium glucose co-transporter 2 (SGLT2) inhibitors

Dapagliflozin, canagliflozin, empagliflozin and ertugliflozin are licensed for use in adults. They improve glycaemic control by blocking the glucose co-transporter SGLT2, which is found on the epithelial cells of the proximal tubule. Approximately 90% of glucose is reabsorbed by SGLT2 (the remaining 10% is reabsorbed under the influence of SGLT1). Inhibiting this action results in a significant increase in the amount of glucose excreted via the urine. With the excretion of large volumes of glucose, effects of weight loss, dehydration and tiredness may be experienced, and genito-urinary infections can be precipitated. The weight loss is usually welcomed by patients, who are very often over their desired weight. The diuretic effect manifests in a secondary benefit of a reduction in blood pressure.

The mode of action is dependent on renal function and this should therefore be determined before an SGLT2 inhibitor is prescribed, and should be checked at least annually thereafter. An eGFR of > 60ml/minute/1.73m^2 is required before drug initiation and so, currently, it is not recommended for those aged over 75 years and the advice is to monitor renal function 2–4 times a year. However, more recent evidence indicates that SGL2 inhibitors are reno-protective, as well as having benefits in people with heart disease (ADA 2019).

This class of drugs can be used as monotherapy or in combination with other oral anti-diabetic drugs or with insulin. When used in combination with insulin or a sulfonylurea, a lower dose of insulin or the sulfonylurea may be required to reduce the risk of hypoglycaemia. SGLT2 inhibitors have been associated with diabetic ketoacidosis (DKA) and are contraindicated in patients with a history of ketoacidosis. Patients who are started on a SGLT2 inhibitor should be informed of the signs of ketoacidosis and be tested for ketones (blood ketones level is advised, rather than urine) even if their plasma glucose levels are near normal (MHRA 2016).

SGLT2 inhibitors are once-daily drugs. Dapagliflozin has one prescribed dose of 10mg daily for type 2 diabetes. A once-daily 5mg dose is licensed for use in type 1 diabetes as an adjunct to insulin in those who are overweight. Canagliflozin can be started at 100mg and can be increased to 300mg daily if required. Empagliflozin has a starting dose of 10mg. When tolerated and tighter glycaemic control is required, it can be increased to 25mg. Ertugliflozin has a starting dose of 5mg daily that can be increased to 15mg daily if required and if tolerated.

Empagliflozin and ertugliflozin, with limited experience of their usage, will be subject to additional monitoring under the inverted black triangle system. Nurse prescribers will be aware that all black triangle adverse reactions should be reported to the Medicines and Healthcare Products Regulatory Agency (MHRA), using the Yellow Card Scheme.

Canagliflozin, dapagliflozin and empagliflozin are all available as compound drugs with the addition of either 850mg or 1g metformin.

The incretin effect

The incretin effect concept was developed after observations that insulin secretion was significantly greater following oral glucose, compared to intravenous glucose. The hormone incretin is secreted from endocrine cells of the small intestine epithelium in response to an increase in glucose. Gastric inhibitory polypeptide, also known as glucose-dependent insulinotropic peptide (GIP), and glucagon-like peptide-1 (GLP-1) are the two primary incretin hormones secreted. Following secretion, both GLP-1 and GIP are rapidly broken down and inactivated by the enzyme dipeptidylpeptidase-4 (DPP-4) (Russell-Jones & Gough 2012).

Incretin hormones play an integral role in glucose homoeostasis, lowering blood glucose through an increase of insulin secretion as well as an inhibition of glucagon and thus a reduction in hepatic glucose production. GLP-1 also delays stomach emptying so glucose absorption is extended and hyperglycaemia is limited. In type 2 diabetes, the incretin effect is diminished, less GLP-1 is secreted and the beta cells are less responsive to GIP. This diminished effect explains the high post-prandial glucose levels seen in those with diabetes. The incretin-based therapies have a role to play in reducing this post-meal hyperglycaemia.

GLP-1 has a very short half-life – 1.5 minutes following intravenous glucose – so drug therapy has been developed around GLP-1 receptor agonist and DPP-4 inhibitors. There are two classes of incretin-based therapies, dipeptidylpeptidase-4 (DPP-4) inhibitors and glucagon-like peptide (GLP-1) receptor agonists. Both classes of drugs work by increasing insulin secretion in a glucose-dependent way.

Glucagon-like peptide (GLP-1) receptor agonists

The GLP-1 receptor agonists are also known as incretin mimetics. Like the DPP-4 inhibitors, they are glucose dependent and less likely to cause hypoglycaemia than sulfonylureas.

GLP-1 receptor agonists must be given by subcutaneous injection. For many people, this will be their first injected therapy. Nurse prescribers should consider the skills required in initiating injection-based therapies, including the fear some individuals may have and the support they may need to self-manage their injections.

When used in combination with oral anti-diabetic drugs, GLP-1 agonists are highly effective at reducing HbA1c levels, although sulfonylureas may need dose reduction when combined with a GLP-1 agonist. In addition to glycaemic effects, GLP-1-based therapies have a beneficial effect on weight because of their action in slowing gastric emptying, increasing the feeling of fullness and reducing appetite (Gaspari, Welungoda, et al. 2013). There are cardiovascular benefits from this class of drugs (Sheahan, Wahlberg & Gilbert 2019) and the American Diabetes Association has now incorporated this consideration into its 2019 guidelines on diabetes treatment. GLP-1 agonists (or an SGLT2) is the ADA's first choice of combination therapy, in individuals who do not achieve their target glucose levels with metformin alone, when presenting with arteriosclerotic cardiovascular disease (ADA 2019). In the UK, NICE continues to reserve the GLP-1 agonists for adults with type 2 diabetes who have a BMI of 35kg/m^2 or higher, or in whom obesity and weight loss require significant management (NICE 2019).

There are some concerns regarding reported pancreatitis with GLP-1 agonists and prescribers should alert patients to the signs and symptoms, including abdominal pain, nausea and vomiting (MHRA 2009).

Exenatide and liraglutide are licensed for use with metformin or a sulfonylurea or both, or with pioglitazone or with metformin and pioglitazone. Semaglutide is licensed for use with metformin or alone and has shown some good results for reducing cardiovascular risk in those with type 2 diabetes (Leiter, Bain, *et al*. 2019). Prescribers should be alert to the costs versus benefits of combination therapy and adhere to national and local guidelines.

Prescribers are directed to the safety information from the MHRA, which is clearly outlined in the BNF, when prescribing or administering GLP-1 agonists. Life-threatening diabetic ketoacidosis has been reported in those with type 2 diabetes who are on a combination of a GLP-1 receptor agonist and insulin, specifically after a rapid dose reduction of insulin. Any reduction in insulin dose should be done in a stepwise manner and the patient informed of the risks, the signs of DKA and the need to seek medical help (MHRA 2019).

Dipeptidylpeptidase-4 (DPP-4) inhibitors (gliptins)

DPP-4 inhibitors are types of anti-diabetic medication that block the DPP-4 enzymes, thus increasing incretin levels. As incretin production is glucose-dependent, hypoglycaemia is less likely than with the traditional sulfonylureas.

DPP-4 inhibitors have a weight-neutral effect, making them acceptable to patients and useful in obesity-related type 2 diabetes. They have been found to have a low incidence of hypoglycaemia when used as monotherapy or in combination with metformin or pioglitazone. A slight increase in hypoglycaemic events has been shown when they are combined with a sulfonylurea. The dose of the sulfonylurea should therefore be reduced when a DPP-4 inhibitor is prescribed.

DPP-4 inhibitors may be added to metformin or a sulfonylurea, or to both, if blood glucose levels are above target.

Currently, no DPP-4 inhibitor has shown superiority, and prescribers should be guided by NICE guidelines and local policies.

Thiazolidinediones (glitazones)

If an individual's blood glucose cannot be maintained at a desirable level with diet, exercise and metformin, combination therapy may be offered. NICE (2019) has authorised the use of thiazolidinediones (TZDs), as well as sulfonylureas, and DPP-4 inhibitors, to reduce blood glucose by lowering insulin resistance in the liver and peripheral tissues and reducing hepatic glucose output. The HbA1c for those taking pioglitazone should be measured at 3–6 monthly intervals.

Pioglitazone is currently the only TZD licensed in the UK. There have been concerns related to cardiovascular events and TZDs. The PROactive study showed that pioglitazone can reduce the risk of secondary macrovascular events, in those individuals who have established macrovascular disease (Erdmann, Song, et al. 2014). TZDs are not recommended for combined use with insulin, if the person has heart failure or is at higher risk of fracture (MHRA 2014).

Pioglitazone carries a small risk for bladder cancer and should be avoided in those with a current or past history (MHRA 2011). However, a six-year follow-up on findings from the PROactive study found no difference in bladder malignancy between the pioglitazone and placebo group (Erdmann, Song, et al. 2014). Pioglitazone is associated with an increased risk of bone fractures (Viscoli, Inzucchi, et al. 2017). The nurse prescriber should therefore adhere to advice in the BNF and carefully evaluate all their patients on this drug, specifically the frail and elderly.

Pioglitazone does not have any pharmacological effect on metformin or sulfonylureas and can be used in combination with both. However, blood glucose levels must be carefully monitored with an increased risk of hypoglycaemia, particularly if combined with a sulfonylurea.

Sulfonylureas

Sulfonylureas act by binding to the potassium channel on the cell membrane of the beta cells. This triggers a series of intracellular responses, notably an influx of calcium that leads to the secretion of insulin from the cells. These drugs can cause hypoglycaemia and individuals receiving them should be advised of this risk. Due to the risk of hypoglycaemia and the weight gain associated with sulfonylureas, they are rarely prescribed, and should be avoided in older adults.

When prescribing or administering sulfonylureas, information should be given on maintaining regular mealtimes and adhering to usual exercise patterns. An imbalance in ingested carbohydrates and energy expenditure through exercise will increase the risk of an adverse hypoglycaemic event. Prescribers should regularly review those receiving sulfonylureas, with 3–6-monthly HbA1c checks, and adjust the dose if mild hypoglycaemia is reported. Severe hypoglycaemia with neuroglycopaenic symptoms, such as confusion or slurred speech, requires urgent hospital treatment. Suffering one or more episodes of severe hypoglycaemia has been linked to cardiovascular complications and death in the next five years (Lee, Warren, et al. 2018, ADVANCE study 2008).

The therapeutic effect of sulfonylureas can be expected to diminish over time. This may be due to the progressive nature of the disease or to a reduced response to the drug, known as secondary failure.

The long-acting sulfonylurea glibenclamide should be avoided in the elderly and in those with renal impairment. Glipizide should also be avoided in individuals with renal and hepatic impairment. Tolbutamide can be used in renal impairment, as can gliclazide, as it is predominantly metabolised in the liver. Generally, self-testing is not advised (for the NICE 2019 criteria on when self-testing may be appropriate, see the answer to Activity 16.2) but all individuals will need to be counselled regarding the signs of hypoglycaemia. All individuals taking sulfonylureas require regular blood glucose testing.

Meglitinides

Repaglinide and nateglinide bind to potassium channels on the cell membrane of the beta cells, in a similar way to sulfonylureas, but not as strongly. They stimulate insulin release and they therefore have the potential to cause hypoglycaemia.

Repaglinide and nateglinide have a rapid onset of action and a short duration of action. Therefore, they should be given pre-prandially, before each main meal. If meals are skipped (or added), those taking the medication should be advised to omit (or add) a dose. Doses are titrated over 1–2 weeks.

Repaglinide can be administered as monotherapy or with metformin but there is an increased risk of hypoglycaemia. Nateglinide is licensed only in combination with metformin.

The drugs are primarily excreted via the bile and therefore can be prescribed, with caution, in renal disorders. The drugs should be avoided in severe hepatic impairment.

Acarbose

Acarbose acts by inhibiting alpha glucosidase, an enzyme of the intestine that releases glucose from complex carbohydrates. This inhibitory action reduces the rate of digestion of the carbohydrates, decreasing the amount of glucose that is absorbed and moderately reducing blood glucose levels.

The mode of action requires that acarbose is taken with the first bite of the main meal, and its action will depend on the amount of complex carbohydrates eaten. Acarbose inhibits the enzymes needed to digest carbohydrates and the undegraded carbohydrates pass into the colon. The carbohydrates are then acted upon by bacteria, and unpleasant side effects of flatulence and diarrhoea are commonly reported.

Case study: Diabetic drug adherence

Mr Edmund Wilson is a 75-year-old retired post office worker. He has never been married and lives alone with social support from neighbours and family. He is a past smoker and likes a beer each evening. He denies taking any recreational drugs and does not take any over-the-counter (OTC) remedies. He reports no allergies. He is not overweight. His father died of a heart attack aged 65. Past medical history includes hypertension diagnosed over twenty years ago and a myocardial infarction two years ago. He was diagnosed with type 2 diabetes ten years ago. Current medication is metformin, gliclazide, atorvastatin and ramipril. At the most recent review, 2 weeks earlier, HbA1c was 7mmol.

Activity 16.2 (Case study)

On closer questioning, it seems that Mr Wilson stopped taking his anti-diabetic drugs several weeks ago as he was feeling generally unwell.

1. Applying your knowledge of anti-diabetic drugs and with reference to the BNF and other supporting documentation, consider the review of Mr Wilson's anti-diabetic drug therapy now required in view of the low HbA1c test result.
2. Consider what actions you need to take to improve adherence to prescribed treatment.
3. With reference to Mr Wilson's current medication, are there any interactions that should be noted? Where in the BNF would you look for interactions?

Summary

Type 2 diabetes is a complex condition, and nurse prescribers have a major role to play in preventing or reducing the burden of diabetes-related complications by managing blood glucose, as well as blood pressure and lipids.

Structured education, patient involvement and self-care underpin all effective healthcare management. Changes to diet and lifestyle modification form the cornerstone of diabetes care, augmented by pharmacological therapies.

On average, a person with diabetes requires twice as much healthcare expenditure as someone without diabetes (International Diabetes Federation 2017). The RPS Competency Framework makes it quite clear to the nurse prescriber that any prescribing decision must be based on a holistic assessment and prescribers should not practise outside their competencies (RPS 2016). Medication must be prescribed based on the patient's clinical need (RPS 2016) and must be reviewed for tolerability and adherence and for effectiveness (NICE 2019). Working collaboratively and following guidelines and protocols will ensure that nurse prescribers meet these expectations and deliver evidence-based, effective diabetes care.

Answers to activities

Activity 16.1 (Case study)

1. Consider Mrs Aswad's risk factors for a possible diagnosis of type 2 diabetes.

Risk factors that should be considered are raised BMI (> 25), increasing age, ethnicity, family history, hypertension and smoking. If the blood tests are negative, Mrs Aswad should still be regularly monitored and counselled about her risk factors. There are no criteria as to how many or which combination of risk factors constitute a severe risk of developing diabetes, so all are equally weighted. A QDiabetes risk assessment could be carried out (QDiabetes 2019).

2. Outline the tests that Mrs Aswad needs to have, in order to confirm a diagnosis of type 2 diabetes.

The test would be a HbA1c. A HbA1c greater than 48mmol/mol (6.5%) would be indicative of diabetes.

3. Draw on your knowledge of the complications associated with type 2 diabetes and consider what mutually agreed goals you could set, to minimise progression of any diabetes-related complications.

Goal-setting should be a shared approach and achievable. Telling someone they have diabetes means breaking bad news and requires well-developed communication skills. Review some of the work from the Health Foundation on the Co-creating Health initiative for guidance on how to set goals and motivate those with long-term conditions (Health Foundation 2020).

The opportunity to receive support on diet and exercise needs to be discussed, and referral to a diabetes educational programme should take place as soon as possible. NICE recommends starting someone newly diagnosed with type 2 diabetes on a three-month diet and exercise programme. There is a continuing debate on the effects of any delay in reducing hyperglycaemia and optimising blood glucose levels, and the risk to the legacy effect. Any management plan should therefore be discussed and agreed with the patient and should be in line with the most up-to-date evidence and departmental protocols.

Target blood glucose levels (as well as blood pressure and lipids and weight) should be agreed by the practitioner and the patient, and should be reviewed and adjusted as necessary. When managed by diet and lifestyle alone, or on a single anti-diabetic drug that is not associated with hypoglycaemia, such as metformin, the target is usually 48mmol/mol (6.5%). If target blood glucose levels cannot be maintained on single therapy (generally considered a HbA1c above 58mmol/mol/7.5%), then combination therapy may be required. When two or more anti-diabetic drugs are prescribed, the aim would be for the HbA1c to be 53mmol/mol (7.0%). However, there should be a case-by-case approach to target HbA1c, and the target might be relaxed for some individuals (e.g. older and frail patients or those at a high risk of hypoglycaemia).

Activity 16.2 (Case study)

1. Applying your knowledge of anti-diabetic drugs and with reference to the BNF and other supporting documentation, consider the review of Mr Wilson's anti-diabetic drug therapy now required in view of the low HbA1c test result.

A patient-centred approach should be used to guide the choice of an anti-diabetic agent. Considerations must include comorbidities (atherosclerotic cardiovascular disease, heart failure, chronic kidney disease), hypoglycaemic risk, impact on weight, cost, risk for side effects, and patient preferences (ADA 2019).

Any medication that causes hypoglycaemia should be avoided in the elderly. Sulfonylureas secrete insulin and therefore induce hypoglycaemia. In the elderly this can be frightening and dangerous and should be avoided. Sulfonylureas are no longer the mainstay of hyperglycaemia reduction. As such, any prescriber could be held accountable for issuing a prescription that falls outside national and/or local guidelines and is not in keeping with the evidence. Prescribers can be called to account for any acts of negligence and this is increasingly important where there is team prescribing and the nurse prescriber may be issuing a repeat prescription.

Generally, in patients taking metformin and not achieving their target HbA1c, the prescriber should consider dual therapy. However, de-prescribing and simplification of drug regimens should be considered in older adults. With an HbA1c of 42mmol/mol (6.0%), and given his age, Mr Wilson may require discontinuation of the sulfonylurea and to continue solely with metformin plus diet, exercise and regular review. You need to find out if he has changed his diet or exercise routine recently or has taken any OTC or prescribed medication that could potentiate his anti-diabetic medication. His weight could be checked if there is any indication he is not eating – and to ensure safe prescribing.

If his HbA1c is found to be elevated at the next review, Mr Wilson has established atherosclerotic cardiovascular disease, so an anti-diabetic drug with demonstrated cardiovascular disease benefit may be added (possibly a SGLT2 inhibitor). But it should be prescribed with caution and his renal function should be checked before commencing any combination of anti-diabetic drugs.

2. Consider what actions you need to take to improve adherence to prescribed treatment.

Non-adherence to drug regimens is multi-factorial. Mr Wilson could be experiencing frequent hypoglycaemic events and his decision to stop taking the gliclazide may in fact be a well-informed decision, prompted by his recognition of the signs of hypoglycaemia.

The nurse prescriber should be alert to an expected degree of autonomic neuropathy, a complication of long-standing diabetes. It can affect the nerves that control the heart and regulate blood pressure and blood glucose. Some people can also have diminished recognition of the symptoms of hypoglycaemia, so-called 'hypoglycaemic unawareness'. Mr Wilson may feel hungry and tired and generally unwell but without the specific signs of hypoglycaemia.

While nurse prescribers have a duty of care to promote effective blood glucose management, they should also be alert to the implications of tight blood glucose control. Hypoglycaemia is possibly the most feared side effect for those individuals requiring pharmacological management of diabetes. Effective prescribing in diabetes necessitates patient education and self-management. In Mr Wilson's case, his age and HbA1c of 2 weeks ago, is an indication of hypoglycaemia and all advice is to avoid drugs that induce hypoglycaemia (ADA 2019).

Self-monitoring of blood glucose levels is an option but it is not routinely recommended unless:
- The person is on insulin
- There is evidence of hypoglycaemic episodes

- The person is on oral medication that may increase their risk of hypoglycaemia while driving or operating machinery
- The person is pregnant or planning to become pregnant (NICE 2019).

Older people with diabetes have a higher than average incidence of dementia or cognitive decline. All older adults should be screened for cognitive impairment as well as for depression, as both can result in non-adherence.

To aid patient-centred agreed targets, and promote adherence, communication with the wider health and social care team and regular review is also required.

3. With reference to Mr Wilson's current medication, are there any interactions that should be noted? Where in the BNF would you look for interactions?

Ramipril is an ACE inhibitor. Older people taking ACE inhibitors should be monitored for hypotension and their renal function should be checked.

Caution is advised in the use of statins with the elderly. There is a risk of hyperglycaemia and HbA1c must be regularly monitored. A full lipid profile is required and liver enzymes must be regularly checked.

Sulfonylureas are likely to induce hypoglycaemia and the current regimen is not in line with the recommended oral anti-diabetic agents (ADA 2019).

The BNF gives specific instructions on prescribing for the elderly. Polypharmacy increases the chance of adverse drug reactions and interactions. Non-pharmacological interventions should be considered for all, but especially with the elderly who may have altered pharmacokinetics. Prescribers are directed by the BNF to the STOPP/START criteria. These evidence-based criteria are used to review medication regimens in elderly people. In the elderly, drug regimens should be reviewed regularly and monitoring carried out as per the drug monograph and/or local protocols.

Consideration should be given to potential cognitive decline with any prescribed medication in the elderly and older individuals should be reviewed regularly.

Drug interactions are found under each monograph in the online BNF or the App or in Appendix 1 of the hard copy BNF.

References and further reading

ACCORD Study (2008). Action to Control Cardiovascular Risk in Diabetes Study Group. *New England Journal of Medicine*. **358**, 2545–59.

Adler, A.L., Stevens, R.J., Manley, S.E., Bilous, R.W., Cull, C.A. & Holman, R.R. (2003). Development and progression of nephropathy in type 2 diabetes: the United Kingdom Prospective Diabetes Study (UKPDS 64).

ADVANCE study (Action in Diabetes and Vascular Diseases: Preterax and Diamicron Modified Release Controlled Evaluation) Collaborative Group (2008). *New England Journal of Medicine*. **358**, 2560–72.

American Diabetes Association (ADA) (2019). Classification and diagnosis of diabetes: Standards of medical care in diabetes – 2019. *Diabetes Care*. **42**, S13–S28.

Diabetes Prevention Program Research Group (2002). Reduction in the incidence of type 2 diabetes with lifestyle intervention or metformin. *New England Journal of Medicine*. **346**, 393–403.

Diabetes UK (2018). *Diabetes Prevalence 2018*. https://www.diabetes.org.uk/professionals/position-statements-reports/statistics/diabetes-prevalence-2018 (Last accessed 2 November 2020).

Diabetes UK (2020). Latent Autoimmune Diabetes in Adults (LADA). Available at: https://www.diabetes.org.uk/diabetes-the-basics/other-types-of-diabetes/latent-autoimmune-diabetes. (Accessed: 20 October 2020).

Erdmann, E., Song, E., Spanheimer, R., van Troostenburg de Bruyn, A.R. & Perez, A. (January 2014). Observational follow up of the PROactive study: a 6 year update. *Diabetes, Obesity and Metabolism*. **16** (1), 63–74, doi: 10.1111/dom.1280. Epub 2013 Aug 19.

Gaspari, T., Welungoda, I., Widdop, R.E., Simpson, R.W. & Dear, A.E. (2013). The GLP-1 receptor agonist liraglutide inhibits progression of vascular disease via effects on atherogenesis, plaque stability and endothelial function in an ApoE-/- mouse model. *Diabetes and Vascular Disease Research*. **10** (4), 353–60. doi: 10.1177/1479164113481817. Epub 2013 May 14.

Health Foundation (2020). Co-creating Health. https://www.health.org.uk/funding-and-partnerships/programmes/co-creating-health (Last accessed 2 November 2020).

Insel, R.A., Dunne, J.L., Atkinson, M.A., Chiang, J.L., Dabelea, D., Gottlieb, P.A., Greenbaum, C.J., Herold, K.C., Krischer, J.P., Lernmark, A., Ratner, R.E., Rewers, M.J., Schatz, D.A., Skyler, J.S., Sosenko, J.M. & Ziegler, A.G. (2015). Staging presymptomatic type 1 diabetes: A scientific statement of JDFR, the Endocrine Society, and the American Diabetes Association. *Diabetes Care*. Oct; **38** (10), 1964–74. doi: 10.23337/dc15-1419.

International Diabetes Federation (IDF) (2017). *IDF Diabetes Atlas*. 8th edn. Brussels, Belgium: International Diabetes Federation. http://www.diabetesatlas.org (Last accessed 2 November 2020).

Kohner, E.M., Aldington, S.J., Stratton, I.M., Manley, S.E., Holman, R.R., Matthews, D.R. & Turner, R.C. (1998). The United Kingdom Prospective Diabetes Study (UKPDS), 30: diabetic retinopathy at diagnosis of non-insulin-dependent diabetes mellitus and associated risk factors. *Archives of Ophthalmology*. **116** (3), 297–303.

Laiteerapong, N., Ham, S., Gao, Y., Moffet, H.H., Liu, J.Y., Huang, E.S. & Karter, A.J. (2019). The legacy effect in Type 2 Diabetes: Impact of early glycemic control on future complications (The Diabetes & Aging Study). *Diabetes Care*. **42** (3), 416–26.

Lean, M.E., Leslie, W.S., Barnes, A.C., Brosnahan, N., Thom, G., McCombie, L., Peters, C., Zhyzhneuskaya, S., Al-Mrabeh, A., Hollingsworth, K.G., Rodrigues, A.M., Rehackova, L., Adamson, A.J., Sniehotta, F.F., Mathers, J.C., Ross, H.M., McIlvenna, Y., Stefanetti, R., Trenell, M., Welsh, P., Kean, S., Ford, I., McConnachiem, A., Sattar, N., & Taylor, R. (2018). Primary care-led weight management for remission of type 2 diabetes (DIRECT): an open-label, cluster-randomised trial. *The Lancet*. **391** (10120), 541–51.

Lee, A.K., Warren, B., Lee, C.J., McEvoy, J.W., Matsushita, K., Huang, E.S., Sharrett, A.R., Coresh, J. & Selvin, E. (2018). The association of severe hypoglycemia with incident cardiovascular events and mortality in adults with type 2 diabetes. *Diabetes Care*. **41** (1), 104–11.

Leiter, L.A., Bain, S.C., Hramiak, I., Jodar, W., Madsbad, S., Gondolf, T., Hansen, T., Holst, I. & Lingvay, I. (2019). Cardiovascular risk reduction with once-weekly semaglutide in subjects with type 2 diabetes: a post hoc analysis of gender, age, and baseline CV risk profile in the SUSTAIN 6 trial. *Cardiovascular Diabetology*. **18** (73). doi: 10.1186/s12933-019-0871-8.

Lindström, J., Peltonen, M., Eriksson, J.G., Ilanne-Parikka, P., Aunola, S., Keinänen-Kiukaanniemi, S., Uusitupa, M., & Tuomilehto, J. (2013). Improved lifestyle and decreased diabetes risk over 13 years: long-term follow-up of the randomised Finnish Diabetes Prevention Study (DPS). *Diabetologia*. **56**, 284–93

Medicines and Healthcare Products Regulatory Agency (MHRA) (2009). Exenatide (Byetta ▼): risk of severe pancreatitis and renal failure. https://www.gov.uk/drug-safety-update/exenatide-byetta-risk-of-severe-pancreatitis-and-renal-failure (Last accessed 2 November 2020).

Medicines and Healthcare Products Regulatory Agency (MHRA) (2011). New advice on risk of bladder cancer with the anti-diabetic drug pioglitazone (Actos ▼, Competact ▼). Available at: https://webarchive.nationalarchives.gov.uk/20150110162352/http://www.mhra.gov.uk/Safetyinformation/Safetywarningsalertsandrecalls/Safetywarningsandmessagesformedicines/CON123285 (Accessed: 12 February 2021).

Medicines and Healthcare Products Regulatory Agency (MHRA) (2014). Insulin combined with pioglitazone: risk of cardiac failure. https://www.gov.uk/drug-safety-update/insulin-combined-with-pioglitazone-risk-of-cardiac-failure (Last accessed 2 November 2020).

Medicines and Healthcare Products Regulatory Agency (MHRA) (2016). SGLT2 inhibitors: updated advice on the risk of diabetic ketoacidosis. https://www.gov.uk/drug-safety-update/sglt2-inhibitors-updated-advice-on-the-risk-of-diabetic-ketoacidosis (Last accessed 2 November 2020).

Medicines and Healthcare Products Regulatory Agency (MHRA) (2017). SGLT2 inhibitors: updated advice on increased risk of lower-limb amputation (mainly toes). https://www.gov.uk/drug-safety-update/sglt2-inhibitors-updated-advice-on-increased-risk-of-lower-limb-amputation-mainly-toes (Last accessed 2 November 2020).

Medicines and Healthcare Products Regulatory Agency (MHRA) (2019). GLP-1 receptor agonists: reports of diabetic ketoacidosis when concomitant insulin was rapidly reduced or discontinued. https://bnf.nice.org.uk/drug/exenatide.html#nationalFunding (Last accessed 2 November 2020).

Medicines and Healthcare Products Regulatory Agency (MHRA) (2020). SGLT2 inhibitors: monitor ketones in blood during treatment interruption for surgical procedures or acute serious medical illness. March 2020. https://www.gov.uk/drug-safety-update/sglt2-inhibitors-monitor-ketones-in-blood-during-treatment-interruption-for-surgical-procedures-or-acute-serious-medical-illness (Last accessed 2 November 2020).

NHS England. (2020). The NHS Diabetes Prevention Programme (NHS DPP). https://www.england.nhs.uk/diabetes/diabetes-prevention/ (Last accessed 2 November 2020).

National Institute for Health and Care Excellence (NICE) (2019). Type 2 Diabetes: The management of type 2 diabetes. Clinical guideline NG28, published Dec 2015, updated Aug 2019. https://www.nice.org.uk/guidance/ng28 (Last accessed 2 November 2020).

QDiabetes (2019). https://qdiabetes.org/ (Last accessed 2 November 2020).

Royal Pharmaceutical Society (RPS) (2016). A Competency Framework for all Prescribers. https://www.rpharms.com/Portals/0/RPS%20document%20library/Open%20access/Professional%20standards/Prescribing%20competency%20framework/prescribing-competency-framework.pdf (Last accessed 2 November 2020).

Russell-Jones, D. & Gough, S. (2012). Recent advances in incretin-based therapies. *Clinical Endocrinology*. **77**, 489–99.

Sasso, F.C., Chiodini, P., Carbonara, O., De Nicola, L., Conte, G., Salvatore, T., Nasti, R., Marfella, R., Gallo, C., Signoriello, S., Torella, R. & Minutolo, R. (2012). High cardiovascular risk in patients with Type 2 diabetic nephropathy: the predictive role of albuminuria and glomerular filtration rate. The NID-2 Prospective Cohort Study. *Nephrology Dialysis Transplantation*. **27** (6), 2269–74.

Scheen, A.J. & Paquot, N. (2013). Metformin revisited: A critical review of the benefit-risk balance in at-risk patients with type 2 diabetes. *Diabetes and Metabolism*. **39** (3), 179–90.

Semiz, S., Dujic, T. & Causevic, A. (2013). Pharmacogenetics and personalized treatment of type 2 diabetes. *Biochemia Medica*. **23** (2), 154–171.

Sheahan, K.H., Wahlberg, E.A. & Gilbert, M.P. (2019). An overview of GLP-1 agonists and recent cardiovascular outcomes trials. *Postgraduate Medical Journal*. **96**, 156–61. doi:10.1136/postgradmedj-2019-137186.

Stratton, M., Adler, A.I., Neil, H.A., Matthews, D.R., Manley, S.E., Cull, C.A., Hadden, D., Turner, R.C. & Holman, R.R. (2000). Association of glycaemia with macrovascular and microvascular complications of type 2 diabetes (UKPDS 35): prospective observational study. *British Medical Journal*. **321**, 405–12.

Tuomilehto, J., Lindström, J., Eriksson, J.G., Valle, T.T., Hämäläinen, H., Ilanne-Parikka, P., Keinänen-Kiukaanniemi, S., Laasko, M., Louheranta, A., Rastas, M., Salminen, V. & Uusitupa, M. (3 May 2001). Prevention of type 2 diabetes mellitus by changes in lifestyle among subjects with impaired glucose tolerance. *New England Journal of Medicine*. **344** (18), 1343–50.

Vergès B. (2015). Pathophysiology of diabetic dyslipidaemia: where are we? *Diabetologia*. **58**, 886–99.

Viscoli, C.M., Inzucchi, S.E., Young, L.H., Insogna, K.L., Conwit, R., Furie, K.L., Gorman, M., Kelly, M.A., Lovejoy, A.M. & Kernan, W. (2017). Pioglitazone and risk for bone fracture: Safety data from a randomized clinical trial. *Journal of Clinical Endocrinology & Metabolism*. **102** (3), 914–22. doi: 10.1210/jc.2016-3237.

World Health Organisation (WHO) (2019). *Classification of Diabetes Mellitus 2019*. Geneva: WHO.

17

Pharmacological case studies: Mental illness

Herbert Mwebe
Mental health senior lecturer, Independent Prescriber,
SFHEA, B.Sc, PG Dip, AdvDip, PGCert HE, MSc, Mprof, Doctoral student

This chapter:

- Debates the proposed causal factors for mental illness
- Discusses the mechanism of action of antipsychotics and antidepressants
- Discusses the adverse effects of antipsychotics and antidepressants
- Examines the recommended monitoring checks in people taking psychotropic medications.

Introduction

This chapter provides the reader with an overview of commonly prescribed psychotropic medications used in the treatment and management of mental health conditions including schizophrenia, major depressive disorder, anxiety and bipolar affective disorder. The discussions are based on examples of the medications given in the chapter: examining the mechanism of action, indications and recommended dose ranges, therapeutic benefits of usage and common side effects (iatrogenic health problems) associated with the use of these medications in clinical practice (Mwebe 2018a). As the use of psychotropic medications is increasingly being linked to the incidence of metabolic syndrome (hyperlipidaemia, diabetes, glycaemic abnormalities, obesity and cardiovascular complications) in users of mental health services (Mental Health Taskforce NHS England 2016), obligatory physical health monitoring checks are discussed. In addition, the role of the mental health professional (including mental health nurses, nurse prescribers, social workers, psychiatrists and psychologists) in ensuring safe practice is considered (Royal Pharmaceutical Society 2016, Stahl 2017).

It is of course impossible to incorporate all accessible information about any individual medication in this short chapter. The information given is therefore by no means comprehensive; it is simply intended to act as an introductory guide, offering practical clinical information and advice on how to use these medications in mental health settings.

Mental illness

A mental illness or disorder is a behavioural, psychological or emotional presentation associated with subjective distress, anguish or disability that occurs in the course of someone's life but which is not viewed as part of normal development or culture. In mental illness, symptoms may be linked to a mixture of cognitive, behavioural, perceptual and affective difficulties.

The exact cause of mental illness is not known but several factors and theories have been put forward to explain the origin, process and associated symptoms of mental and physical ill health (Pilgrim 2017). Sullivan (2009) argues that mental illness emerges from the interaction of genetic vulnerabilities with environmental-psychosocial stress. According to stress-vulnerability models, when stress factors (such as poverty, loss of employment, bereavement, poor housing, financial worries, poor social connections, difficult interpersonal dynamics, vulnerability due to chronic physical illness, and genetics) interact beyond a certain threshold, mental ill health emerges (Cohen & Brown 2010). Individuals with a background of traumatic experiences (such as physical and psychological injuries including traumatic brain injuries) are at greater risk of developing poor mental health.

There is also a strong link between complex mental illness in adulthood and abuse (physical, emotional and/or sexual), and emotional or psychological trauma in early years (Megele 2015). In biopsychiatry, genetic factors contribute significantly to the course of mental illness and this has been demonstrated by twin, family and adoption studies (Gejman, Sanders & Duan 2010). The risk of developing mental illness increases in relatives of patients with a history of mental illness (Mwebe 2018a; Albert 2015; Bogren, Brådvik & Holmstrand 2018). A study by Rasic, Hajek et al. (2014) found that the offspring of parents with serious mental illness (SMI) had a 32% probability of developing SMI themselves.

Neuroscience research has implicated abnormalities in neurotransmitter circuit systems of dopamine, glutamate, serotonin, gamma-Aminobutyric acid, adrenaline and glutamate (Stahl 2017). The biopsychiatric model (disease model) which focuses on absence or presence of symptoms dominates most psychiatry-led interventions (psychiatric medications) in mental health settings. In addition, the recovery model (or social model) is commonly applied alongside the disease model and looks at wider determinants of health (Marmot, Goldblatt & Allen 2010). Psychosocial interventions e.g. self-help groups, peer support, counselling, psychotherapy, individual and group therapy, family therapy, mindfulness and cognitive behavioural therapies are often used alongside psychiatric medications (Holland, Floyd & Soames 2018; Taylor, Paton & Kerwin 2015).

Antipsychotics
Dopamine theory of schizophrenia

The dopamine hypothesis is the oldest and most recognised of the schizophrenia theories. In the early 1950s it was discovered that when individuals used amphetamines, they reported symptoms like those displayed in psychosis (Stahl 2018). The use of recreational substances (such as amphetamines and cannabis) causes an increase in dopamine in the brain. Dopamine influences functions in the brain including decision-making, thinking, fine muscle movements, integration of emotions and thought processes. The dopamine hypothesis proposes that an excess of dopamine in the mesolimbic pathway is linked to positive symptoms of schizophrenia (such as delusions, auditory hallucinations and paranoia), whereas hypoactivity of dopamine neurotransmission in the mesocortical pathway is linked to negative symptoms of schizophrenia (including flattening of affect, apathy, poverty of speech, anhedonia and social withdrawal).

The glutamate hypothesis of schizophrenia, which first emerged in the 1980s and has gained much wider support, postulates that hypofunction glutamate levels at the glutamate receptor (N-Methyl-D-aspartate or NMDA) in the brain can result in positive psychotic symptoms in healthy individuals and in patients with schizophrenia (Hu, MacDonald, *et al.* 2015; Yang & Tsai 2017).

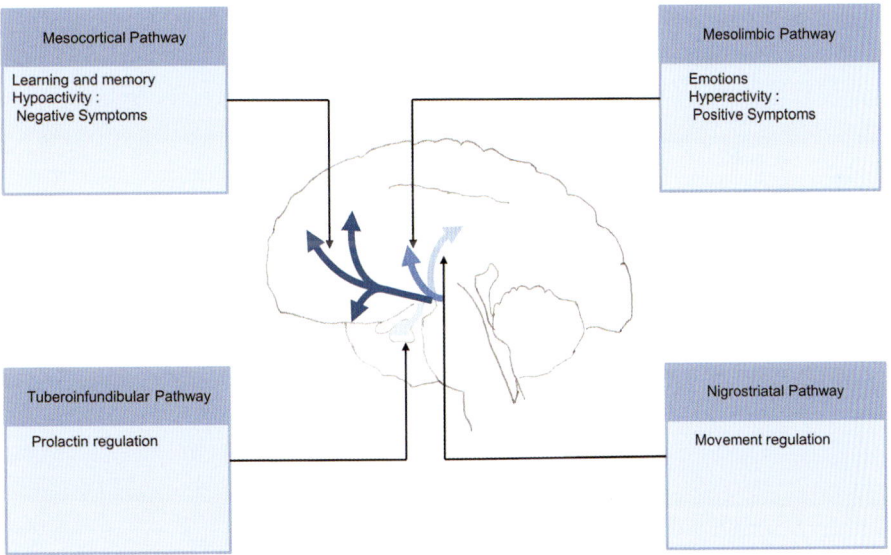

Figure 17.1: Four of the dopamine pathways in the brain, showing their position and function. The dopamine hypothesis suggests that hyperactivity of dopamine in the mesolimbic pathway produces psychotic symptoms, and hypoactivity in the mesocortical pathway produces negative symptoms.

Mechanism of action of antipsychotics

All antipsychotic medications block dopamine neurotransmission in the brain in one way or another. Some antipsychotic drugs interfere with the release of dopamine at the presynaptic cell; others block postsynaptic dopamine receptors and stop postsynaptic neurones from recognising dopamine. By blocking excess dopamine production in the mesolimbic pathway, it has been reported that the positive symptoms of schizophrenia can be reduced. Antipsychotics are further divided into two different families: the typical medications, first-generation antipsychotics (FGAs), and atypical second-generation antipsychotics (SGAs), according to their propensity to produce extrapyramidal side effects (drug-induced movement disorders).

Typical antipsychotics (FGAs) and side effects

The typical antipsychotic medications (haloperidol and others) mainly target dopamine 2 (D2) receptors, histamine 1 (H1), muscarinic 1 (M1) and alpha 1 (α1) (Mwebe 2018a, Mutsatsa 2015). The administration of typical medications interferes with normal dopaminergic neurotransmission in the substantia nigra and tuberoinfundibular pathways in the brain; dopamine release in these areas is responsible for motor co-ordination and modulatory functions in prolactin release, respectively. The antipsychotic's block on dopamine neurotransmission in the tuberoinfundibular pathways leads to higher prolactin levels (see Figure 17.2), resulting in side effects such as sexual dysfunction, gynaecomastia, galactorrhoea, and amenorrhoea.

Dopamine release in the nigrostriatal dopamine pathway helps to modulate the release of acetylcholine, an excitatory neurotransmitter responsible for stimulating muscles, regulating movement and aiding memory function. Blocking dopamine significantly increases acetylcholine, and this action results in motor effects (abnormal movements, sometimes referred to as extra-pyramidal side effects or EPSEs). Examples of EPSEs include akathisia, tardive dyskinesia, and dystonia (Mwebe 2018a). Strong affinity for D2 receptors by typical drugs increases the liability to cause EPSEs, particularly where D2 receptor drug occupancy exceeds 75% (Stahl 2017, Mwebe 2018a). For this reason, typical antipsychotics are not usually recommended as first-line treatment options (NICE 2019). The mechanism of action by typical medications on H1, M1 and α1 receptors (see Figure 17.3) results in cardiovascular, antihistamine and muscarinic side effects (Mwebe 2018a).

Pharmacological case studies: Mental illness

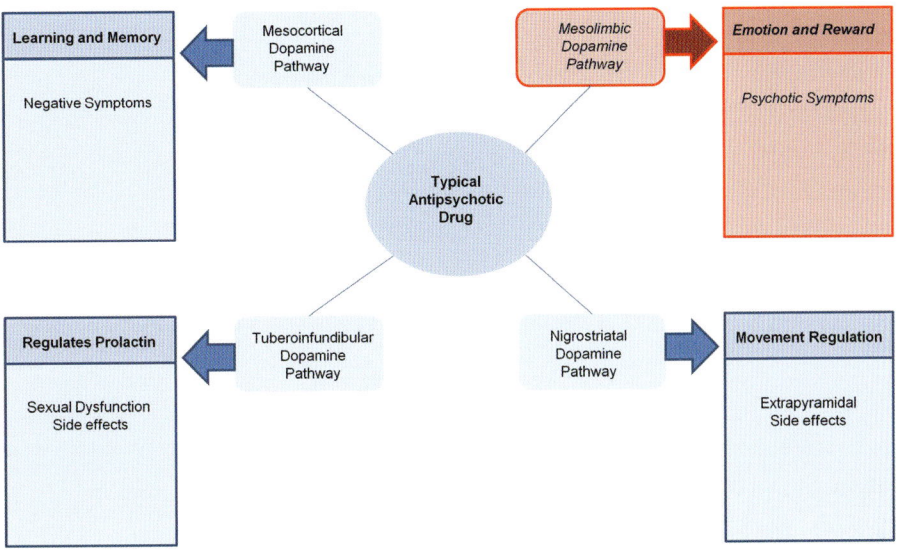

Figure 17.2: D2 antagonism in the tuberoinfundibular and nigrostriatal pathways by antipsychotic medications is associated with sexual dysfunction and movement disorders.

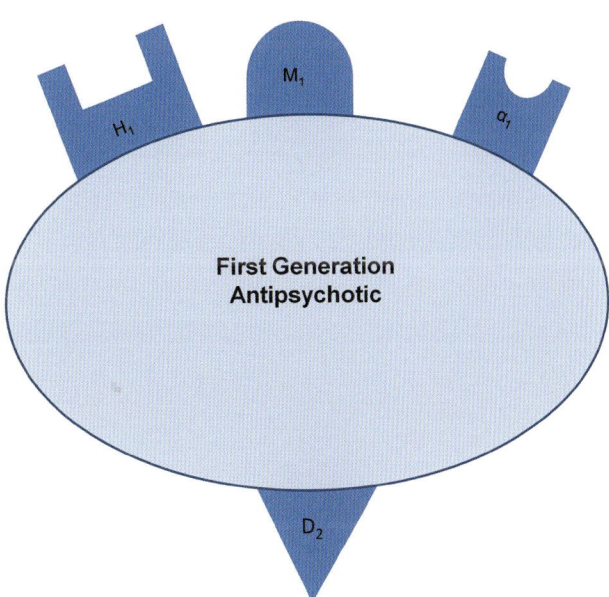

Figure 17.3: The receptor profile of typical antipsychotics (FGAs). Understanding the effects of these receptors can help the mental health practitioner predict the side effects that are likely to occur.

Case study: Medication management

Tom, aged 48, presents with flat affect, appears indifferent to his surroundings, and says that he has no sense of pleasure in life. Tom is also overweight and reports disturbed sleep. He complains that he hears voices which command him to shout at people. He is admitted to the acute psychiatric ward where he is given an antipsychotic drug X. After treatment, his hallucinations and paranoia resolve, but he complains that he has a tremor, stiff neck, akathisia, gets dizziness and cannot move about quickly. After a change in his medication to drug D, all these symptoms eventually improve. Tom does not need to have weekly blood tests.

A. Zuclopenthixol Clozapine

B. Haloperidol Olanzapine

C. Risperidone Sertraline

D. Citalopram Clozapine

E. Quetiapine Paroxetine

Activity 17.1 (Case study)

Identify drug X (from list A to E above) and explain the side effects Tom suffered after taking drug X and how they are managed in practice.

Atypical or second-generation antipsychotics (SGAs) and side effects

Atypical antipsychotics are known to be particularly effective against negative symptoms. They are better tolerated and have a lower risk of causing EPSEs – except for risperidone, which can cause motor side effects especially at high doses. Most atypical drugs act on other receptors, such as serotonin (5-HT2a, 5HT1a and 5-HT2C); dopamine D1, D2, D4; and histamine (H1), muscarinic (M1) and adrenergic (alpha-1 and alpha-2) receptors. This appears to be particularly true for amisulpride, clozapine, olanzapine, risperidone, and quetiapine (Stahl 2013; Kapur, Remington, et al. 1995).

SGAs are also commonly known as dopamine-serotonin antagonists (Stahl 2013). This action results in increased dopaminergic neurotransmission in the nigrostriatal pathway and might explain the lower risk of EPSEs associated with atypical drugs. It has been suggested that 5HT2a blockade enhances dopamine release in the prefrontal cortex (PFC) and thus leads to improvement in negative symptoms of schizophrenia. For instance, a medication such as clozapine, which is routinely used in treatment-resistant presentations, has high affinity for 5HT2a receptors but a relatively lower affinity for D2 receptors in comparison to typical antipsychotics (Mwebe 2018a).

Understanding the atypical profile of SGAs requires an understanding of the pharmacology of 5HT2a receptors and the importance of the effects of 5HT2a receptor antagonism by SGAs. The 5HT2a receptors are present in many brain regions, and they are mostly excitatory and enhance glutamate release. Glutamate is a powerful excitatory neurotransmitter that is released by nerve cells in the brain. Glutamate activation stimulates or blocks 5HT2a receptors, thereby also helping to regulate dopamine release. Thus far, 5HT2a receptors in the nigrostriatal pathway act as brakes on dopamine release. In the nigrostriatal pathway, antagonism of 5HT2a receptors by SGAs acts to reverse the effects of D2 antagonism, to enhance dopamine neurotransmission and therefore reduce the risk of EPSEs (Stahl 2017). As well as reducing motor side effects, 5HT2a antagonism by SGAs in other cortical brain regions contributes to enhanced dopamine release, possibly improving cognitive and affective symptoms.

Researchers have also found that atypical antipsychotics achieve their effects through rapid dissociation from D2 receptors, which may explain the lower incidence of extra-pyramidal side effects. In comparison to FGAs (which have a high affinity for D2 receptors), SGAs have low potency and a reduced affinity to D2 receptors and therefore disassociate very quickly from them. Rapid disassociation from D2 receptors by SGAs allows for natural dopamine stimulation of D2 post-synaptic receptors, enabling neurotransmission. Some SGAs can act as 5HT1a agonists. This effect enhances dopamine release in the prefrontal cortex, an action which leads to improvement in negative symptoms in patients taking drugs like clozapine and quetiapine.

Aripiprazole is the only atypical antipsychotic drug that reduces dopaminergic neurotransmission through D2 partial agonism and not D2 antagonism. As a partial agonist at D2 receptors, aripiprazole modulates dopaminergic transmission in both the mesolimbic and mesocortical pathway, an action which decreases and increases activity of dopamine in both pathways to improve positive and negative symptoms of schizophrenia (Mailman & Murthy 2010, Stahl 2017). Most SGAs bind with muscarinic and histamine receptors (M1 and H1) and this can result in side effects including increased appetite (which is linked to weight gain in patients) and cholinergic (dry mouth for which patients should be encouraged to keep hydrated), blurred vision, drowsiness, urine retention and others (Mwebe 2018a).

Figures 17.4, 17.5 and 17.6 (below) reflect the receptor binding profiles of the atypical (second-generation) antipsychotics.

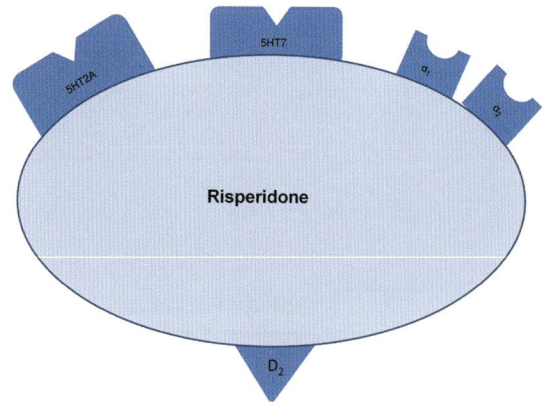

Figure 17.4: The receptor binding profile of risperidone.

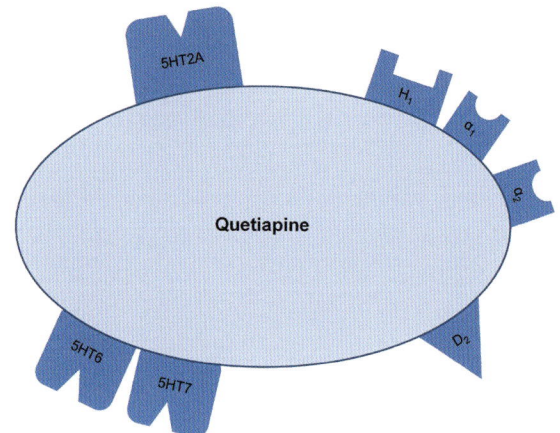

Figure 17.5: The receptor binding profile of quetiapine.

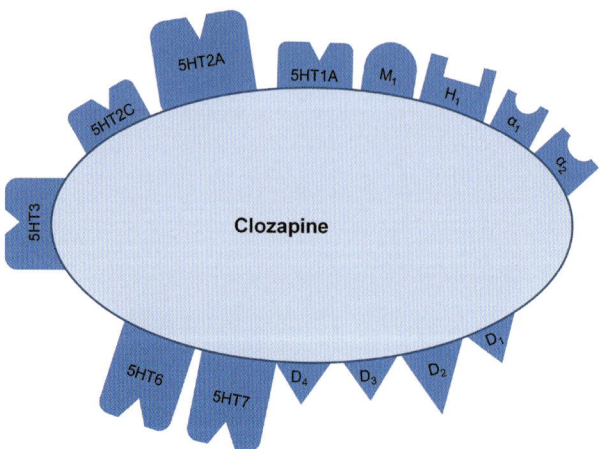

Figure 17.6: The receptor binding profile of clozapine.

Case study (continued)

Tom, aged 48, presents with flat affect, appears indifferent to his surroundings, and says that he has no sense of pleasure in life. Tom is also overweight and reports disturbed sleep. He complains that he hears voices which command him to shout at people. He is admitted to the acute psychiatric ward where he is given an antipsychotic drug X. After treatment, his hallucinations and paranoia resolve, but he complains that he has a tremor, stiff neck, akathisia, gets dizziness and cannot move about quickly. After a change in his medication to drug Y, all his symptoms improve. Tom does not need to have weekly blood tests.

F. Zuclopenthixol Clozapine

G. Haloperidol Olanzapine

H. Risperidone Sertraline

I. Citalopram Clozapine

J. Quetiapine Paroxetine

Activity 17.2 (Case study)

Which one of the above pairs (F to J) most likely corresponds to drug X and drug Y?

Weight gain monitoring

There is a significantly high risk of weight gain in all individuals taking any type of antipsychotic medication. Weight gain occurs soon after initiating treatment and may be difficult to reverse. However, weight gain should not only be attributed to pharmacological interventions; the nature and degree of mental illness can be linked to increased appetite and weight gain. Research evidence suggests that histaminergic transmission is involved in energy homeostasis (Ballon, Pajvani, et al. 2018). This effect appears to be relevant to the adverse effects of antipsychotics, as the extent of histamine H1 receptor antagonism by antipsychotic medication was the best predictor of the degree of weight gain in clinical studies by Ballon, Pajvani, et al. (2018). In addition, 5-HT2a and 5-HT2c have a major role in the control of body weight and food intake (Nasrallah 2008). Most SGAs, including clozapine and olanzapine, are potent 5-HT2c antagonists, and the action on this receptor has also been implicated in antipsychotic-induced weight gain (Freyberg & McCarthy 2017; Balt, Galloway, et al. 2011; Manu, Dima, et al. 2015).

Weight gain is associated with increased risk of hyperlipidaemia, insulin resistance, hyperglycaemia and diabetes in patients (Lipscombe, Austin, et al. 2014; Stubbs, Vancampfort et al.

2015). To date, several medications have been trialled, with some success in tackling antipsychotic-induced metabolic side-effects. Metformin, amantadine, reboxetine and topiramate have been shown to be effective in reducing antipsychotic-induced weight gain, with metformin having the most promising effects on weight loss (Baptista, Uzcátegui, *et al.* 2008; De Silva, Suraweera, *et al.* 2016).

Management of weight gain:
- Obtain baseline personal and family history of diabetes, obesity, dyslipidaemia, hypertension and cardiovascular disease
- As a general rule, monitor weight/BMI/waist circumference before initiation of treatment, at 3 months and annually after
- Provide dietary and lifestyle advice (refer for social prescribing, smoking cessation, physical activity)
- Refer to NICE guideline CG43 (NICE 2006) and Lester tool for best practice and management (Lester, Shiers & Rafi 2012)
- Refer to British Association of Psychopharmacology Guidelines (BAP 2016)
- Discuss the results of any monitoring with the patient and jointly agree on an action plan.

Glucose monitoring

Increases in glucose may occur early on after starting treatment with antipsychotics and may be difficult to reverse. For glucose homeostasis, the binding action of SGAs on M2 and M3 receptors (situated on the pancreatic beta cells) seems relevant. This is because M3 receptors help to control and regulate cholinergic-dependent insulin release from the pancreas into the circulatory system (Molina, Rodriguez-Diaz, *et al.* 2014). It has been suggested that antipsychotics, including clozapine and olanzapine, might impair both cholinergic and glucose-dependent insulin secretion from pancreatic beta cells. The high affinity for M3 receptor (which applies to both drugs) appears to be the most convincing evidence and predictor of a propensity for glucose dysregulation and development of type 2 diabetes mellitus (Chen, Huang, *et al.* 2017).

The major complication of diabetes is heart disease; and individuals suffering from schizophrenia who are taking antipsychotics are at an increased risk of developing type 2 diabetes (Stubbs, Vancampfort, *et al.* 2015). Metabolic effects associated with antipsychotics, including glycaemic abnormalities, diabetes and dyslipidaemia, have a devastating impact on quality of life for people taking these medications (Lin, Chen, *et al.* 2014; Wu, Tsai, *et al.* 2015). Regular screening and monitoring should be conducted for patients taking psychotropics and at risk of diabetes, including where polypharmacy is evident, a past family history of diabetes, sedentary behaviour, and weight gain problems.

Management of fasting glucose/HbA1c:

- Obtain baseline personal and family history of diabetes, obesity, dyslipidaemia, hypertension and cardiovascular disease
- As a general rule, monitor blood glucose (fasting glucose/HbA1c) before starting treatment, at 3 months and annually thereafter
- Long-term blood glucose can be monitored using HbA1c (glycated haemoglobin)
- Provide dietary and lifestyle advice (refer for social prescribing, smoking cessation and physical activity)
- Refer to NICE guidelines NG 28 (NICE 2015) and Lester tool for monitoring (Lester, Shiers & Rafi 2012)
- Refer to British Association of Psychopharmacology Guidelines (BAP 2016)
- Discuss results of any monitoring with the patient and jointly agree on an action plan.

Lipid monitoring

Initiating antipsychotics can increase cholesterol and triglycerides; and levels can rise over the longer term if not managed properly in high-risk patients, especially those taking antipsychotic medication. In a randomised controlled trial of healthy volunteers treated with olanzapine, iloperidone or placebo for 28 days, Ballon, Pajvani, et al. (2018) found that gains in body weight and adipose mass in olanzapine-treated subjects were associated with increased caloric intake, which unsurprisingly was further associated with development of dyslipidaemia (hypertriglyceridaemia and high total/LDL cholesterol). Evidence shows that dyslipidaemia in people with serious mental illness is higher than in people without mental illness; and those taking antipsychotics are at greater risk of developing lipid abnormalities (WHO 2018). While affinity for the muscarinic M3 receptor correlates with an increased risk of diabetes, the drug receptor-binding mechanisms that underlie dyslipidaemia remain poorly understood (Cox 2017, Foley, Mackinnon, et al. 2014).

Management of lipid checks and monitoring:

- As a general rule, monitor blood lipids (total cholesterol, non-HDL, HDL, triglycerides) before starting treatment, at 3 months and annually thereafter
- Provide dietary and lifestyle advice (refer for social prescribing, smoking cessation, physical activity)
- Refer to NICE guidelines CG 181 (NICE 2014) and Lester tool for monitoring (Lester, Shiers & Rafi 2012)
- Refer to British Association of Psychopharmacology Guidelines (BAP 2016)
- Discuss results of any monitoring with the patient and jointly agree on an action plan.

Activity 17.3 (Case study, see p. 332)
1. Explain Tom's weight gain.
2. How would you help Tom to manage his weight gain?
3. How would you check Tom's cardiovascular health?

Management of people taking antipsychotic medications:
- Obtain baseline personal and family history of diabetes, obesity, dyslipidaemia, hypertension, and cardiovascular disease
- As a general rule, monitor blood lipids (total cholesterol, non-HDL, HDL, triglycerides), blood glucose, BMI, waist circumference before starting treatment, at 3 months and annually thereafter
- The simple guidance on screening for cardiometabolic risk in serious mental illness (Lester Cardiometabolic Tool) should be used to screen for cardiovascular disease (CVD) risk (Lester, Shiers & Rafi 2012)
- The QRISK®3 calculator (QRISK 2018) is a validated prediction CVD risk assessment tool commonly used in primary care to estimate the 10-year risk of CVD in men and women (Collins & Altman 2012)
- The JBS3 (Joint British Societies for prevention of cardiovascular disease) risk tool (2014) can be used alongside QRISK3. The JBS3 tool estimates CVD risk over a lifetime and it can help inform strategies to screen for CVD risk and interventions (lifestyle and medication therapies) to manage CVD (British Cardiovascular Society 2019). The JBS3 includes the 10-year risk estimation but has also been developed to include CVD risk over time
- ECG monitoring is advised before and at least once a year during treatment, depending on the needs of the individual patient
- Physical examinations (blood pressure, pulse, temperature and respirations) should be offered to individuals taking psychotropic medications
- Watch out for clozapine-induced myocarditis, which is potentially fatal. Rare side effects may require immediate discontinuation of clozapine treatment (elevated CRP and troponin levels appear to have more diagnostic significance)
- Provide dietary and lifestyle advice (refer for social prescribing, smoking cessation, physical activity)
- Refer to British Association of Psychopharmacology Guidelines (BAP 2016)
- Discuss results of any monitoring with the patient and jointly agree on an action plan.

Depression

The World Health Organisation estimates that more than 300 million people worldwide suffer from depression. In the UK, about 90% of people with depression are treated in primary care (Ferenchick, Ramanuj & Pincus 2019). Primary healthcare services play a fundamental role as gatekeepers in the early screening and management (including routine follow-up) of depression and other common mental disorders (including anxiety, substance use disorders, eating disorders and panic disorders).

In England, 4–10% of individuals will experience depression in their lifetime (Ferenchick, Ramanuj & Pincus 2019). Depression is characterised by cognitive, mental, functional disability; persistent sadness and reduced activity; disturbed thinking, poor concentration, and sleep; dysregulated appetite; and feelings of apathy and rejection. Hopelessness and suicidal thoughts may be a complication of severe depression. Possible causes of depression include genetic factors; early object relations, including parental behaviours towards siblings; psychological and sexual abuse, neglect and traumatic life events (such as loss and bereavement); menopause; co-morbid physical/medical conditions; and socio-economic challenges in recent migrant populations (Khushboo 2017).

Antidepressants are routinely used in the treatment and management of moderate–severe depressive disorders. The most common type of depression is major depressive disorder (MDD), also known as clinical depression. Bipolar disorder (BD), which is characterised by intermittent episodes of mania or hypomania, is sometimes interwoven with depressive episodes. Clinical depression usually includes symptoms such as loss of interest and pleasure, reduced energy, severe low mood, insomnia, excessive feelings of worthlessness and guilt, hopelessness, anxiety, and weight loss or gain.

People experiencing a major depressive episode or major depressive disorder are at significantly increased risk of suicide (Stone, Laughren, *et al.* 2009). Encouraging them to seek help and treatment from healthcare professionals can dramatically reduce the risk of suicide or self-harm if evident. Routinely, remember to ask about suicidal ideations and thoughts when conducting an initial assessment at baseline, and at any agreed review points during disease management. It is always useful to involve the patient and their family/carers in order to improve clinical decision-making about their care (Courtet & Lopez-Castroman 2017).

Diagnosing depression

For a diagnosis of depression to be made, symptoms including persistent low mood, persistent sadness, and significant loss of pleasure and interest, must occur most days and times in the preceding two weeks. In addition, two or three of the associated symptoms below must be present:

- Disturbed sleep
- Poor concentration or indecisiveness
- Low self-confidence
- Poor or increased appetite
- Suicidal thoughts/acts
- Agitation
- Guilt or self-blame.

The severity of the depressive disorder is determined by both the number and severity of symptoms, as well as the degree of functional impairment (Goldberg, Prisciandaro & Williams 2012). For a formal diagnosis of depression, the ICD-11 requires four out of ten symptoms to be evident. At least five out of nine symptoms are required for the DSM-V (Gaebel, Zielasek & Reed 2017; Goldberg 2019). A compressive assessment of the patient's symptoms and difficulties should be made, considering evidence of any functional impairment, alongside other symptoms, to inform diagnosis. Living with depression can be significantly debilitating for sufferers. They may experience challenges in maintaining meaningful social connections/networks and may lose interest in socialising with others, and in seeing their friends or families (Mwebe 2018a; NICE 2018; Holland, Floyd & Soames 2018).

Treating depression

While antidepressants are the first-line treatment to manage major depressive disorder, in practice it is not uncommon to augment them with antipsychotics, benzodiazepines and/or lithium. For example, with antipsychotic medication such as risperidone, quetiapine may be added as an adjunct intervention, alongside antidepressants for an individual diagnosed with psychotic depression with active psychotic symptoms such as hallucinations (Stahl 2017). Other adjunct non-pharmacological interventions may include cognitive therapies such as CBT, self-help programmes, family and group therapies, and counselling.

Monoamine theory of depression

In addition to the sociological and psychological factors that can help to explain the causes of depression, biological influences have been proposed in relation to the role of monoamine neurotransmitters (serotonin, dopamine, and adrenaline) in the brain. Abnormalities in production and function of these neurotransmitters led to the formulation of the monoamine theory of depression. The depletion of serotonin (5HT), dopamine (DA) and noradrenaline (NA) underlies depressive pathology. The strongest evidence supporting this theory is that antidepressants work by increasing levels of these chemicals in the areas of the brain that influence mood, emotions, behaviour, and cognitive functioning. Monoamine chemicals play various roles in the body, including mood and emotional regulation, sleep, memory, food intake and social behaviour (Kring, Davidson & Neale 2013). Stahl (2013) suggests that symptoms of serotonin deficiency can include anxiety, panic, phobia, obsessive compulsive disorder (OCD) and food craving/bulimia. Noradrenaline deficiency may result in depressed mood, with impaired cognitive functioning and psychomotor retardation.

Alongside the monoamine theory of depression, the neurotrophic theory of depression proposes that symptoms of depression are linked to reduced brain derived neurotrophic factor (BDNF) levels and that antidepressant medications improve depressive symptoms by increasing BDNF levels (Lee & Kim 2010). BDNF is a gene that is responsible for ensuring the viability and functioning of neurones. It is proposed that in people with clinical symptoms of depression (including stress reactions) BDNF levels may become suppressed due to stress. This can lead to atrophy or death of neurones. Treating stress can therefore help to reverse neuronal loss (Phillips and Fahimi 2018; Goldberg, Reed, et al. 2016).

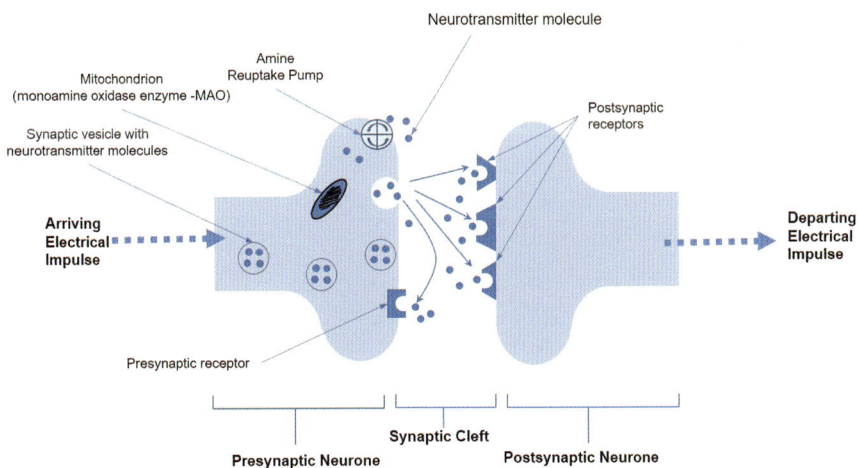

Figure 17.7a: Events (or physiological processes) that occur at the synapse. Action potentials (electrical signals) travel along the axon, stimulate the presynaptic nerve terminal, causing presynaptic vesicles containing neurotransmitters* (amines) to fuse with the neuronal membrane, releasing its contents into the synaptic cleft. These amines bind to postsynaptic receptors, stimulating a response. Neurotransmitters are then removed from the synapse by reuptake pump and monoamine oxidase (MAO) enzyme degrades presynaptic amines.

*The neurone can make and release either noradrenaline, dopamine, or serotonin neurotransmitter.

Key points:

- Have you conducted a thorough enquiry of modifiable and non-modifiable risk factors to gain an understanding of the process of ill health and related causal factors before making any prescribing decision?
- Steps should be taken to develop the patient's understanding of risk factors linked to poor mental and physical health.
- The use of antidepressant medications is part of a range of the many other tools (self-guided help, counselling, CBT, group therapy, psychotherapy, yoga, physical activity, healthy eating) used to treat depression.
- The use of pharmacological products in mental health settings should not define the patient nor the role of mental health professionals but what is required is a collaborative effort between the patient, healthcare professional and carers to jointly work towards supporting and enabling the patient towards optimum function and a degree of autonomy.

Case study: Depression 1

Jane has gone to see her general practitioner in the company of her husband. Jane is 35 and works as an accountant but has not been at work for more than a month. On presentation, Jane appears tearful and visibly low in mood, her hair is messy, and her blouse looks stained. Jane speaks very softly, with long pauses in between sentences, to the GP. She informs the GP that she left her job about five weeks ago because she could not cope any more. She explains that for the last 6–7 weeks, she has been experiencing extremes of low mood, loss of energy, loss of appetite, insomnia, and loss of pleasure in activities. Jane reports that her husband is worried about her, and he has encouraged her to book today's visit.

Activity 17.4 (Case study)

1. Based on the diagnostic criteria for depressive disorder (ICD-11), do you think the GP would be correct to diagnose Jane with a depressive episode?
2. What would a comprehensive health assessment look like for Jane?

Antidepressants

Since the introduction of antidepressants in the 1950s, their pharmacotherapeutic benefits have dominated and influenced treatment and management of moderate to severe cases of depression across the world. Alongside antidepressants, psychosocial interventions (including CBT, counselling, and self-help activities) have been shown to improve outcomes in people with depression (Mwebe 2018a). Psychological therapies have been found to be as effective as medication and are better tolerated, with no adverse metabolic effects associated with the use of psychotropic medications. As discussed earlier, the pathology of depression is strongly linked with functional deficiency and alterations of catecholamines, especially noradrenaline, serotonin (5HT) and dopamine. Antidepressants inhibit reuptake of neurotransmitters through selective receptors (see Figure 17.7b), and this action helps to increase the concentration of specific neurotransmitters in the synaptic space in the brain (Khushboo 2017).

There are four main types of antidepressant medications. While each one may work slightly differently, it is true to say that they all generally work by influencing the levels of serotonin, noradrenaline, and dopamine in the brain (see Figure 17.8, p. 344). Nevertheless, the exact mechanism of antidepressant activity remains unclear. Although neurotransmitter levels rise within hours of taking an antidepressant, the real effect on symptoms of clinical depression usually takes longer – between 2–6 weeks (Holland *et al.* 2018). And non-response at 2–6 weeks is usually a good predictor of overall response. During this period, continue treatment and assess for a further 2–3 weeks, before reviewing whether the patient reports overall improvement in mood.

The absence of any improvement at week 3–4 should normally trigger a change in treatment. Poor response to one drug does not necessary predict response to another drug class or another drug within the same class. It is important to discuss any prescribing decisions with the patient and offer a holistic review of their health needs. Interventions should follow an integrated approach, including self-help activities, advice around self-hygiene, improving social networks, healthy eating, and physical activities, as well as psychological interventions.

Antidepressants are associated with worsening of anxiety, agitation, and increased suicide thoughts at initiation (1–2 weeks) and patients should be informed of this risk before starting these medications. Ask about risk of suicide at first review, and when stopping, the doses should be tapered gradually over 1–2 weeks to minimise discontinuation symptoms, including anxiety, agitation, insomnia, and nightmares (NICE 2018).

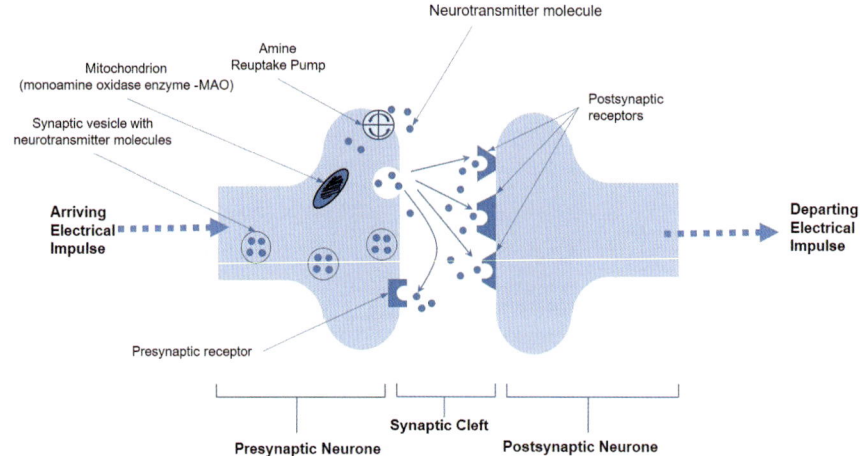

Figure 17.7b: Reuptake and breakdown of noradrenaline by monoamine oxidase (MAO) and catecho-O-methyl transferase (COMT) enzymes. COMT, produced by neurones in the brain, deactivates neurotransmitters such as noradrenaline and dopamine.

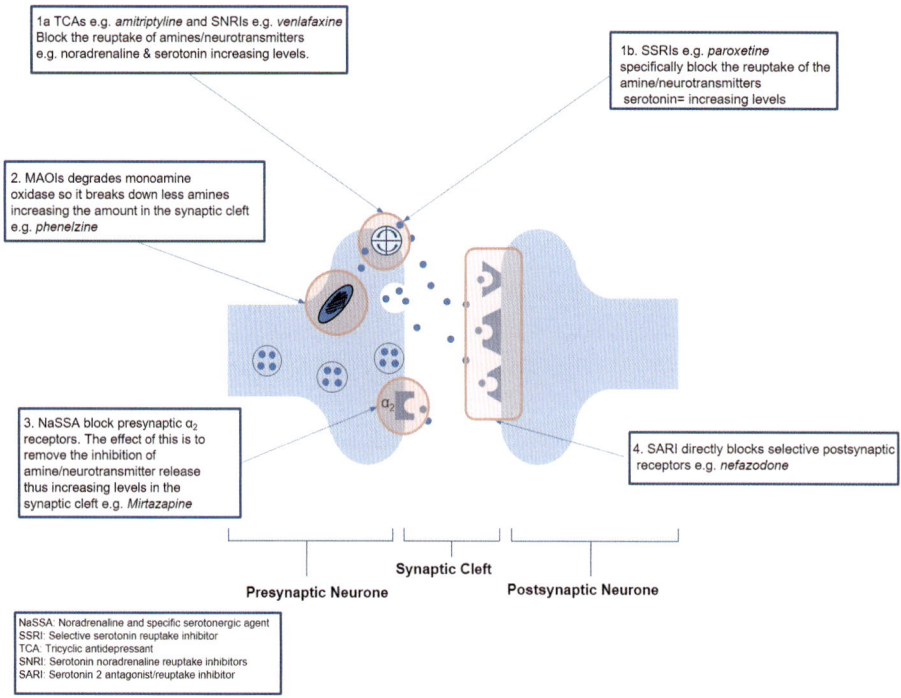

Figure 17.8: Mechanism of action of different groups of antidepressants, showing the proposed effects of different groups of antidepressant medication at the adrenergic nerve terminal.

MAO (found in the presynaptic nerve cell) and COMT transferase (situated in the synapse) enzymes are responsible for the breakdown of MAO neurotransmitters (dopamine and serotonin). In depressed patients, this means that there is a relative deficiency of MAO neurotransmitters, including serotonin, noradrenaline and dopamine.

Tricyclic antidepressants (TCAs)

Tricyclic antidepressants block the reuptake of noradrenaline (NA) and serotonin (5HT). TCAs, which include amitriptyline, desipramine, clomipramine, imipramine, nortriptyline, and others, have also been reported to block muscarinic, alpha 1 and histamine receptors. Alpha 1 blockade can cause side effects such as postural hypotension, light-headedness, and dizziness. Encourage the patient to move slowly when assuming an upright position, from sitting or lying down. The symptoms can also be improved through a gradual slow titration.

Muscarinic receptor blockade causes side effects including dry mouth, blurred vision, photophobia, constipation, urinary retention, and tachycardia. Slow titration can also help to relieve these symptoms and/or a dose reduction may be required. Blockade of histamine 1 receptors can cause weight gain and sedation. To counter daytime sedation, give the dose at bedtime and the sedative effects may then be of clinical benefit for patients with problematic insomnia and agitation. However, sedating TCAs (such as amitriptyline) should be avoided, if possible, in patients with severe psychomotor retardation or hypersomnia.

TCAs are lethal in overdose and can cause cardiac complications, including long QRS interval, convulsions, cardiotoxicity, arrhythmias and cardiac arrest. Severely depressed patients with prominent suicidal symptoms (including imminent risk to self), clear intent and plans to act on thoughts, should not be given more than a week's prescription of TCA medications.

Case study: Depression 2

John, aged 40, has a long history of major depressive illness. At the age of 17, John was sexually abused and physically attacked by his stepfather. John disclosed these events to his mother, but she did not believe him. Instead John was branded by her as a troubled and evil child. John's relationship with two of his older siblings has been fractured over the years. John failed to complete school because of bullying and lack of support from teachers. He was excluded from high school on various occasions for problematic behaviours, including violence towards his peers. At the age of 22 John reconnected with his biological father but in the same year John lost his mother to depression. John walked into his mother's room and found that she had hanged herself. John was distraught about this incident – he blames himself for his mother's death, partly because he feels that if he had got to her earlier, she would still be alive.

John also feels that her untimely death robbed him of her apology and that she needed to say sorry for all the traumatic events she had put him through while he was growing up.

John's relationship with his biological father has remained rocky, as he blames his father for abandoning the family. John has struggled to hold down jobs over the past 15 years; he says he has a problem with people telling him what to do. He has struggled financially over the past 10 years, seeking comfort from alcohol and cannabis, as these substances help to numb his pain and help him forget the past and the bad memories.

For the past 8 years, John has been taking 100mg amitriptyline in divided doses daily. John has recently been transferred to an inpatient psychiatric facility, following an overdose of 8 tablets of amitriptyline (50mg each) after spending a month on a general medical ward.

Amitriptyline is one of the TCA medications. Based on what you have learnt so far about the side effects of TCAs, an overdose of amitriptyline would almost certainly expose John to some of the toxic side effects of TCAs, particularly if a medication is taken outside the recommended daily dose range

Activity 17.5 (Case study)

1. Based on what you have read so far about depression, what are the most likely triggers and underlying factors in the development of John's depressive disorder?
2. What are the possible side effects John suffered?

Case study (continued)

At a ward review meeting, the prescribing psychiatrist (who has not previously been known to John) discusses John's care with the clinical team in John's presence. He advises John that he is considering changing his medication to another type of antidepressant, called a selective serotonin reuptake inhibitor (SSRI). The doctor informs John that SSRIs have fewer and less toxic side effects compared to his current medication and that John is very lucky to have survived the overdose. John informs the team that he did not intend to kill himself and that the overdose was accidental. He does not want to die because of his dog and a very supportive friend called Monica.

1. The team agree to reduce John's daily dose of 100mg amitriptyline gradually, over the following 1–2 weeks, before commencing him on citalopram, which is an SSRI. SSRIs are generally better tolerated than TCAs or MAOIs.
2. The clinical team also agree with John that he should be allocated a nurse who will monitor his daily mental state. This allocated nurse will give John an outlet to express his thoughts, fears and worries.
3. A referral to the drug service is deemed necessary but John is not ready for this and declines to engage. The team will need to revisit this later when John is ready to address it.
4. John's sleep and food intake are monitored.
5. Participation in activities on and off the ward is encouraged, to improve John's functioning.
6. He is discouraged from using alcohol or other recreational substances, both on and off the ward.
7. The team specifically work with John and support him to engage in activities of interest, hobbies etc.

Serotonin and noradrenaline reuptake inhibitors (SNRIs)

Venlafaxine is a commonly used antidepressant classified as an SNRI. SNRIs inhibit both serotonin and noradrenaline reuptake. Venlafaxine has little or no anticholinergic (dry mouth, constipation, blurred vision), histaminergic (sedation) or alpha-adrenergic effects. Rarely, the use of venlafaxine has been associated with akathisia and this is often dose dependent as higher doses are more likely to induce akathisia. Regular blood pressure monitoring is recommended in patients taking venlafaxine; and in patients with known secondary hypertension, it is advisable to control the hypertension before starting venlafaxine.

Common side effects reported include nausea, loss of appetite, raised blood pressure, sight problems, sleepiness, sexual dysfunction, irregular bleeding, and a 'pins and needles' sensation.

Alpha 2 antagonist (noradrenaline and specific serotonergic antidepressant)

Mirtazapine is a noradrenergic and serotonergic antidepressant because it blocks receptors that regulate the release of these neurotransmitters. Increase in noradrenaline neurotransmission is achieved by blocking alpha-2 presynaptic receptors in the noradrenergic neurons while increase in serotonin neurotransmission is achieved by blocking alpha-2 adrenergic presynaptic receptors on serotonergic neurons. Mirtazapine also blocks other serotonin receptors (5HT2A, 5HT2C and 5HT3) and histamine receptors (H1). This causes effects such as sedation, increased appetite, weight gain, improved cognitive function and concentration. Due to very strong sedative effects, it is recommended to prescribe the medication as a single dose before bedtime (Mwebe 2018a).

Common side effects, in addition to those discussed above, include dry mouth, constipation, dizziness, abnormal dreams, hypotension, changes in urinary function and anxiety.

Selective serotonin reuptake inhibitors (SSRIs)

Selective serotonin reuptake inhibitors (SSRIs) are known to act by inhibiting the reuptake of serotonin into the serotonin presynaptic neurone. It is also true that SSRIs and others (SNRIs, TCAs, MAOIs) are not just antidepressants, as these medications are often used in clinical practice to treat and manage other conditions, apart from depression (Stahl 2017, British National Formulary 2020). Generally, all SSRIs selectively inhibit serotonin transport and are indicated in the treatment and management of psychiatric presentations such as depression, panic disorder, generalised anxiety disorders, post-traumatic stress disorder, social anxiety and obsessive-compulsive disorder. Examples of SSRIs include fluoxetine (Prozac), paroxetine (Paxil), sertraline (Zoloft), citalopram (Celexa, Cipramil) and escitalopram (Lexapro).

The action of SSRIs at the synaptic junction results in an increase in serotonin (5HT) within the somatodendrite area of the serotonergic nerve cell, which causes downregulation (desensitisation) of the somatodendrite 5HT1A auto-receptors on the presynaptic serotonergic neurone (Stahl 2013). This increases neuronal impulse (message) flow and results in increased production of 5HT (serotonin) from the nerve terminals which desensitises the post-synaptic nerve receptors. These actions (especially the desensitisation of the receptors) are thought to contribute to the therapeutic actions of SSRIs as well as iatrogenic side effects associated with their use in clinical practice. The onset of the therapeutic action of all antidepressants is usually not immediate, but often takes between 2 and 4 weeks. Psychopharmacologist Professor Stahl argues that a review of the patient's antidepressant treatment regime may be required if there is no reported clinical benefit for the patient after 6–8 weeks.

It is thought that the toxicity of the 5-HT2 and 5-HT3 receptors of certain serotonergic pathways (due to increases in serotonin concentrations at receptors in the brain and other areas in the body) may be responsible for the side effects of SSRIs.

Common side effects associated with the use of SSRIs include anxiety, sleep disturbances, sexual dysfunction (decreased libido and reduction in arousal), dizziness, nausea, bloating, vomiting, diarrhoea, fatigue, irritability, and insomnia headaches. While most side effects may be immediate, they often subside with time. It is important to reassure patients, as non-concordance within the first 1–2 weeks of antidepressant treatment may often be due to occurrence of side effects.

SSRIs are not addictive, but care should be taken when using them. Patients should also be reminded to seek medical advice and not to stop treatment abruptly, as this can cause discontinuation symptoms (e.g. dizziness, 'pins and needles', nausea, vomiting, irritability and flu-like features).

SSRIs are safer than TCAs and MAOIs in overdose and are associated with less serious side effects. SSRIs are also tolerated better by older adults. For all patients assessed and requiring a pharmacological intervention, it's advisable to start by choosing a generic SSRI as recommended by NICE CG90 (NICE 2018) while also considering any risk of drug interactions and the patient's lifestyle choices (such as recreational drug use) and medical comorbidities. For mild depressive symptoms, NICE guidelines (NICE 2018) recommend that psychological interventions including, cognitive therapy, cognitive behavioural therapy, self-help, problem-based therapy, mindfulness-based cognitive therapy, and counselling should be offered in place of medications.

Key points about the use of antidepressants in depression

- The initial consultation should explore the patient's personal and family history of both mental and physical illness, current psychosocial stress factors (e.g. recent loss, bereavement, and financial stress), medication history, recreational drug use. It should also cover the use of objective clinical tools (PHQ-9, two 5-item depression and anxiety scales etc.) and include assessment of symptom severity, as well as physical health examinations and checks including blood tests (full blood count, liver function tests, thyroid function tests, urea and electrolytes, ferritin, Vitamin D).
- Have you discussed with the patient their drug choice and the non-pharmacological interventions that are available?
- Discuss the drug of choice in view of any existing comorbid psychiatric/medical disorders such as OCD, anxiety, diabetes, or heart conditions.
- Explore patients' expectations from treatment and discuss with them the likely outcomes – for example, gradual improvement/relief of depressive symptoms over several weeks.
- Prescribe a dose of antidepressant (after titration, if necessary) that is likely to be effective.
- Review patients at least every 1 or 2 weeks after commencing treatment, including assessment of side effects, adherence, and suicidal risk.
- Consider review of diagnosis and/or dose increase and/or stopping the antidepressant if there is no clinical improvement after 2–4 weeks.
- For swapping and stopping advice, refer directly to the Maudsley Prescribing Guidelines 12th edition (Taylor, Paton & Kerwin 2015) or contact your local pharmacy team for advice.
- If there is clinical improvement after 3–4 weeks, continue treatment for at least 6–9 months after resolution of symptoms (those at risk of relapse should continue for at least 2 years).
- Antidepressants should be withdrawn gradually, and patients should always be informed of the risk and nature of discontinuation symptoms.
- SSRIs have been linked to increased risk of internal GI bleeding so gastro-protective drugs

(such as omeprazole) should be prescribed, especially in vulnerable patients such as older adults taking NSAIDs or aspirin.
- Citalopram has been associated with abnormal changes in the electric activity of the heart when prescribed at doses greater than 40mg. It is therefore recommended to avoid prescribing above this range.
- TCAs are most toxic in overdose. SSRIs are therefore preferred as first-line treatment and drug of choice when prescribing, apart from citalopram which is the most toxic of SSRIs in overdose (and can lead to coma, seizures, and arrhythmia).
- Fluoxetine, fluvoxamine, and paroxetine have a higher propensity for drug interactions.
- Citalopram and sertraline have a lower risk of drug interaction and should therefore be considered in patients with multi-morbidities and in polypharmacy.
- Physical health monitoring (including weight/BMI checks, full blood count, liver function tests, lipids, glucose checks, blood pressure and pulse) is recommended at least annually in patients taking antidepressants.

Summary

In this chapter, the role played by psychotropics (including antipsychotics and antidepressants) in the treatment and management of schizophrenia, depression and other related psychiatric comorbidities has been examined. The use of these drugs has revolutionised psychiatric intervention over the past few decades, with wider acknowledgement of the benefits – including symptom reduction and a return to baseline functioning. As discussed, the use of psychotropics is also associated with iatrogenic and toxic cardiometabolic side effects which, in addition to the challenges of living with complex and severe psychiatric illnesses (such as paranoid schizophrenia, bipolar affective disorder and major depressive disorder) can lead to premature mortality and a reduced lifespan in users of mental health services. Due to an increased risk of developing metabolic complications (such as weight gain, obesity, glycaemic abnormalities, dyslipidaemia, diabetes and cardiovascular complications), regular physical health assessments and examinations (including blood pressure, pulse, weight/BMI, blood glucose, and lipid checks) should form part of the patient's care plan and be offered at least every 6 to 12 months.

Answers to activities

Activity 17.1 (Case study)

Identify drug X (from list A to E above) and explain the side effects Tom suffered after taking drug X and how they are managed in practice.

The side effects (tremor, stiff neck, and Tom's difficulties with movement) are usually associated with typical antipsychotics (FGAs) but can also occur with atypical (SGAs) drugs such as risperidone. As discussed earlier, movement disorders usually result from an increase in acetylcholine (a neurotransmitter responsible for neuromuscular movement and memory functioning). Dopamine plays a modulatory role in the substantia nigra when antipsychotic drugs (e.g. haloperidol) block the effects of dopamine in this area of the brain. This action interferes with the modulatory role of dopamine over acetylcholine, resulting in extra-pyramidal side effects (EPSEs). We can conclude that drug X is most likely to be a typical antipsychotic or an atypical antipsychotic with relatively strong D2 receptor affinity in the substantia nigra.

In clinical practice, treatment, and management of EPSEs normally includes anticholinergics, benzodiazepines, and propranolol. Anticholinergics work by blocking the actions and effects of excess acetylcholine. Commonly used anticholinergics include procyclidine, orphenadrine and benzhexol. The overuse of procyclidine should be monitored in patients who are at risk of developing constipation or in those where constipation is a problem (particularly as constipation can also be a side effect associated with antipsychotics). Therefore, chronic use of procyclidine should be avoided and a discussion with the patient about potential side effects should always be part of their care plan.

Side effects rating scales are very useful tools to screen for the presence, severity, and duration of drug-induced side effects in clinical practice. For example, with guidance from the health professionals, the Liverpool University Side Effects rating scale (LUNSERS) and Glasgow Antipsychotic Side Effects Scale (GASS) (Waddell & Taylor 2008) can be self-administered by the patient (Mwebe 2018a).

In patients where other cholinergic side effects are suspected (e.g. blurred vision and dry mouth), the nurse should encourage the patient to remain hydrated and to limit the consumption of stimulants, i.e. coffee and high-energy sugary drinks, as these can exacerbate dehydration. The prescriber should consider adjusting the dose, if the risks outweigh the benefits in individual cases, and the treating team should consider stopping the drug. In situations where constipation and/or weight gain is problematic, encourage healthy eating (foods rich in fibre, fruits, vegetables) and promote participation in physical activity activities (consider social prescribing referrals via the patient's General Practitioner).

Tom complained of dizziness while taking drug X and this is not uncommon in people taking psychotropic medication, due to the blocking effects by both typical and atypical antipsychotics on alpha-1 and alpha-2 adrenergic muscarinic receptors. The receptor binding profile of most of the antipsychotics on these receptors results in cardiovascular side effects including dizziness and hypotension. This is discussed later in Activity 17.3, 'Cardiovascular effects' (Mwebe 2018a, Stahl 2017).

Activity 17.2 (Case study)

Which one of the above pairs (F to J) most likely corresponds to Drug X and Drug Y?

Drug X is most likely to have a relatively higher affinity for D2 receptors. As discussed earlier in this chapter, FGAs are notorious for binding too tightly to D2 receptors. This action does not allow naturally occurring dopamine to bind with the D2 receptors. In the course of treatment, while there might be improvement in a patient's positive symptoms (such as hallucinations, delusions and paranoia), increased block on D2 receptors is associated with increased risk of EPSEs. Therefore, the correct drug pair here for (Drug X and Y) is Haloperidol and Olanzapine.

Tom's movement disorders gradually improved after his medication was changed to a low potent antipsychotic drug that has a low affinity to D2 receptors and theoretically disassociates briefly from the D2 receptor but long enough to allow dopamine neurotransmission across the synapse. This action is commonly associated with atypical antipsychotics. Olanzapine, a commonly used atypical antipsychotic in adult psychiatry, is associated with increased appetite and weight gain in patients. Regular checks including weight measures, full blood count, blood pressure, ECGs and pulse will need to be conducted regularly.

We are told that Tom does not need to have a weekly blood test. As clozapine is the only atypical antipsychotic where individuals taking this medication are required to have a blood test either weekly, fortnightly or every 4 weeks, as a safety precaution, we can rule clozapine out as the correct answer. Options H (Risperidone Sertraline) and J (Quetiapine Paroxetine) have an antidepressant added, which rules them out.

Regular blood monitoring (including full blood count and white blood cell count) is a mandatory intervention in all individuals taking clozapine. Full blood count (FBC), BMI, pulse, blood pressure and ECG must be conducted at baseline before starting clozapine or any antipsychotic medication. A weekly FBC should be carried out for the first 18 weeks of clozapine treatment, then fortnightly for 12 months and 4-weekly thereafter. (This monitoring regime can be reviewed if there are dose changes, non-concordance issues or other treatment issues are identified.)

Clozapine therapy has been known to cause a drop in white blood cell count; and a fall in larger amounts of neutrophils (agranulocytosis) can be serious and should be monitored closely via a blood test. Both agranulocytosis and neutropenia may occur in the first 18 weeks of treatment and/or when the individual is taking other medications which can affect white cell count or physical/medical conditions which can induce both conditions. Symptoms to look out for in patients suspected of being neutropenic include sore throat, fever and a rash.

In view of all this, clozapine is usually prescribed and dispensed to patients after a blood test has been completed and deemed to be within normal parameters. A traffic light monitoring system is used to ensure that clozapine is used safely:

- **Red** (stop clozapine)
- White cell count less than 3×10^9/L OR absolute neutrophil count less than 1.5×10^9/L
- Stop taking clozapine, monitor white cell count daily and look for signs of infection

- Patients who develop signs of infection, such as sore throat and raised temperature, should be advised to contact their doctor (GP, Responsible Clinician) or a member of the mental health team.
- 🟠 **Amber** (proceed with precaution, patient might require additional monitoring)
- White cell count 3.0-3.5 × 109/L OR absolute neutrophil count 1.5-2.0 × 109/L
- Continue taking clozapine and monitor white cell count twice a week until it recovers
- Proceed with caution, patient might require additional monitoring (temperature, blood pressure, pulse, clinical observations).
- 🟢 **Green** (proceed with clozapine normally but both patient and healthcare professional must remain vigilant and ensure that the required monitoring is done)
- Blood test is within usual parameters and so clozapine can be taken.

Activity 17.3 (Case study)

1. Explain Tom's weight gain.

The relationship between mental illness and weight gain is a complex one. It is argued that weight gain can contribute to the development of mental illness and, similarly, people with mental and physical/medical conditions are at increased risk of weight gain. The problems with weight in this scenario may be a direct consequence of living and suffering with a complex mental illness but, equally, the administration of psychiatric drugs is associated with a range of metabolic side effects. All the psychotropic drugs listed under the different treatment options have an associated risk of weight gain and other cardiometabolic effects.

Some of the symptoms Tom reports are consistent with depression (including flat affect, appearing indifferent to his surroundings, having no sense of pleasure in life, being overweight and experiencing insomnia). Individuals with depression and anxiety are particularly prone to weight gain. Authors of a systematic review of a longitudinal study concluded that there was a bi-directional relationship between depression and weight gain. They found that 'overweight persons had a 55 per cent increased risk of developing depression over time, while depressed persons had a 58 per cent increased risk of becoming obese' (Luppino, de Wit, et al. 2010, p. 225). In people with severe mental illness, the mean weight is significantly greater than those without mental illness (Cooper, Reynolds, et al. 2016). Poor mental health can lead to poor decision making, unhealthy lifestyle choices including unhealthy diets, substance abuse and sedentary behaviour. As discussed in earlier text, medication side effects can make it difficult for the individuals with mental illness to avoid weight gain (Markowitz et al,. 2008; Nash 2011, Mwebe 2018a).

2. How would you help Tom to manage the weight gain?

Discuss health concerns with Tom, gain his consent and jointly agree a plan of action:
- Screen Tom for depression and anxiety
- Offer counselling/CBT and/or an antidepressant as a last resort if Tom agrees

- Consider an antidepressant with less propensity to induce weight gain (such as citalopram or fluoxetine)
- Offer advice on healthy eating, physical activity and smoking cessation (Mwebe 2018b)
- Screen for recreational drug use (cannabis, stimulants, alcohol) and refer to appropriate services
- Consider weekly weight/BMI monitoring if Tom continues to take olanzapine
- Or discontinue olanzapine and start Tom on another antipsychotic with weight-neutral effects (such as aripiprazole, lurasidone, asenapine, paliperidone or amisulpride)
- Blood tests for glucose (HbA1c) and lipid checks to be conducted regularly during treatment
- Offer Tom an ECG every 6 to 12 months
- Carry out vital checks regularly, including blood pressure, pulse, temperature, and respiration.

3. How would you check Tom's cardiovascular health?

In individuals taking psychiatric medication (antipsychotics, antidepressants and mood stabilisers), cardiovascular risk is significantly increased. Cardiovascular effects are common at commencement of treatment. Dizziness usually resolves within a few days after initial administration and does require the patient to be monitored (blood pressure pulse assessments at least twice daily). However, if the patient finds the side effects intolerable, it may be advisable to reduce the dose or stop the drug.

The patients at highest risk are those on polypharmacy and those with a family history of heart problems (diagnosed or undiagnosed), overweight patients, recreational drug misusers, older adults, and those on high-dose antipsychotic treatment regimens. In a study by Correll, Solmi, et al. (2017), individuals with serious mental illness were found to have a significantly increased risk of developing cardiovascular disease (CVD) over time and CVD-related deaths compared to those without mental illness. According to the British Heart Foundation (2018), individuals of Asian and African-Caribbean heritage are at greater CVD risk than the general population. This population group should therefore be regularly screened and monitored for CVD risk.

Psychiatric medications can directly or indirectly increase cardiometabolic effects and risks (Kahl, Westhoff-Bleck & Kruger 2018; Walker, McGee & Druss 2015). Most antipsychotics, particularly SGAs, can escalate the risk of developing obesity, weight gain complications including type 2 diabetes and dyslipidaemia (Tosh, Clifton, et al. 2014). In serious mental illness, the rates of metabolic syndrome, a cluster of conditions (high systolic blood pressure, large waist circumference, raised glycaemic levels, dyslipidaemia, insulin resistance and obesity associated with increased risk of developing heart disease, diabetes and stroke) are greater than in the general population (Mutsatsa 2015, Mwebe & Roberts 2019).

You will need to screen Tom's CVD risk by asking about his family history, smoking status, weight checks and recreational substance use. You should also offer advice around healthy alcohol use and eating (Stoner 2018).

Activity 17.4 (Case study)

1. Based on the diagnostic criteria for depressive disorder (ICD-11), do you think the GP would be correct to diagnose Jane with a depressive episode?

Yes, simply due to the duration of Jane's symptoms (6–7 weeks). This is more than the 4 weeks stipulated by both ICD-11 and DSM-5 (WHO 2020). In addition, we can see that Jane is presenting with more than 5 out of 10 core symptoms, which again is the requirement for diagnosing depressive disorder in both diagnostic taxonomies (Chakrabarti 2018).

2. What would a comprehensive health assessment look like for Jane?

You will need to gather information in the following areas:

- History/current presentation, including symptoms, duration, triggers and physical health concerns (including pain, systemic infection, fever, etc.)
- Complete past and current medical history (include medical, psychiatric and surgical history)
  - Is there a history of mental illness in Jane's family? Parents, siblings, aunts and uncles?
- Family history – does Jane have any siblings? Does she have good relations with them? Do Jane and her husband have any children?
- Lifestyle factors (sexual health, drug and alcohol use, nutrition, activity levels, sleep)
  - Jane's appetite has changed. Is this new and does it link in with the current symptoms and presentation? What is she able to eat? What about her fluid intake? Does she use alcohol or other recreational drugs? If yes, is this a problem? Tools including Audit-C (alcohol screening) and pack years (smoking screening) can be used to assess the severity of the problem.
- Current medication (prescribed or non-prescribed – for example, bought on the internet or over the counter, recreational drugs). Has Jane used antidepressants or other medications before? Is there a history of stopping treatment without medical advice? Has she suffered from any major medication side effects or allergies?
- Social history, including hobbies, employment history, money (does Jane have any worries about money?), social networks
- Screening history (breast and cervical)
- Mental state examination will include:
  - Appearance and behaviour
  - Speech
  - Mood/thoughts/affect (is there evidence of psychotic or manic/hypomanic symptoms?)
  - Cognitive checks (memory, learning, concentration)
  - Does Jane have any insight into her current situation?
  - Detailed suicide risk screening, including whether Jane has made any active plans, intent and probable chance of carrying plans out. Are there any risk to others, especially if the couple have dependants under the age of 16?
  - Depression and anxiety screening tools can help to assess degree of severity (PHQ-9, GAD-

7, 5-item depression scale, 5-item anxiety scale) (Goldberg 2019, Goldberg & Fawcett 2012)
- Physical examination (these tests can be conducted by the GP or practice nurse)
  - Temperature, pulse, blood pressure, weight, height, body mass index, urinalysis
- Blood tests can include thyroid function tests, full blood count, vitamins D and B12, folate, urea and electrolyte, liver function tests, glucose checks (HbA1c) and lipid panel if patient risk factors are present (e.g. overweight, history of heart disease and hyperlipidaemia in family, smoker, harmful use of alcohol, history of diabetes and hypertension, unhealthy diet and sedentary lifestyle)
  - General physical assessment and examination could also include the cardiovascular, respiratory, genitourinary, gastrointestinal and neurological systems.

Activity 17.5 (Case study)

1. Based on what you have read so far about depression, what are the most likely triggers and underlying factors in the development of John's depressive disorder?

- John's young age of 17 when he experienced traumatic abusive events (approximately half of all lifetime mental disorders in most studies start by the mid-teens and three-quarters by the mid-twenties)
- Psychological, emotional, and sexual abuse
- Problematic relational dynamics with parents probably led to John feeling abandoned
- Physical violence at the hands of his stepfather created feelings of resentment, fear, and issues of self-image for John
- Distrust towards mother, probably made worse when John confided in her and she failed to recognise and acknowledge his fear, worries and concerns
- Difficult relationship with siblings
- Bullying at school, defiance, and failure to develop and maintain meaningful social relationships/friendships
- Social isolation: cessation of school activities probably made John feel more isolated
- Poor locus of control; tendency to lash out, and physical violence towards others, probably suggestive of emotional dysregulation and poor impulse control
- Loss, death and bereavement
- Unemployment compounded with financial stress and worries
- Problematic substance use (alcohol and cannabis).

Amitriptyline is a TCA medication. Based on what you have learnt so far about the side effects of TCAs, an overdose of amitriptyline would almost certainly expose John to some of the toxic side effects of TCAs, particularly if a medication is taken outside the recommended daily dose range.

2. What are the possible side effects John suffered?

- Cardiac arrhythmias due to cardiovascular toxicity potential of TCAs
- Orthostatic hypotension (alpha 1 blockade)
- Diaphoresis – sweating, especially to an unusual degree
- Elevated mood – mania due to increased serotonergic activity at the synaptic space
- Anxiety, apathy, confusion, akathisia,
- Dry mouth, blurred vision, photophobia
- Constipation, urinary retention
- Tachycardia
- Increased sedation.

References and further reading

Albert, P.R. (2015). Why is depression more prevalent in women? *Journal of Psychiatric Neuroscience*. **40** (4), 219–21.

American Psychiatric Association (2013). *Diagnostic and Statistical Manual of Mental Disorders*. 5th edn. Washington, DC: American Psychiatric Publishing.

Ballon, J.S., Pajvani, U.B., Mayer, L.E., et al. (2018). Pathophysiology of drug induced weight and metabolic effects: Findings from an RCT in healthy volunteers treated with olanzapine, iloperidone, or placebo. *Journal of Psychopharmacology*. **32** (5), 533–40.

Balt, S.L., Galloway, G., Baggot, M., et al. (2011). Mechanisms and genetics of antipsychotic-associated weight gain. *Clinical Pharmacology and Therapeutics*. **90** (1), 179–83.

Baptista, T., Uzcátegui, E., Rangel, N., El Fakih, Y., Galeazzi, T., Beaulieu, S. & de Baptista, E.A. (2008). Metformin plus sibutramine for olanzapine-associated weight gain and metabolic dysfunction in schizophrenia: a 12-week double-blind, placebo-controlled pilot study. *Psychiatry Research*. **159** (1–2), 250–53. doi: 10.1016/j.psychres.2008.01.011. Epub. PMID: 18374423.

Bogren, M.L., Brådvik, C. & Holmstrand, L. (2018). Gender differences in subtypes of depression by first incidence and age of onset: a follow-up of the Lundby population. *European Archives of Psychiatry and Clinical Neuroscience*. **268** (2), 179.

British Association of Psychopharmacology (BAP) (2016). BAP guidelines on the management of weight gain, metabolic disturbances and cardiovascular risk associated with psychosis and antipsychotic drug treatment. https://www.bap.org.uk/pdfs/BAP_Guidelines-Metabolic.pdf (Last accessed 11 November 2020).

British Cardiovascular Society (BCS) (2019). JBS3: Lifetime Risk: Concept of lifetime risk in the JBS3 Report. http://www.jbs3risk.com/pages/lifetime_risk.htm (accessed 3 July 2020).

British Heart Foundation (BHF) (2018). CVDT Statistics – BHF UK Factsheet. https://www.bhf.org.uk/what-we-do/our-research/heart-statistics/heart-statistics-publications/cardiovascular-disease-statistics-2018 (Last accessed 11 November 2020).

British National Formulary (BNF) (2020). https://bnf.nice.org.uk/ (Last accessed 15 November 2020).

Chakrabarti, S. (2018), Mood disorders in the international classification of Diseases-11: Similarities and differences with the *Diagnostic and Statistical Manual of Mental Disorders* 5 and the international classification of diseases – 10. *Indian Journal of Social Psychiatry*. **34** (5), 17–22.

Chen, J., Huang, X. F., Shao, R., Chen, C. & Deng, C. (2017). Molecular mechanisms of antipsychotic drug-induced diabetes. *Frontiers in Neuroscience*. **11**, 643. https://doi:10.3389/fnins.2017.00643 (Last accessed 11 November 2020).

Cohen, J. & Brown, C.S. (2010). *John Romano & George Engel. Their Lives and Work*. Rochester, NY: University of Rochester Press and Suffolk, UK: Boydell and Brewer Limited.

Collins, G.S. & Altman, D.G. (2012). Predicting the 10-year risk of cardiovascular disease in the United Kingdom: independent and external validation of an updated version of QRISK2. *British Medical Journal*. **344**, e4181. https://doi:10.1136/bmj.e4181 (Last accessed 11 November 2020).

Cooper, S.J., Reynolds, G.P., Barnes, T., et al. (2016). BAP guidelines on the management of weight gain, metabolic disturbances and cardiovascular risk associated with psychosis and antipsychotic drug treatment. *Journal of Psychopharmacology*. **30** (8), 717–48.

Correll, C.U., Solmi, M., Veronese, N., et al. (2017). Prevalence, incidence and mortality from cardiovascular disease in patients with pooled and specific severe mental illness: a large-scale meta-analysis of 3,211,768 patients and 113,383,368 controls. *World Psychiatry*. **16** (2), 163–80.

Courtet, P. & Lopez-Castroman, J. (2017). Antidepressants and suicide risk in depression. *World Psychiatry: Official Journal of the World Psychiatric Association (WPA)*. **16** (3), 317–18. https://doi:10.1002/wps.20460 (Last accessed 11 November 2020).

Cox, C.E. (2017). Role of physical activity for weight loss and weight maintenance. *Diabetes Spectrum*. **30** (3), 157–60.

De Silva, V.A., Suraweera, C., Ratnatunga, S.S., et al. (2016). Metformin in prevention and treatment of antipsychotic induced weight gain: a systematic review and meta-analysis. *BMC Psychiatry*. **16**, 341.

Electronic Medicines Compendium (eMC). Up-to-date, easily accessible information about medicines licensed for use in the UK [Online resource]. https://www.medicines.org.uk/emc (Last accessed 11 November 2020).

Ferenchick, E., Ramanuj, P. & Pincus, H.A. (2019). Depression in primary care: diagnosis and management. *The British Medical Journal*. **365** (8205), 463–504.

Foley, D.L., Mackinnon, A. & Morgan, V.A. (2014). Predictors of type 2 diabetes in a national sample of adults with psychosis. *World Psychiatry*. **13**, 176–83.

Freyberg, Z. & McCarthy, M.J. (2017). Dopamine D2 receptors and the circadian clock reciprocally mediate antipsychotic drug-induced metabolic disturbances. *NPJ Schizophrenia*. **3**, 17. https://doi.org/10.1038/s41537-017-0018-4 (Last accessed 11 November 2020).

Gaebel, W., Zielasek, J. & Reed, G.M. (2017). Mental and behavioural disorders in the ICD-11: Concepts, methodologies, and current status. *Psychiatria Polska*. **51**, 169–95.

Gejman, P., Sanders, A. & Duan, J. (2010). The role of genetics in the etiology of schizophrenia. *Psychiatric Clinics of North America*. **33** (1), 35–66.

Goldberg, D. (2019). Are official psychiatric classification systems for mental disorders suitable for use in primary care? *British Journal of General Practice*. **69** (680), 108–109.

Goldberg, D. & Fawcett, J. (2012). The importance of anxiety in both major depression and bipolar disorder. *Depression and Anxiety*. **29** (6), 471–78.

Goldberg, D., Prisciandaro, J.J. & Williams, P. (2012). The primary health care version of ICD-11: the detection of common mental disorders in general medical settings. *General Hospital Psychiatry*. **34** (6), 665–70.

Goldberg, D.P., Reed, G.M., Robles, R. et al. (2016). Multiple somatic symptoms in primary care: A field study for ICD-11 PHC, WHO's revised classification of mental disorders in primary care settings. *Journal of Psychosomatic Research*. **91**, 48–54.

Goldberg, D.P., Wittchen, H.U., Zimmermann, P., Pfister, H. & Beesdo-Baum, K. (2014). Anxious and non-anxious forms of major depression: familial, personality and symptom characteristics. *Psychological Medicine*. **44** (6), 1223–34.

Holland, L., Floyd, E. & Soames, S. (2018). *The Nurse's Guide to Mental Health Medicines*. London: SAGE Publishers.

Hu, W., MacDonald, M.L., Elswick, D.E. & Sweet, R.A. (2015). The glutamate hypothesis of schizophrenia: Evidence from human brain tissue studies. *Annals of the New York Academy of Sciences*. **1338** (1), 38–57.

Joint British Societies for the prevention of cardiovascular disease (JBS3) (2014). http://www.jbs3risk.com/ (Last accessed 11 November 2020).

Joseph, J. (2003). *The Gene Illusion: Genetic Research in Psychiatry and Psychology Under the Microscope*. Herefordshire: PCCS Books.

Kahl, G.K., Westhoff-Bleck, M. & Kruger, T.H.C. (2018). Effects of psychopharmacological treatment with antipsychotic drugs on the vascular system. *Vascular Pharmacology*. **100**, 20–25.

Kapur, S., Remington, G., Zipursky, R.B., Wilson, A.A., et al. (1995). The D2 dopamine receptor occupancy of risperidone and its relationship to extrapyramidal symptoms: a PET study. *Life Sciences*. **57** (10), PL103–107.

Khushboo, S.B. (2017). Antidepressants: mechanism of action, toxicity and possible amelioration. *Journal of Applied Biotechnology & Bioengineering*. **3** (5), 437–48.

Kring, A.M., Davidson, G.C. & Neale, J.M. (2013). *Abnormal Psychology*. London: John Wiley and Sons.

Lee, B.H. & Kim, Y.K. (2010). The roles of BDNF in the pathophysiology of major depression and in antidepressant treatment. *Psychiatry Investigation*. **7** (4), 231–35. https://doi.org/10.4306/pi.2010.7.4.231 (Last accessed 11 November 2020).

Lester, H., Shiers, D. & Rafi, I. (2012). *Positive Cardiometabolic Health Resource: An Intervention Framework for Patients with Psychosis on Antipsychotic Medication*. London: Royal College of Psychiatrists.

Lin, S.T., Chen, C.C., Tsang, H.Y., Lee, C.S., Yang, P., Cheng, K.D. & Yang, W.C. (2014). Association between antipsychotic use and risk of acute myocardial infarction: a nationwide case-crossover study. *Circulation*. **130**, 235–43.

Lipscombe, L.L., Austin, P.C., Alessi-Severini, S., Blackburn, D.F., Blais, L., Bresee, L., et al. (2014). Atypical antipsychotics and hyperglycaemic emergencies: multicentre, retrospective cohort study of administrative data. *Schizophrenia Research*. **154**, 54–60.

Luppino, F.S., de Wit, L.M., Bouvy, P.F., et al. (2010). Overweight, obesity, and depression: A systematic review and meta-analysis of longitudinal studies. *Archives of General Psychiatry*. **67** (3), 220–29.

Mailman, R.B. & Murthy, V. (2010). Third generation antipsychotic drugs: Partial agonism or receptor functional selectivity? *Current Pharmaceutical Design*. **16**, 488–501.

Manu, P., Dima, L., Shulman, M., Vancampfort, D., et al. (2015) Weight gain and obesity in schizophrenia: epidemiology, pathobiology, and management. *Acta Psychiatrica Scandinavia*. **132**, 97–108

Markowitz, S., Friedman, M.A. & Arent, S.M. (2008). Understanding the relation between obesity and depression: Causal mechanisms and implications for treatment. *Clinical Psychology: Science and Practice*. **15** (1), 1–20.

Marmot, M., Goldblatt, P. & Allen, J. (2010). *Fair Society, Healthy Lives: The Marmot Review*. London: Institute of Health Equity. http://www.instituteofhealthequity.org/resources-reports/fair-society-healthy-lives-the-marmot-review (Last accessed 11 November 2020).

McGlinchey, J.B., Zimmerman, M., Young, D. et al. (2006). Diagnosing major depressive disorder VIII: are some symptoms better than others? *Journal of Nervous and Mental Disease*. **194**, 785–90.

Megele, C. (2015). *Psychosocial and Relationship-based Practice*. London: Critical Publishing.

Mental Health Taskforce to the NHS England (2016). The Five Year Forward View for Mental Health. [online] http://www.england.nhs.uk/wp-content/uploads/2016/02/Mental-Health-Taskforce-FYFV-final.pdf (Last accessed 11 November 2020).

Molina, J., Rodriguez-Diaz, R., Fachado, A., Jacques-Silva, M.C., Berggren, P.O. & Caicedo, A. (2014). Control of insulin secretion by cholinergic signaling in the human pancreatic islet. *Diabetes*. **63** (8), 2714–26.

Mutsatsa, S. (2015). *Physical Healthcare and Promotion in Mental Health Nursing*. London: SAGE Publishers.

Mwebe, H. (2018a). *Psychopharmacology: A mental health professional's guide to commonly used medications*. London: Critical Publishing Ltd.

Mwebe, H. (2018b). Serious mental illness and smoking cessation. *British Journal of Mental Health Nursing*. **7** (1), 39–46.

Mwebe, H. & Roberts, D. (2019). Risk of cardiovascular disease in people taking psychotropic medication: a literature review. *British Journal of Mental Health Nursing*. https://www.magonlinelibrary.com/doi/full/10.12968/bjmh.2018.0033 (Last accessed 11 November 2020).

Nash, M. (2011). *Physical Health and Well-Being in Mental Health Nursing: Clinical Skills for Practice*. London: Open University Press.

Nasrallah, H.A. (2008). Atypical antipsychotics-induced metabolic side effects: insights from receptor binding profiles. *Molecular Psychiatry*. **13** (1), 27–35.

National Institute for Health and Care Excellence (NICE) (2006). Obesity prevention. https://www.nice.org.uk/guidance/cg43 (Last accessed 12 November 2020).

National Institute for Health and Care Excellence (NICE) (2014). Cardiovascular disease: risk assessment and reduction, including lipid modification. https://www.nice.org.uk/guidance/cg181 (Last accessed 12 November 2020).

National Institute for Health and Care Excellence (NICE) (2015). Type 2 diabetes in adults: management. https://www.nice.org.uk/guidance/ng28 (Last accessed 12 November 2020).

National Institute for Health and Care Excellence (NICE) (2018). Depression in adults: recognition and management. Clinical Guidance 90. [online] https://www.nice.org.uk/guidance/cg90 (Last accessed 12 November 2020).

National Institute for Health and Care Excellence (NICE) (2019). Psychosis and schizophrenia in adults: prevention and management. Clinical Guidance 178. [online] https://www.nice.org.uk/guidance/cg178 (Last accessed 12 November 2020).

NHS Specialist Pharmacy Service (SPS) (2020). [Online resource]. https://www.sps.nhs.uk/ (Last accessed 12 November 2020).

Phillips, C. & Fahimi, A. (2018). Immune and neuroprotective effects of physical activity on the brain in depression. *Frontiers in Neuroscience*. **12**. https://doi.org/10.3389/fnins.2018.00498 (Last accessed 12 November 2020).

Pilgrim, D. (2017). *Key Concepts in Mental Health*. 4th edn. London: Sage Publishers.

QRisk (2018). https://qrisk.org/three/ (Last accessed 12 November 2020).

Rasic, D., Hajek, T., Alda, M. et al. (2014). Risk of mental illness in offspring of parents with schizophrenia, bipolar disorder, and major depressive disorder: A meta-analysis of family high-risk studies. *Schizophrenia Bulletin*. **40** (1), 28–38.

Royal Pharmaceutical Society (RPS) (2016). *Prescribing Framework: A Competency Framework for all Prescribers*. London: RPS.

Stahl, S.M. (2013). *Stahl's Essential Psychopharmacology: Neuroscientific Basis and Practical Applications*. New York: Cambridge University Press.

Stahl, S.M. (2017). *Stahl's Essential Psychopharmacology: Prescriber's Guide*. 6th edn. New York: Cambridge University Press.

Stahl, S.M. (2018). Beyond the dopamine hypothesis of schizophrenia to three neural networks of psychosis: dopamine, serotonin, and glutamate. CNS Spectrums **23**: 187-91. Cambridge University Press. doi:10.1017/S1092852918001013.

Stone, M., Laughren, T., Jones, M.L., et al. (2009). Risk of suicidality in clinical trials of antidepressants in adults: analysis of proprietary data submitted to US Food and Drug Administration. *British Medical Journal*. **339**, b2880.

Stoner, S.C. (2018). Management of serious cardiac adverse effects of antipsychotic medications. *Mental Health Clinician*. **7** (6), 246–54. https://doi.org/10.9740/mhc.2017.11.246 (Last accessed 12 November 2020).

Stubbs, B., Vancampfort, D., De Hert, M., & Mitchell, A.J. (2015). The prevalence and predictors of type two diabetes mellitus in people with schizophrenia: a systematic review and comparative meta-analysis. *Acta Psychiatrica Scandinavica*. **132**, 144–57.

Sullivan, L.E. (2009). *The SAGE Glossary of the Social and Behavioural Sciences*. London: SAGE Publications.

Taylor, D., Paton, C. & Kerwin, R. (2015). *The South London and Maudsley & Oxleas NHS Foundation Trusts Prescribing Guidelines*. 12th edn. London: Wiley-Blackwell.

Tosh, G., Clifton, A.V., Xia, J. & White, M.M. (2014). General physical health advice for people with serious mental illness. *Cochrane Database of Systematic Reviews*. Issue 3. Art. No: CD008567. https://doi.org/10.1002/14651858.CD008567.pub3 (Last accessed 12 November 2020).

Waddell, L. & Taylor, M. (2008). GASS-Glasgow Antipsychotic Side-effect Scale. *Journal of Psychopharmacology*. **22** (3), 238–43.

Walker, E.R., McGee, R.E. & Druss, B.G. (2015). Mortality in mental disorders and global disease burden implications: a systematic review and meta-analysis. *JAMA Psychiatry*. **72** (4), 334–41.

World Health Organisation (WHO) (2018). Premature Death Among People with Severe Mental Disorders: Information Sheet. [online] https://www.who.int/mental_health/management/info_sheet.pdf (Last accessed 12 November 2020).

World Health Organisation (WHO) (2020). *ICD-11: International Classification of Diseases for Mortality and Morbidity Statistics*. 11th edn. Geneva: WHO. https://icd.who.int/browse11/l-m/en (Last accessed 12 November 2020).

Wu, C.S., Tsai, Y.T. & Tsai, H.J. (2015). Antipsychotic drugs and the risk of ventricular arrhythmia and/or sudden cardiac death: a nation-wide case-crossover study. *Journal of the American Heart Association*. 4:e001568. doi: 10.1161/JAHA.114.001568

Yang, A.C. & Tsai, S.J. (2017). New targets for schizophrenia treatment beyond the dopamine hypothesis. *International Journal of Molecular Sciences*. **18** (8), 1689. https://doi.org/10.3390/ijms18081689 (Last accessed 12 November 2020).

18

Pharmacological case studies: Eye problems

Donna Scholefield
MSc, BSc (Hons), RN, PGDip HE; Cardiac Nursing (254);
OND.Senior Lecturer, Health and Education, Middlesex University, London

This chapter has been revised and updated by Donna Scholefield. It is based on work originally produced by **Mahesh Seewoodhary** BSc (Hons), OND (Hons), RN, DN, FETC 730, ENB 100, RCNT, RNT, Cert Ed; Senior Lecturer in Ophthalmic Nursing and Adult Nursing, University of West London, London

This chapter:

- Gives an overview of ocular anatomy, physiology and common eye conditions
- Explains how to classify the ophthalmic medications used to manage ocular conditions
- Discusses the pharmacokinetics and pharmacodynamics of ophthalmic medications used in ocular disorders
- Applies pharmaceutical knowledge to clinical case studies.

Introduction

A sound understanding of the management of common eye conditions is essential as, according to a report by the Royal National Institute for the Blind (RNIB 2016), the UK's healthcare cost linked to eye health is estimated to be at least £3 billion, with over £380 million spent on prescriptions. Therefore the aim of this chapter is to give an insight into commonly prescribed medications used in the management of ophthalmic conditions. The chapter has several sections relating to the healthcare practitioner's role in ensuring safe practice. Ophthalmic medications are administered both topically and systemically. Due care must be exercised both by the healthcare worker and the patient (NMC 2018). Four selected case studies are presented on specific conditions – blepharitis, conjunctivitis, glaucoma, and contact lens-related eye problems. To begin with, a basic understanding of the anatomy and physiology of the eye is essential.

Ocular structure and physiology

The eye is the organ of sight, which is situated in the bony orbit, surrounded by orbital fats. It is about 24mm in diameter. The eye starts developing within two weeks of gestation. It reaches its mature size by the age of 13, and vision goes on developing until the age of 7. The eye consists of many parts, which are all important for visual health. The anatomy of the eye and its various structures is shown in Figure 18.1 (below).

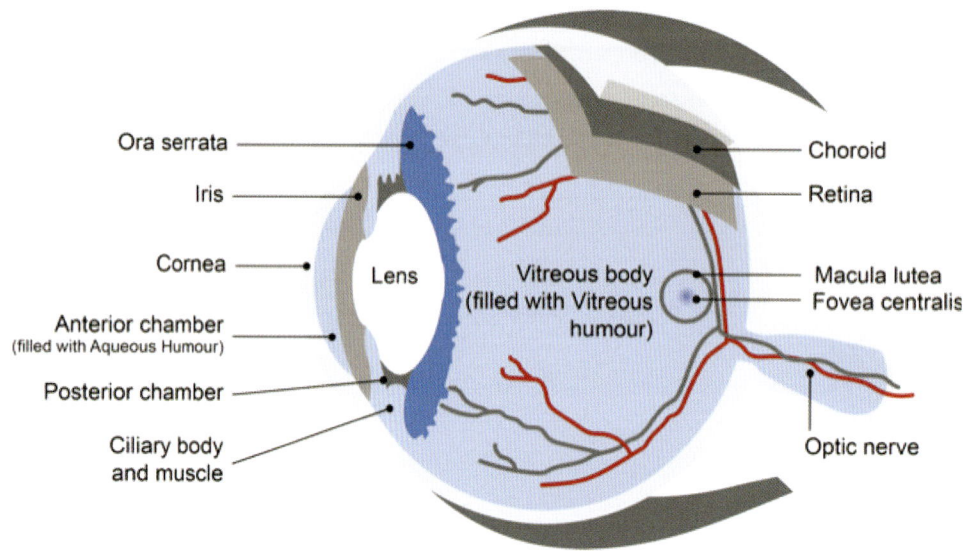

Figure 18.1: Anatomy of the eye.

The cornea is the clear surface of the outer eye. It is about 0.5mm thick and consists of five layers: the epithelium, Bowman's membrane, stroma, Descemet's membrane and the endothelium layer. It has two main functions. Firstly, it acts as a barrier, preventing micro-organisms, dirt and other harmful material from entering the eye. Secondly, the cornea acts as a window that controls and focuses the entry of light into the eye. The cornea contributes 70% of the eye's total focusing power. The cornea refracts incoming light onto the lens. Its surface is covered by a thin tear film, which is essential for corneal metabolism and corneal clarity. The tear film provides nourishment and has antimicrobial properties.

The iris gives the eye its colour. It is made up of connective tissues and muscle fibres. Its main function is to control the amount of light entering the eye through the pupil. The pupil changes its size in response to light levels. In bright light, the pupil constricts. In dim light, the pupil dilates, allowing more light into the eye.

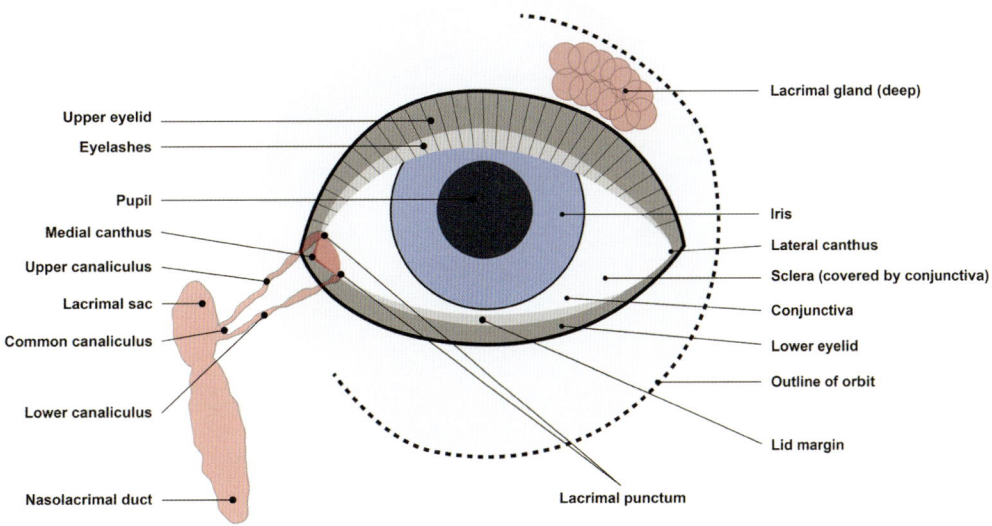

Figure 18.2: External features and accessory structures of the eye.

The lens is a transparent structure about 5mm thick, with a diameter of about 9mm. It is positioned directly behind the iris. It is made of proteins called crystallins. Its function is to focus light onto the retina. The lens is flexible and its curvature is controlled by the oculomotor nerve. Changing the curvature of the lens allows the eye to focus on objects at different distances, a process known as accommodation. The lens is encased in a capsule and suspended within the eye by zonule fibres.

The vitreous humour is a clear substance that fills the centre of the eye. It is mainly composed of water and makes up approximately two-thirds of the eye's volume, giving it form and shape. It also contains hyaluronic acid and collagen molecules to give it a jelly-like structure. It keeps the retina in place.

The choroid is an extensive network of capillaries containing melanocytes. It is attached to the outer layer of the retina and covered by the sclera. It is this network of capillaries that delivers nutrients and oxygen to the retina.

The aqueous humour is a clear watery fluid that is produced continuously by the ciliary body, which is a thickened, extended region of the choroid. The main function of the aqueous humour is to nourish the structures in the anterior region of the iris (anterior chamber) as well as helping to maintain the shape of the eye and position of the retina by means of the pressure it exerts. As mentioned earlier, the aqueous fluid is continually being renewed. It flows from the ciliary body through the pupil into the anterior chamber, then into a network of connective tissue (trabecular meshwork) at the base of the iris. The fluid then enters a passageway that surrounds the eye called Schlemm's Canal, and from here it drains into the scleral veins and back into the general circulation (see Figure 18.3 below). Obstruction of this fluid can lead to raised intraocular pressure and a condition called glaucoma.

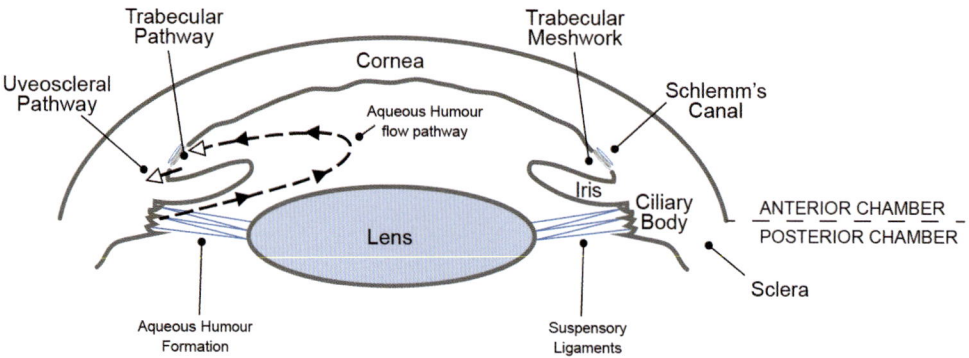

Figure 18.3: The contents of the aqueous humour are constantly being refreshed by a flow of fluid produced by the ciliary body.

The retina is a multi-layered sensory tissue of neural cells that lines the back of the inside of the eye. It contains three layers of nerve cells, including the outermost layer of sensory photoreceptor cells. These cells capture light rays and convert them into electrical impulses, which are transmitted by the optic nerve to the brain. There are two types of photoreceptors: rods and cones. Each retina comprises approximately 125 million rods. These are responsible for peripheral vision and function best in dim light. There are approximately 7 million cones in a human eye and these are more concentrated in the macula, most densely in the fovea. Cones are essential for vision in bright light and for seeing colours. The outer layer of the retina is known as the retinal pigment epithelium layer. This layer nourishes the photoreceptor cells.

The macula is situated at the centre of the retina. It is the focus for incoming light and is responsible for central vision and the ability to see detail. It has a diameter of approximately 1.5mm.

The fovea centralis is a small pit of around 0.3mm, near the centre of the macula. The fovea has the highest concentration of cone cells and is free of rod cells.

The optic nerve transmits visual information, in the form of electrical impulses, from the retina to the brain. It connects to the back of the eye, near the macula. The retinal photoreceptor cells are not present in the optic nerve. As a result, there is a blind spot in our field of vision. This is not normally noticeable because the vision of one eye overlaps with that of the other.

Ophthalmic pharmacodynamics and pharmacokinetics

There are many factors that influence the absorption and thus bioavailability (amount reaching the circulation) of ophthalmic drugs. These factors include the drug formulation, its strength, pH, volume, frequency of instillation and of course patient compliance. All these factors should therefore be considered in order to enhance the efficacy of ophthalmic medication.

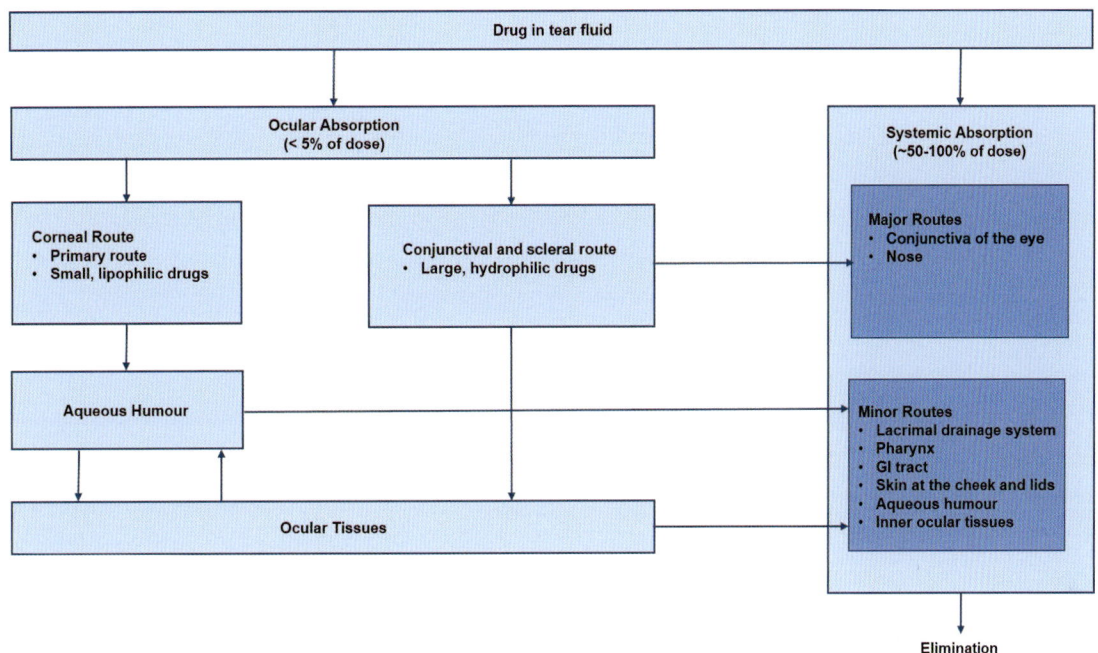

*Figure 18.4: Destination of drugs instilled onto the surface of the eye.
(Source: Jűnemann, Chorągiewicz, et al. 2016)*

Topically applied drugs are absorbed by crossing anatomical barriers to enter the eye, and often have poor bioavailability. Pharmacologists and drug delivery scientists therefore need to find strategies to overcome the restrictions imposed on drug absorption by the structure and physiology of the eye. There are multiple routes, including through the conjunctiva, sclera and cornea (see Figure 18.4). These structures vary in their permeability to lipophilic and hydrophilic drugs. However, the corneal epithelium is thought to be more permeable to lipophilic drugs than the conjunctiva and the sclera. Indeed, the cornea is considered the main way for locally applied drugs to enter the anterior chamber of the eye, although hydrophilic drugs can access the sclera and conjunctiva more readily (Jünemann, Chorągiewicz, et al. 2016).

Most topical eye medication (drops or ointment) is either instilled or applied in the lower conjunctival sac (lower fornix), which is exposed by gently pulling the lower eyelid down (see Figures 18.5 and 18.6, p. 383). Only a fraction of the drop instilled into the lower conjunctival sac will be absorbed. In fact, some sources suggest only about 5% of a drug from a drop instilled gets to the ocular structure (Jünemann, Chorągiewicz, et al. 2016). The average eye dropper holds 50 microlitres, with an average drop size of 39 microlitres, so a drop can overload the conjunctival sac. Some droppers have a tip that can dispense a smaller drop. However, the conjunctival sac can only accommodate approximately 25 microlitres and so it is important to remember to instil only one drop at a time. If two different eye drops are to be administered at the same time of day, there should be a 5-minute interval to avoid dilution and overflow (Joint Formulary Committee 2020).

Sometimes after/during instillation there is rapid tear secretion and aqueous solutions will be diluted or drained into the tear duct, leading to some systemic absorption. This can be reduced by applying gentle pressure near the lacrimal punctum (see Figure 18.2, p. 364) for approximately one minute after the drop is instilled. Nevertheless, systemic absorption of some ophthalmic drugs via the nasolacrimal route can lead to adverse systemic effects.

Because so little of a drug instilled in the eye gets through the corneal barrier, other strategies need to be employed to increase the bioavailability of the drug. These strategies may include more frequent administration but this is very dependent on patient compliance. Other strategies include improving the form in which the drug is delivered. For example, eye ointments increase the bioavailability of the drug. Drugs may also be administered into the conjunctival sac by impregnating them into thin gelatin discs or plastic devices; they are held under the eyelid and gradually release the drug as they dissolve. Innovative approaches to improve ocular drug delivery are continually being developed, piloted and/or marketed. Examples of some of these approaches include the use of nanotechnology, contact lenses, microneedles, in situ thermosensitive gels (Patel, Cholkar, et al. 2013) and mydriasert pellets containing two mydriatic agents such as phenylephrine and topicamide.

The eye can withstand a pH range of 4.5–10 but a range of 6.6–9 is considered optimal to avoid ocular irritation. In addition, some medications are only physiologically active at a particular pH range so buffers, such as borates, acetates, citrates, bicarbonates and phosphates, are used to regulate pH.

In summary, administering ocular medication is a challenge, as each drug has to overcome a number of structural and anatomical barriers to reach its site of action. These anatomical barriers vary in their permeability so the drug's physicochemical properties will determine the route used to access the anterior chamber of the eye. Interaction of the drug within its environment determines its physicochemical properties, e.g. its ability to dissolve and cross biological membranes within the eye.

Two key challenges to overcome, in order to facilitate effective ocular delivery of drugs, are absorption across the cornea and patient adherence; and these in turn depend on other factors.

Factors affecting absorption and bioavailability in topically applied drugs:
- Physicochemical structure of drug (e.g. pH, size, lipophilic, hydrophilic)
- Drug concentration and drug formulation
- Drop instilled
- Administration technique
- Patient adherence
- Ocular structures (eye-related factors).

Classification of ophthalmic medications

For patients receiving eye medications, it is important for the healthcare practitioner to understand the classification of ophthalmic medications, their mode of action and their side effects, in order to provide safe practice.

Table 18.1: Classification of ophthalmic medications

Classification	Modes of action	Examples	Indications for use
Mydriatic (adrenergic)	• Direct action on the dilator muscle of the iris by mimicking the neurotransmitter nor-adrenaline. • It does not paralyse lens accommodation, and thus has no cycloplegic properties. • It causes pupil dilatation.	• Phenylephrine	• Fundoscopy for retinal examination • Pre-operative cataract surgery
Cycloplegic	• Blocks the action of sphincter pupillae and ciliary muscles by interfering with muscarinic receptor sites. • It causes pupil dilatation and loss of accommodation.	• Tropicamide	• Fundoscopy • To alleviate ciliary spasm when treating patients with acute iritis due to corneal abrasion
Beta-blocker	• Reduces intraocular pressure, possibly due to blockade of beta-adrenergic receptors in the ciliary processes, which inhibits the formation of aqueous humour.	• Timolol • Carteolol • Levobunolol	• Primary open angle glaucoma
Prostaglandin analogue	• Increases the amount of aqueous humour that leaves the eye through the uveoscleral outflow route (iris root and ciliary body), thus reducing intraocular pressure.	• Latanoprost • Tafluprost	• Ocular hypertension or primary open angle glaucoma
Carbonic anhydrase inhibitor	• Reduces the production of aqueous humour, thus reducing intraocular pressure.	• Acetazolamide • Dorzolamide	• As an adjunct in the treatment of glaucoma • Acetazolamide – systemic administration (oral or intravenous), generally short-term • Dorzolamide – (topical), long-term

(table continued overleaf)

Table 18.1 continued

Classification	Modes of action	Examples	Indications for use
Miotic	• Stimulates the parasympathetic nervous system and excites the sphincter pupillae and ciliary muscles, resulting in pupil constriction. • Enhances aqueous humour drainage through the trabecular meshwork.	• Pilocarpine	• Primary acute angle closure glaucoma
Anti-infective agent	• Antibiotic • Anti-viral • Anti-fungal	• Chloramphenicol • Aciclovir • Amphotericin-B	• Bacterial conjunctivitis • Herpetic keratitis • Fungal keratitis
Local anaesthetic	• Works by stabilising cell membranes, thus preventing nerve impulse conduction.	• Tetracaine	• To facilitate eye irrigation following chemical burns • For removal of corneal foreign body
Dye	• Stains damaged corneal epithelial cells as in abrasion or dry eyes.	• Fluorescein • Rose bengal	• Corneal abrasion • Investigation of dry eye symptoms
Lubricant Tear replacement	• Non-medicated viscous solution used to moisten the ocular surface. • Used to provide optimum comfort.	• Carmellose • Hypromellose • Carbomer 980 (polyacrylic acid) • Polyvinyl alcohol • Liquid paraffin	• Replacement therapy for management of dry eyes • Promotion of corneal healing following abrasions or chemical injury
Irrigation solution	• To neutralise or dilute chemical splash	• Normal saline • Sterile water	• Chemical eye injury
Corticosteroid	• Anti-inflammatory • Reduces activity to T cells	• Dexamethasone	• To reduce post-operative inflammatory reactions
Non-steroidal anti-inflammatory drug	• Inhibits the enzyme cyclooxygenase, which is involved in the conversion of arachidonic acid to prostaglandins and thromboxane	• Diclofenac sodium	• Inhibition of pre-operative miosis during cataract surgery • Treatment of post-operative inflammation

| Anti-allergic | • Inhibits the release of inflammatory mediators by stabilising mast cells | • Sodium cromoglicate | • Useful in vernal seasonal conjunctivitis |

The importance of taking a good medical history

It is very important to obtain and record details of the patient's medical history to identify and record any pre-existing diseases. Indeed, assessment of the eyes should always form part of a holistic patient assessment, as many aspects of the patient's general physical condition and ability to carry out activities of daily living are related to having good eyesight. For example, diabetes, hypertension and retinopathy all significantly affect eyesight; and falls in the older person are frequently linked to impaired vision. In addition, the healthcare professional should also be aware and record any potential adverse reactions following the administration of eye medications. Table 18.2 provides examples of systemic diseases and possible drug interactions.

Table 18.2: Systemic diseases and drug interactions

Systemic disease	Possible drug interactions
Hypertension	Phenylephrine may raise systemic blood pressure and affect the cardiovascular system.
Diabetes mellitus	Mannitol may affect glucose metabolism.
Depression	Acetazolamide may worsen the symptoms of depression.
Thyroid disease	Use of systemic beta-blocker may make thyroid medications less effective.
Asthma	Use of beta-blockers may precipitate an asthma attack.
Herpes simplex-related infection	Use of corticosteroids may cause secondary corneal infection in herpes keratitis.

Any history of allergies to eye medications, or the preservatives contained within them, should be documented. Similarly, if the patient wears contact lenses, details should be obtained as to whether the lenses are hard, soft or gas-permeable. Drugs and their preservatives can be absorbed through contact lenses and this will increase toxicity to the corneal epithelium, which could result in toxic keratitis.

In order to ensure that the correct diagnosis is made, and correct medication is prescribed, it is important to assess the patient thoroughly and record details of the onset, duration and severity of the presenting clinical signs and symptoms as well as current eye medication. As mentioned previously, a comprehensive patient assessment is essential to ensure that the correct diagnosis is made and medications are prescribed correctly. A history of pregnancy should also be documented, since ocular medications absorbed systemically can cross the placental barrier. Similarly, a breastfed baby may be affected by drugs such as corticosteroids and antibiotics

Indications for the instillation of eye medications

The instillation of eye drops and ointment is an important skill for many healthcare practitioners. They should be aware of the implications of using eye medications for the preservation of sight during the healing process. Indications for the instillation of eye drops and ointment are outlined in Table 18.3.

Table 18.3: Indications for the instillation of eye medications

Indications	Examples
Diagnostic procedures	• Cycloplegic eye drop for fundoscopy • Fluorescein dye to diagnose a corneal abrasion
Emergency use	• Anaesthetic eye drop before eye wash • Eye irrigation for chemical burns
Promoting corneal wound healing	• Potassium ascorbate for severe chemical injury
Lubrication and replacement therapy (artificial tears, e.g. Sjogren's disease)	• Hypromellose for dry eyes, to promote comfort, and prevent recurrent corneal erosions
Pain relief	• Local anaesthetic for eye examination for contact lens-related corneal abrasion
Pre- and post-operative ophthalmic surgery	• Pupil dilatation to allow viewing of the retina during surgery
Prophylaxis	• Sodium cromoglicate for seasonal conjunctivitis
Surgery	• Local anaesthetic for cataract surgery
Therapeutic	• Beta-blocker eye drop to reduce intraocular pressure in glaucoma • Antibiotic to fight an infection such as in blepharitis or conjunctivitis

Eye medications are governed by the same controls as medications administered by other routes. This emphasises the legal aspects of the practitioner's role. One-fifth of all clinical negligence litigation in the UK arises from errors in the use of prescribed medications. The law requires that medicines should be given to the right person, at the right time, in the correct form, using the correct dose and via the correct route (RPS 2019). Ophthalmic medications are important for the patients who need them, and healthcare practitioners should exercise caution to avoid drug errors.

Use of lubricants

Lubricants are tear substitutes, which are prescribed to promote comfort in patients presenting with conditions such as dry eyes, blepharitis and corneal abrasion. Lubricants also provide ocular lubrication when wearing hard or gas-permeable contact lenses. Examples of commonly used lubricants include hypromellose, carbomers, polyvinyl alcohol and carmellose.

Many artificial tear products contain preservatives, such as benzalkonium chloride and cetrimide, and mainly consist of non-medicated solutions. The choice of artificial tears is subjective, with little evidence for the advantage of one product over another. The effects of carbomers persist longer than those of simpler lubricants such as hypromellose so less frequent administration is required. Mucolytics, such as acetylcysteine, can be combined with hypromellose. Healthcare practitioners must take care not to instil artificial tears containing preservatives in patients who are allergic to the preservatives.

Preservatives and active ingredients

Preservatives are used to prolong the shelf-life of the medication as well as protecting against in-use contamination. Examples of preservatives include benzalkonium chloride 0.01%, phenylmercuric nitrate 0.004%, thiomersal 0.001% or chlorhexidine acetate 0.01% in drops.

The concentrations of preservatives used, and of active ingredients, are listed as percentage concentrations. Eye drops are expressed as percentage weight in volume, whereas eye ointments and other solids are listed as percentage weight in weight. In general, minims preparations are preservative-free and unit dose. Preservative-free products may contain buffers that can cause allergic reactions. Therefore, those who wear contact lenses need to take special care. All eye drops should be discarded after 4 weeks and preservative-free preparations after 7 days unless otherwise stated or if dispensed as unit doses. In hospitals ocular preparations are often allocated shorter in-use shelf-lives of 1–2 weeks.

Case study: Contact lens hypersensitivity

Miss Sunita Patel is a 24-year-old law student who attends the ophthalmic outpatient clinic saying that she has had bilateral red eyes and ocular discomfort for the previous two days. She has been wearing soft contact lenses for the past three years. She is studying for her final year written examination.

While studying, she has neglected her contact lens eye care. She ran out of contact lens cleaning solution and used her friend's (Julie's) solution to clean her lenses. Soon after inserting her lenses, she experienced severe discomfort, watery eyes and photophobia. Her vision has been reduced and she describes it as 'misty'.

When she comes to the clinic, she is still wearing her contact lenses in both eyes. She is accompanied by Julie. Sunita is myopic and has a pair of glasses, which she has not used for the past four months. Her health is otherwise good and she takes contraceptive pills.

She appears very distressed. The ophthalmologist attends to Sunita as a priority case, and a diagnosis of hypersensitivity reaction to contact lens solution is made. The doctor also notes a small infective left corneal ulcer. Antibiotic eye drops and cycloplegics are prescribed. She is to stop wearing contact lenses until both eyes have settled. She is to be reviewed in two days' time in the corneal clinic.

Activity 18.1 (Case study)

1. Explain the dangers associated with using someone else's cleaning solution.
2. Why has Sunita's vision become misty?
3. What eye complications may have occurred?
4. How would you care for Sunita on arrival?
5. What advice would you give Sunita before she leaves the clinic?

Drugs used to manage blepharitis

Blepharitis is an inflammation and infection of the eyelid margins. There are two types of blepharitis: squamous (non-ulcerative) and ulcerative. The two types of blepharitis are also commonly referred to as anterior and posterior blepharitis.

The squamous type is characterised by hyperaemia of the lid margins, some swelling and redness of the eyelids, and fine powdery deposits or scales on the lashes. It can be both acute and chronic. The abnormal changes are accentuated by a tendency to rub the eyelids. It is essentially a seborrhoeic condition – hence its increased incidence in childhood, particularly in early adolescence, but it may be induced by exposure to irritants such as smoke or cosmetics.

The occurrence of secondary infection, usually caused by a Staphylococcal bacterial group, increases the severity of the condition, with obvious signs of inflammation in the region of the eyelashes. It can lead to in-turning of lashes. These offending lashes will rub on the cornea and cause corneal abrasions and ulcerations.

The ulcerative type is more common in unsanitary surroundings and in conditions of malnutrition, or in association with other diseases, such as eczema and diabetes mellitus. Due to their lower resistance to infection, the ulcerative type is more prevalent among these individuals.

A hypersensitive response to Staphylococcus may occur in some individuals. Staphylococcal blepharitis is treated with antibiotic eye ointment applied to the lid margins daily. Warm compresses and lid hygiene are recommended to promote healing. Artificial tear solution should be used, as it promotes ocular comfort.

The most common signs and symptoms of blepharitis are:
- Eyelid irritation
- Redness
- Swelling and discomfort
- Crusts on the eyelashes
- Burning sensation
- Itching.

Complications of blepharitis include chronic infection of the lid and conjunctiva, loss of eyelashes, trichiasis (ingrowth of the eye lashes), conjunctivitis, dry eyes, corneal ulceration and eyelid scarring.

Activity 18.2

Drawing on your knowledge of the causes of blepharitis, list five predisposing factors besides those identified above.

The management of patients with blepharitis mainly involves lid hygiene and antibiotic therapy to treat the infection and to promote ocular comfort.

Case study: Blepharitis

Mr Williams is a 55-year-old car mechanic who has been complaining of bilateral sore eyes and redness for the past two months. He lives in a crowded two-bedroom flat with his wife and three teenage daughters. He is a heavy smoker and also drinks daily with work colleagues in the local pub. He is diabetic, for which he takes metformin 500 mg twice daily. He does not eat healthily. He has financial worries and is in rent arrears.

He has been referred to the eye clinic by his GP, as his eyes have not responded to chloramphenicol 0.5% eye drops, 1 drop 4-hourly, for the past five days. His symptoms feel much worse. His right vision is reduced and he has a constant 'foreign body sensation' in the right eye. His eyes are sticky on waking up. He also complains of a dry burning sensation in both eyes.

The ophthalmologist assesses his eyes and notes that he has severe crust on the lid margins. A diagnosis of Staphylococcal blepharitis is made. There is also a small ulcer near his right cornea. He is very worried about his sight and also about taking time off work.

Activity 18.3

1. Can you suggest why Mr Williams is experiencing these symptoms despite having been on chloramphenicol eye drops prescribed by his GP?
2. Why do you think he has developed pain in his right eye?
3. What specific health advice would you give Mr Williams?
4. Outline the ophthalmic medications that may be prescribed for Mr Williams, and explain why they would be prescribed.

Glaucoma

Glaucoma refers to a group of eye conditions that damage the optic nerve head and cause visual field loss, with open angle glaucoma accounting for the majority of cases. Key clinical signs and symptoms include: raised intraocular pressure (IOP), although not in all cases; as well as visual field abnormalities, reduced visual acuity, and pallor and cupping of the optic disc. In most cases, this is a silent disease that results in impairment and/or loss of vision. It is a leading cause of blindness worldwide, causing sight loss in over 4.5 million people and accounting for about 12% of global blindness (WHO 2020). However, many individuals with the condition remain undiagnosed.

In the UK, glaucoma management makes up a significant proportion of ophthalmologists' workload and it is estimated that there are over a million glaucoma-related NHS appointments annually (King, Azuara-Blanco & Tuulonen 2013). It is also one of the most common reasons for patients to register as visually impaired – and is therefore a major cause of disability. All this evidence indicates that glaucoma has significant social and economic costs to society. However, early intervention can halt the progress of the disease, thus preventing loss of vision.

There are several types of glaucoma, which are classified according to the age of onset, the anterior chamber angle; how rapidly the condition develops, or due to primary or secondary causes.

Two of the most common types of glaucoma are primary open angle glaucoma (POAG) and acute angle closure glaucoma (AACG).

Primary open angle glaucoma

In this type of glaucoma, the angle between the iris and cornea appears normal but the aqueous outflow (see Figure 18.3, p. 365) is blocked. This leads to a gradual increase in IOP, caused by blockage of the drainage system over time or by excessive production of aqueous fluid. This is the most common type of glaucoma in the UK, affecting 2% of the over-40 population, and rising to 10% in those aged over 75 (NICE CKS 2020).

The groups most at risk for open angle glaucoma are individuals with IOP >21mmHg, and those of advancing age, with myopia, diabetes or a family history of glaucoma, and those of black ethnicity (who experience a higher prevalence of the disease). Furthermore, chronic open angle glaucoma is challenging to treat, as many patients are not aware that they have the disease until it has been identified by an optometrist or other eye care specialist during a routine check-up. Unfortunately, by the time they are diagnosed at this late stage, many patients have already lost 70–80% of their optic nerve fibres. However, patients with a family history of glaucoma are usually reviewed regularly and are aware of the seriousness of the disorder and thus seem to benefit from regular monitoring.

A number of strategies are in place to help increase awareness amongst the public, including posters in areas such as GPs' surgeries and pharmacies, and free information leaflets from pharmacies or from the International Glaucoma Association. Furthermore, a Glaucoma Awareness Week, which takes place annually in June, highlights the importance of early diagnosis and treatment. Healthcare professionals can also play a key role in raising awareness and referring patients to their primary eye care professional, particularly if they belong to one of the 'at risk' groups.

Optometrists and other eye care specialist have a key role to play in screening, advising and managing patients as well as their family members – for example, by ensuring that all patients over the age of 40 years have an annual eye check-up. Furthermore, NICE (2017a) set out clear guidelines for the level of expertise that eye healthcare professionals (HCP) should possess in order to manage all types of glaucoma.

Pharmacological management is a key part of the management process, and most medications are designed to reduce raised IOP by either inhibiting aqueous formation or by improving aqueous outflow (see Table 18.4). A comprehensive history and assessment must be carried out before prescribing glaucoma medications and patients must be informed of any potential adverse reactions. For example, prostaglandin analogues are sometimes used to manage primary chronic open angle glaucoma (see Table 18.4) but they can cause pigmentary changes in the eye as well as periorbital fat atrophy, leading to asymmetrical enophthalmos. However, adherence to medication is an important factor in halting the progress of the disease so it is important that a trusting relationship develops between the HCP and the patient, in which the patient is fully informed and involved in all aspects of the management of their condition.

Other forms of management include laser trabeculoplasty, a procedure that involves laser drilling of minute holes in the trabecular meshwork (which promotes the outflow of aqueous humour, thus reducing IOP) and trabeculectomy surgery which involves removal of tissue from the trabecular meshwork (which also has a good success rate in reducing IOP). Current research is focusing on improving the efficacy of pharmacological therapy as well as exploring the use of stem cells to repair damage to the retina and gene therapy to improve the trabecular meshwork outflow (King, Azuara-Blanco & Tuulonen 2013).

Acute angle closure glaucoma

In acute angle closure glaucoma (AACG) the aqueous drainage angle is obstructed by the root of the iris so that the fluid is unable to drain through Schlemm's canal (see Figure 18.3) into the trabecular network, thus raising IOP. The onset of AACG is usually sudden. This type of glaucoma should be suspected in patients who develop an acute painful red eye, with a history of blurred vision, nausea, headaches and seeing halos around lights. There is also a higher incidence of this condition in females, people of Asian ethnic origin and individuals who are long-sighted (NICE CKS 2020).

AACG constitutes an emergency, as the IOP rises acutely due to pupillary block at the iris and cornea border and this can lead to partial or complete loss of vision. The primary aim of management is to reduce the IOP using eye drops, laser treatment or surgery. Specifically, treatment consists of: positioning (lying the patient face up); pharmacological management including analgesia, intravenous acetazolamide 500mg, pilocarpine eye drops (2% in blue eyes or 4% in brown eyes) and beta-blocker eye drops which usually reduce the IOP within half an hour to an hour. The unaffected eye should also be monitored and treated at a later date, as the disease tends to affect both eyes. Patients should be referred to an ophthalmologist or optometrist (NICE 2020).

Table 18.4:
Types of medication that are frequently prescribed for glaucoma

Type of medication	Mode of action	Side effects	Examples	Indications for use
Carbonic anhydrase inhibitor	Reduces aqueous formation from the ciliary body	• Drowsiness • Depression • Diminishes platelet counts • Nausea and vomiting • Agranulocytosis • Metallic taste in mouth • Renal colic and calculi	• Acetazolamide • Dorzolamide	• Primary chronic open angle glaucoma • Acute closed angle glaucoma

Type of medication	Mode of action	Side effects	Examples	Indications for use
Alpha 2 adrenergic agonist	Reduces aqueous humour formation and increases uveoscleral outflow	• Burning • Stinging • Ocular pain and dryness • Tearing • Eyelid erythema • Conjunctival blanching and erosions • Fatigue and drowsiness • Headache	• Brimonidine • Apraclonidine	• Primary chronic open angle glaucoma
Miotic	Constricts pupil by stimulating the sphincter pupillary muscle, to improve aqueous drainage	• Drowsiness • Brow ache	• Pilocarpine	• Primary open angle glaucoma • Acute closed angle glaucoma
Beta-blocker	Blocks beta receptor sites in the ciliary body to reduce aqueous humour production	• Can provoke an acute asthma attack • Loss of libido • Feeling of weakness	• Timolol	• Primary chronic open angle glaucoma
Prostaglandin analogue	Redirects aqueous humour around obstructed meshwork, through the uveoscleral pathway	• Conjunctival redness • Mild punctate corneal erosions • Increased pigmentation of the iris in mixed green-brown or blue/grey-brown eyes	• Latanoprost • Travoprost	• Primary chronic open angle glaucoma
Combination beta-blocker and carbonic anhydrase inhibitor	Reduces aqueous humour production	• Taste disturbance • Respiratory complication • Cardiovascular complication	• Dorzolamide with timolol (Cosopt®)	• Primary chronic open angle glaucoma • Pseudo-exfoliative glaucoma

Case study: Glaucoma

Miss Watson is a 47-year-old Afro-Caribbean patient who has been diagnosed with chronic open angle glaucoma by the ophthalmologist. She has been attending clinic for the past two years. Her visual acuity assessment shows that her left vision has progressively diminished to counting fingers only. Two years ago, her left vision was 6/9 with glasses. This was her best corrective visual acuity with glasses. The normal range of vision is between 6/4 and 6/6 when a Snellen's chart is used. Her right eye has been totally blind due to end-stage glaucoma for the past two years. Following her initial diagnosis two years ago, the ophthalmologist advised a left trabeculectomy. She refused to have surgery. She was initially treated with levobunolol 0.5% and pilocarpine 4% to both eyes, and was on acetazolamide 250mg 4 times a day.

On assessment she appears polite, pleasant but rather withdrawn. She answers only to direct questioning. She has missed two clinic appointments over the past six months and does not wish to explain why. Her intraocular pressures in both eyes are 26mmHg. The range of intraocular pressure varies from one individual to another, and can be between 12mmHg and 21mmHg. Any pressure above that range would cause a healthcare practitioner to suspect glaucoma or ocular hypertension and the individual would need to be referred to an eye clinic for screening. She has no known medical history. She worked as a hospital cleaner but was made redundant a year ago.

She had been prescribed timolol 0.5% for both eyes. One week later, she went to her GP complaining of shortness of breath and wheezing.

When questioned, she said she could not recall the frequency of her drops, any details of her medications or any details of her eye condition.

She tells you that her right eye is blind and that she expects to go blind in her left eye, no matter what the doctor does. Her 80-year-old father is registered blind.

Activity 18.4 (Case study)

1. Discuss the issues and challenges you have identified from the case study.
2. Explain why Miss Watson has progressively lost her vision.
3. What advice would you give Miss Watson about her medications and ocular health?

Eye infections and use of anti-infective agents

Eye infections caused by bacteria, viruses, fungi and amoebae can pose a severe threat to sight. All infections require prompt diagnosis and treatment to improve outcome and reduce morbidity. Simple bacterial conjunctivitis is self-limiting and is commonly seen in childhood. Care must be taken not to spread the disease. The causative bacteria may involve *Staphylococcus aureus* or *Haemophilus influenzae*. Broad-spectrum topical antibiotics, such as ciprofloxacin or chloramphenicol, are the mainstay of treatment and help to shorten the course of the disease. Antibiotic drops to treat gram-negative pathogens, such as *Haemophilus influenzae*, may include ofloxacin 0.3% or ciprofloxacin 0.3%.

Bacterial endophthalmitis is a severe intraocular infection that can enter the eye through a surgical incision or an injury. Pathogens may include *Staphylococcus aureus* or *Staphylococcus epidermidis*. Broad-spectrum intravitreal antibiotics, such as vancomycin 2mg in 0.1ml, together with amikacin 0.4mg in 0.1ml, may be administered by the ophthalmologist. Amphotericin, 5–10mcg in 0.1 ml, is given if fungal infection such as *Candida* is suspected.

Fungal infection of the cornea caused by *Candida* or *Fusarium* can be very difficult to treat. Predisposing factors may include long-term use of topical steroids, a history of ocular surface disease and injury. Microbial confirmation of a fungal infection is important but can take several weeks. Local epidemiological data can be used when deciding on treatment. According to the BNF (Joint Formulary Committee 2020), treatments for fungal infection of the eye are not generally available. Practitioners are therefore advised to refer to a specialist ophthalmology centre such as the Moorfields Eye Hospital for advice on pharmacological management of this type of infection (Moorfields Eye Hospital 2020a).

Acanthamoeba keratitis is a serious corneal infection caused by poor contact lens hygiene, agricultural trauma, and exposure to swimming pool water (e.g. swimming while wearing lenses). The pathogen can exist in two forms: active form (trophozoite) and a resilient dormant form (cyst). Treatment with propamidine 0.1% or polihexanide chlorhexidine 0.02% should be started as soon as possible. The patient should be advised to cease contact lens use immediately in both eyes. After positive microbial investigations, initial treatment is with a combination of anti-amoebic and trophozoicidal drugs, administered hourly day and night for 2 days, then by day only for 3 days. Toxicity is common if dosage at this intensity is maintained. The ophthalmologist will reduce the doses to 3-hourly and then adjust the dosage according to individual patient response.

The viral infection herpes simplex keratitis is a secondary manifestation of herpes simplex infection resulting from reactivation of a dormant virus in the cell bodies of corneal sensory neurons. Topical treatment includes aciclovir 3% eye ointment 5 times daily, continued for at least 3 days after healing; or ganciclovir 0.15% eye gel 5 times a day, reducing to 3 times a day for a further 7 days after healing occurs. Oral medication with aciclovir 200mg 5 times a day for 5 days may also be prescribed. Viral eye infections can be sight threatening if they are not managed effectively. Use of steroid eye drops is not recommended, as this may mask progression of the disease or worsen the condition.

Neonatal conjunctivitis (which presents within the first 28 days of birth) must be given high priority if presented in the Accident and Emergency Department. Pathogens such as *Neisseria gonorrhoea* are very virulent and can perforate the cornea within three days if they are not treated. The parents should be referred to the genitourinary (GUM) clinic for assessment and treatment.

The nurse counsellor plays a key role in reassuring the family that the baby's eyes will be treated and followed up with care by the ophthalmologist. Any baby who presents with neonatal conjunctivitis will be admitted for intensive antibiotic drops, and this is discussed with the family. Health professionals must display sensitivity at all times, and dignity and confidentiality must be maintained. Cefuroxime 5% eye drops every 2 hours and systemic ceftriaxone 25–50mg/kg are prescribed daily for three days. A bacterial swab would be taken on admission for culture and sensitivity. A gram-staining test is carried out as soon as possible to help identify the pathogen so that an appropriate antibiotic can be started without delay. The child's eyes will usually respond well to the treatment within 12 to 24 hours.

Case study: Conjunctivitis

Samanta is a four-year-old girl who attends play school. She is very sociable and likes to play with other children. Her friend Mary has had bilateral bacterial conjunctivitis for the past three days and has been off school for the last two days. Today Samanta comes to school with purulent discharge in both eyes. She also has a sore throat. When you assess Samanta, you note that her eyes are red and sticky, and she feels rather febrile. At lunchtime Samanta's temperature is 38.5 degrees centigrade. Samanta's mother has been advised to come and collect her daughter from school. She is to take her to the GP that evening.

Activity 18.5

1. Name some common pathogens that are responsible for causing infective conjunctivitis.
2. What advice would you give her mother?
3. How is this condition treated?

Administration of ophthalmic medications

Drugs for treatment of ophthalmic conditions are administered in a number of different ways. Medications may be given by various routes, as indicated in Table 18.5.

Table 18.5: Ocular medication routes and their indications

Medication route	Indications
Intravitreal injections into the vitreous humour	• Retinal disease • Wet age-related macular degeneration • Diabetic retinopathy, e.g. Ranibizumab injection

Subconjunctival injections into the space between the conjunctiva and sclera	• For delivery of anti-infectives, mydriatics or corticosteroids in cases where the condition does not respond to topical therapy (BNF 67) • In the management of severe iritis, e.g. betamethasone
Topical drops and ointments instilled directly to the eye	• For delivery of local anaesthetic for eye irrigation, antibiotics to treat conjunctivitis, and steroids to counteract corneal graft rejection
Systemic oral and intravenous medication	• Antibiotics are taken orally, e.g. for infected lid lesions • Some medications are taken intravenously, e.g. acetazolamide to manage primary closed angle glaucoma

Precautionary care by healthcare professionals

A good knowledge of commonly used ophthalmic medications is essential in order to avoid errors. The healthcare professional must always exercise caution by following local protocols and adhering to national medicine management standards (NMC 2018 and RPS 2019).

Observation of the mode of action and possible side effects of medications must be noted and reported. Keeping accurate documentation is of paramount importance for medico-legal reasons. The healthcare practitioner should check whether the patient has been informed and is aware of the purpose of eye medications. All topical antibiotics can cause contact sensitivity, and several days of antibiotic use may lead to clinically significant toxicity. For instance, clarithromycin 2% and gentamicin 0.3% eye drops may cause toxic keratoconjunctivitis and non-healing erosions.

Patients who are prescribed beta-blocker eye drops may develop breathing difficulty. Therefore patients who are asthmatics may need to be prescribed an alternative medication. Precautionary care is also required for patients with cardiac problems.

The occurrence of systemic adverse reactions may be reduced by occlusion of the punctum or by closing the eye for 1 minute following administration. This will reduce systemic absorption.

Patients are advised not to drive if a cycloplegic drop has been applied, as they will be unable to focus clearly. This side effect may last 3 hours or longer, depending on the type of drops and individual patient response. Similarly, if an ointment has been applied, the patient is advised not to drive until the vision is clear. This may take up to an hour.

Adherence

A systematic review by Olthoff *et al.* (2005) indicated that the proportion of patients who deviated from the prescribed medication regimen ranged from 5% to 80%. (See Chapter 5 for more details on adherence.)

The reasons for non-adherence related to patients' lack of knowledge about their eye disorder and their ignorance of the therapeutic benefits of the prescribed medication. Additionally, side effects are common on starting glaucoma medication. For example, the initial application of pilocarpine is painful, due to ciliary spasm and the low pH of the medication. Some older people do experience difficulty in managing their medication due to memory impairment. Thus they are more at risk of non-adherence.

Patients must be made aware that not using their medication as instructed can lead to irreversible loss of sight. This simple strategy may have a profound effect in motivating them. There are also advantages to having an individualised patient education strategy, such as providing a medication information leaflet on their particular eye disorder as part of the discharge care planning initiative (see NICE 2016).

Drug interactions

Drug interactions can arise among patients who are taking ophthalmic medications. The management of some patients with pulmonary disorders may be complicated by beta-blockers, as concurrent use of a beta-blocker and beta-adrenergic agonist may reduce the effect of both drugs. Older people who take antipsychotic, anti-Parkinsonian and antidepressant drugs may develop delirium and confusion if atropine is given. This can be mistaken for an exacerbation of the patient's psychiatric disorder, and treating it by increasing the prescribed medication will only aggravate the situation. (See Chapter 3 for more information on drug interactions.)

Instilling eye drops and ointments

All healthcare practitioners will encounter patients and carers who will need instructions and support when learning how to instil eye medications (Gwenhure & Shepherd 2019, Shaw 2016, Joint Formulary Committee 2020).

The medication should be applied only when the eye is clean to achieve maximum effect, as stickiness and debris may inactivate the active ingredient. The stages of instilling drops and ointments are as follows:

- The patient must be positioned comfortably in a chair, with the head well supported. Adequate lighting is essential. An explanation of the procedure must be given, to increase awareness of the benefits of the medication, before obtaining the patient's consent.
- Check the patient's details from the prescription sheet, and check for any allergy history.
- Check that the correct drops/ointment have been prescribed, at the correct strength, and are being instilled into the correct eye at the correct time.
- When separate bottles are being used for each eye, they must be labelled 'right eye' and 'left eye'.
- Check the expiry date and the clarity of the solution. Ensure the seal is not broken if it is a new bottle or tube.

Pharmacological case studies: Eye problems

- Wash hands before and after instilling ophthalmic medication.

Figure 18.5 (below) shows that the lower lid is pulled down gently and the dropper is held perpendicular to the eye. One drop only is instilled into the middle of the lower fornix (lower conjunctiva sac) from a distance of about 1 inch (2.5cm). Ensure that the dropper does not touch the eyelid or lashes, to avoid contamination.

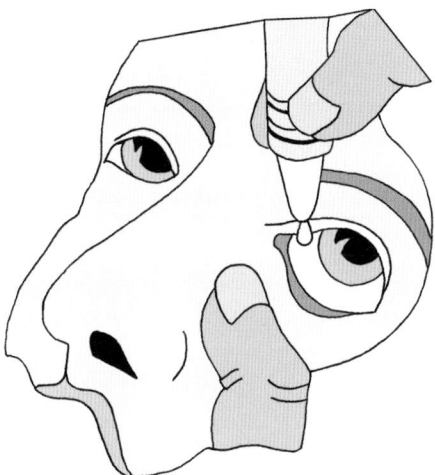

Figure 18.5: Demonstration of eye drop instillation technique.

Figure 18.6 (below) shows application of eye ointment. A thin line of ointment can be squeezed directly from the tube into the conjunctival sac, along the length of the lower fornix, with the patient looking up or behind. Avoid touching the tube with the lashes, to prevent contamination. Finally, close the eye and wipe away any excess with a clean tissue.

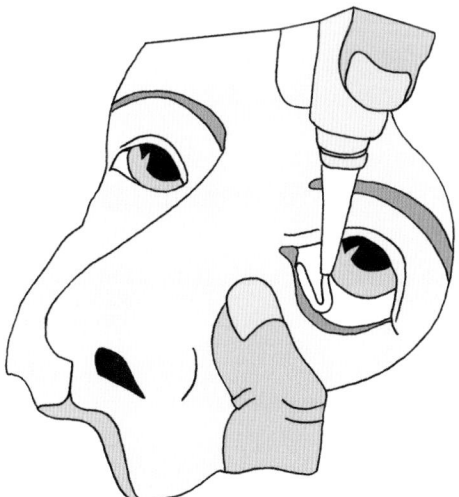

Figure 18.6: Application of eye ointment.

It is important to keep an accurate record of the prescribed medication for medico-legal reasons. The local protocol must be followed. The healthcare practitioner must observe possible side effects from the administered medication, and report and record them appropriately.

If drops are for re-use, they should be labelled (returned to the fridge if required) and kept no longer than one week. Preservative-free drops are often prescribed for patients with an allergic history. All drops, especially those that are preservative-free, are prone to contamination and healthcare practitioners must therefore take precautionary care and observe hygiene principles.

For long-term use of prescribed eye medications at home, the patient should be given appropriate health education to promote self-care and self-administration.

Summary

This chapter has aimed to provide an insight into commonly used ophthalmic medications and the role of the healthcare practitioner. The principles of medication must be applied to promote safe practice. Eye medications are always prescribed for specific conditions, and medications must not be shared with others. Having a thorough knowledge of the actions and side effects of eye medications is important. Patient education and adherence must be encouraged in order to promote healing and prevent sight loss.

Documenting medications is part of the healthcare professional's duty, and local Trust protocols must be followed. Being guided by local policy and working within the law will ensure patient safety. Knowledge and understanding of the legal aspects of the practitioner's role are important since eye medications are legally controlled and it is essential to avoid drug errors. Treating an eye disorder with medications requires the patient or family member to be actively involved. The healthcare practitioner has a duty to ensure safe administration of ophthalmic medication at all times.

Answers to activities

Activity 18.1 (Case study)

1. Explain the dangers associated with using someone else's cleaning solution.
The solution could have expired. It could also be contaminated and toxic. These factors could induce an allergic reaction.

2. Why has Sunita's vision become misty?
Her cornea has become affected, a condition known as toxic epitheliopathy. The cornea could become oedematous due to anoxia and over wear of contact lenses.

3. What eye complications may have occurred?
Possible eye complications are bacterial corneal ulceration and severe corneal toxic epitheliopathy. Secondary iritis is also a possibility if a corneal infection has occurred.

4. How would you care for Sunita on arrival?
Take a thorough history, provide privacy, examine her eyes, ask her to remove her contact lenses and place them safely in their own container. A local anaesthetic eye drop would be required to alleviate her ocular pain as per hospital policy. Record her visual acuity. Examine both eyes using a slit lamp biomicroscope. Document findings and care given.

5. What advice would you give Sunita before she leaves the clinic?
Advise her to use all prescribed drops as instructed. She should also take simple analgesia, wear glasses and not reinsert her contact lenses until advised by her own optometrist. She must not use her friend's solution in future. Inform her that the use of contraceptive pills can reduce tear formation, and ask her to attend for review. Reassure her that her vision will improve.

Activity 18.2

Drawing on your knowledge of the causes of blepharitis, list five predisposing factors besides those identified above.
Dandruff on the scalp, eczema, recurrent styes, acne rosacea and meibomitis.

Activity 18.3 (Case study)

1. Can you suggest why Mr Williams is experiencing these symptoms despite having been on chloramphenicol eye drops prescribed by his GP?
The eyelid crusts act as an irritant, and pathogens can grow and breed in them. This induces an inflammatory response on the eyelid margin, causing soreness, watering eyes, redness and a gritty feeling. The bacteria also affect the quality of the tears, causing a dry, burning sensation. The smoky environment aggravates the symptoms. His working environment also means that adherence to the medication regimen may be poor.

2. Why do you think he has developed pain in his right eye?
Developing pain is a serious ocular complication when there is an on-going episode of blepharitis. This can be caused by the toxin released by *Staphylococcus aureus*. The toxin damages the corneal epithelium and causes small microscopic erosions. As the cornea has an extensive sensory nerve supply from the ophthalmic division of the trigeminal nerve, the pain is usually very marked and severe. Another possible reason for pain is an in-turning eyelash, which can cause a corneal abrasion or ulceration. Ocular pain from blepharitis can also be caused by a marginal corneal ulcer, arising as a result of a hypersensitive reaction to *Staphylococcus aureus*.

3. What specific health advice would you give Mr Williams?
Instruct on lid hygiene twice-daily and advise him to avoid smoky environments and reduce his smoking. He should eat a healthy diet, ideally including two portions of fish per week, as Omega 3 improves tear quality. He must apply the medication as prescribed. He should also take rest and seek advice about his housing and rent arrears.

4. Outline the ophthalmic medications that may be prescribed for Mr Williams, and explain why they would be prescribed.

Mr Williams has a confirmed diagnosis of *staphylococcal* blepharitis and this has been shown to respond to a topical antibiotic, such as chloramphenicol eye ointment for a 6-week period, or fusidic eye drops. If Mr Williams does not respond to this treatment then NICE (2012) suggests a 6-week to 3-month course of an oral antibiotic such as a tetracycline if (as in Mr Williams' case) *staphylococcal* infection is confirmed and eyelid hygiene has failed to address the condition. Blepharitis is a particularly painful condition so Mr Williams may require analgesics. A lubricant such as hypromellose may also be prescribed to address Mr Williams' clinical symptoms of a dry, burning sensation in both eyes. Mr Williams should be encouraged to continue with eyelid hygiene.

Activity 18.4 (Case study)

1. Discuss the issues and challenges you have identified from the case study.

The patient lacks knowledge of glaucoma, she is non-compliant with her medications, her intraocular pressures are not stable, and her optic nerves are severely damaged. She is suffering progressive loss of vision, and has developed side effects from timolol.

2. Explain why Miss Watson has progressively lost her vision.

Her loss of vision could be due to poor compliance and uncontrolled intraocular pressure.

3. What advice would you give Miss Watson about her medications and ocular health?

Miss Watson would benefit from one-to-one health education. She should be informed about what glaucoma is, and the seriousness of her potential vision loss if she does not adhere to the treatment regime. The effects and possible side effects of medications should be explained, e.g. depression associated with acetazolamide. She should be advised to keep a daily diary of her medications, and lifestyle factors such as loss of employment, being a carer for her blind father and also on how she feels. She should attend her clinic appointments, and bring a friend or another family member with her for support.

Activity 18.5 (Case study)

1. Name some common pathogens that are responsible for causing infective conjunctivitis.

Haemophilus influenzae, Staphylococcus aureus, adenovirus.

2. What advice would you give her mother?

She should instil the antibiotic drops as prescribed. The drops must not be shared with other family members. She should wash her hands before and after instilling eye medications, use disposable tissues, not pad the eyes, and keep a separate clean towel for her daughter's use. Simple analgesia can be administered if necessary. Her daughter should not attend school until the infection is cleared.

3. How is this condition treated?

The mainstay of treatment is local antibiotic eye drops during the day and ointment at bedtime.

References and further reading

Gwenhure, T. & Shepherd, E. (2019). Principles and procedure for eye assessment and cleansing. *Nursing Times* [online]; **115** (12), 18–20. https://cdn.ps.emap.com/wp-content/uploads/sites/3/2019/11/191127-Principles-and-procedure-for-eye-assessment-and-cleansing1.pdf (Last accessed 16 November 2020).

International Glaucoma Association (2020). http://www.glaucoma-association.com (Last accessed 16 November 2020).

Jackson, L.T. (ed.) (2019). *Moorfields Manual of Ophthalmology*. 3rd edn. Oxford: JP Medical Ltd.

Joint Formulary Committee (2020). *British National Formulary*. 79th edn. London: BMJ Group.

Jünemann, A.G.M, Chorągiewicz, T., Ozimek, M., Grieb, P. & Rejdak, R. (2016). Drug bioavailability from topically applied ocular drops. Does drop size matter? *Ophthalmology*. **1** (1), 29–35.

King, A., Azuara-Blanco, A. & Tuulonen, A. (2013). Glaucoma. *British Medical Journal*. **346**, f3518. doi: https://doi.org/10.1136/bmj.f3518 (Last accessed 16 November 2020).

Moorfields Eye Hospital (2020a). Common eye condition management. https://www.moorfields.nhs.uk/content/common-eye-condition-management (Last accessed 16 November 2020).

Moorfields Eye Hospital (2020b). Ophthalmic Formulary (Version: 1.29) https://www.moorfields.nhs.uk/sites/default/files/uploads/documents/Ophthalmic%20Formulary%20v1.29%20January%202020.pdf (Last accessed 16 November 2020).

National Institute for Health and Clinical Excellence (NICE) (2009). CG 76. Updated 2019. Medicines adherence: involving patients in decisions about prescribed medicines and supporting adherence. https://www.cntw.nhs.uk/resource-library/medicines-adherence-nice-clinical-guideline-76/ (Last accessed 16 November 2020).

National Institute for Health and Clinical Excellence (NICE) (2012). Blepharitis: Clinical Knowledge Summaries. London: NICE. https://cks.nice.org.uk/topics/blepharitis/ (Last accessed 16 November 2020).

National Institute for Health and Clinical Excellence (NICE) (2016). Medicines adherence. Clinical guideline 76. https://www.cntw.nhs.uk/resource-library/medicines-adherence-nice-clinical-guideline-76/ (Last accessed 16 November 2020).

National Institute for Health and Clinical Excellence (NICE) (2017a). Glaucoma: diagnosis and management. NICE guideline G81. https://www.nice.org.uk/guidance/ng81 (Last accessed 16 November 2020).

National Institute for Health and Clinical Excellence (NICE) (2017b) [KTT 18] Multimorbidity: clinical assessment and management. https://www.nice.org.uk/guidance/ng56/chapter/Recommendations (Last accessed 16 November 2020).

National Institute for Health and Clinical Excellence (NICE) (2020). Clinical Knowledge Summary: Glaucoma. https://cks.nice.org.uk/topics/glaucoma/prescribing-information/ (Last accessed 19 November 2020).

Nursing & Midwifery Council (2018). *The Code: Professional standards of practice and behaviour for nurses, midwives and nursing associates*. Available from http://www.nmc.org.uk/globalassets/sitedocuments/nmc-publications/revised-new-nmc-code.pdf (Accessed: 10 May 2020).

Olthoff, C.M., Schouten, J.S., van de Borne, B.W. & Webers, C.A. (2005). Noncompliance with ocular hypotensive treatment in patients with glaucoma or ocular hypotension an evidence-based review. *Ophthalmology*. **112** (6), 953–61.

Patel, P., Cholkar, P., Agrahari, V. & Mitra, A.K. (2013). Ocular drug delivery systems: An overview. *World Journal of Pharmacology*. **2** (2), 47–64. doi;10.5497/wjp.v2.i2.47.

Rang, H.P., Dale, M.M., Ritter, J.M., Flower, R.J. & Henderson, G. (2012). *Pharmacology*. Edinburgh: Churchill Livingstone.

Royal National Institute for the Blind (RNIB) and Specsavers (2016). *The State of the Nation: Eye Health 2016*. https://www.rnib.org.uk/sites/default/files/RNIB%20State%20of%20the%20Nation%20Report%202016%20pdf.pdf (Last accessed 16 November 2020).

Royal Pharmaceutical Society (RPS) and Royal College of Nursing (RCN) (2019). *Professional Guidance on the Administration of Medicines in Healthcare Settings*. https://www.rpharms.com/Portals/0/RPS%20document%20library/Open%20access/Professional%20standards/SSHM%20and%20Admin/Admin%20of%20Meds%20prof%20guidance.pdf?ver=2019-01-23-145026-567 (Last accessed 16 November 2020).

Salmon, J. (2020). *Clinical Ophthalmology: A Systematic Approach*. 9th edn. US Elsevier.

Shaw, M. (2016). How to administer eye drops and eye ointment. *Nursing Standard*. **30** (39), 34–36.

Sherratt, A. & Needham, Y. (2012). Clinical update–pharmacological issues in ophthalmology. *International Journal of Ophthalmic Practice*. **3** (1), 43–47.

University of Manchester (2018). More than 200 million medication errors occur in the NHS per year, say researchers. https://www.manchester.ac.uk/discover/news/more-than-200-million-medication-errors-occur-in-nhs-per-year-say-researchers/ (Last accessed 16 November 2020).

Waterman, H., Evans, J., Gray, T., Henson, D. & Harper, R. (2013). Interventions for improving adherence to ocular hypotensive therapy. *Cochrane systematic review*. https://www.cochranelibrary.com/cdsr/doi/10.1002/14651858.CD006132.pub3/information [Free Full-text] (Last accessed 16 November 2020).

Watkinson, S. (2010). Improving care of chronic open angle glaucoma. *Nursing Older People*. **22** (8), 18–23.

Watkinson, S. & Seewoodhary, R. (2008). Administering eye medications. *Nursing Standard*. **22** (18), 42–48.

Youngkin, E.Q., Sawin, K.J., Kissinger, J.F. & Israel, D. (eds). (2011). *Pharmacotherapeutics: A Primary Care Clinical Guide*. 2nd edn. Connecticut, USA: Appleton-Lange and Stanford.

World Health Organisation (WHO) (2020). Blindness and vision impairment prevention: Priority Eye Disease. https://www.who.int/blindness/causes/priority/en/index6.htm (Accessed 20 November 2020).

19

Pharmacological case studies: Complex health needs and polypharmacy

Julie Moody
MSc, BSc (Hons), RN, DMS, PGCHE, FAETC/D32/D33,
Registered Practice Educator; Lecturer, Health and Education, Middlesex University, London

This chapter:
- Gives an overview of complex health needs and polypharmacy
- Increases awareness of pharmacokinetic and pharmacodynamic changes in the elderly
- Enhances understanding of physiological changes in older people in relation to prescribing and drug usage
- Applies knowledge of physiological changes in the older person to practice-based case studies.

Introduction

This chapter deals with the formulation and provision of optimum drug therapy for individuals with complex health needs, and focuses in particular on a case study involving an older person with both mental health and physical problems. There are an increasing number of older people in the population today. Living longer raises the chances of developing one or more long-term conditions, alongside other medical conditions that may have been present from an earlier age. This combination can make healthcare needs increasingly complex in environments that can also be challenging. Optimising drug therapy is an essential aspect of caring for such patients.

Age-related pharmacokinetic and pharmacodynamic changes

Normal ageing affects all the body's systems, and the nurse prescriber must be aware of the pharmacological differences that affect this special group. Age is also a risk factor for many conditions that may lead to physiological changes. For example, the greatest risk factor for developing type 2 diabetes is ageing, and – as it is a progressive disease – the many complications of diabetes will develop and worsen over time. These pathophysiological changes will provide challenges for the prescriber. The focus of this section is on the pharmacokinetic and pharmacodynamic changes seen in healthy ageing and in age-related disease.

Older people have variable gastrointestinal pH and this can, in some older individuals, have an effect on the absorption of a drug. However, the solubility and absorption of drugs in older people can also be determined by other factors, including the drug's characteristics, whether the drug is taken with food and the use of proton-pump inhibitors (Abuhelwa, Williams, et al. 2017). Reduced splanchnic blood flow in ageing theoretically affects the rate at which drugs are carried away from the gastrointestinal tract (GI). Diminished absorption capacity of the small intestine is also reported in some older people but this may be due to disease states rather than normal ageing. Reduced gastrointestinal motility and reduced gastric emptying may lead to increased absorption as the drug remains in the GI tract for longer (Khan & Roberts 2018). Nevertheless according to Stillhart and colleagues (2020) there is a lack of agreement in the literature of the ageing process on GI absorption.

Ageing also results in a progressive reduction in total body water and lean body mass, and an increase in fat. A reduction in the volume of distribution of water-soluble drugs, such as cimetidine, leads to higher serum levels. The loading dose of water-soluble digoxin, highly bound to muscle, would need to be lowered to accommodate the reduced volume of distribution and resulting increased plasma concentration seen when lean muscle mass is diminished. With lipid-soluble drugs, such as diazepam, the drugs are deposited into the increased body fat, creating a slow-release reservoir effect, with an increased volume of distribution and an extended half-life (Mangoni & Jackson 2004).

Pharmacokinetic changes include a reduction in hepatic clearance. The liver decreases in weight after the age of 50, with a reduced hepatic blood flow. Liver function tests may not always be affected; however, the production of the protein albumin may be diminished. Protein binding of a drug affects its volume of distribution. Only the unbound or free-drug is distributed throughout the body and is able to exert an effect. In older people with reduced albumin production, the level of the free-drug, such as the highly protein-bound phenytoin, will be increased – with resulting toxicity. Hepatic first-pass drug metabolism is known to decrease in older people. The pharmacokinetic implications for drugs that undergo first-pass metabolism, such as diazepam or propranolol, are increased bioavailability and resulting toxicity. For those prodrugs that are activated through hepatic metabolism, such as the ACE-inhibitor enalapril, whose metabolite enalaprilat exerts its therapeutic effect, diminished hepatic function may lead to a reduced therapeutic outcome.

By the age of 80, the average person has a 70% reduction in the weight and volume of their kidneys as well as a significant decrease in their renal plasma flow. The numbers of glomeruli are also reduced. This is clinically significant for the consequential reduced glomerular filtration rate (GFR), while the plasma creatinine is not reduced due to the age-related loss of muscle mass. Drugs that are excreted via the glomeruli of the kidneys (such as digoxin and penicillin) will therefore have an extended half-life. The extent of reduced filtration and excretion depends on the properties of the drug. Drugs with a narrow therapeutic index may produce adverse effects with only a small reduction in GFR.

Pharmacodynamic changes include an increased sensitivity to drugs. As such, they are dependent on the individual drug and the health status of the older person. For example, warfarin may be potentiated as a greater inhibition of vitamin K clotting is noted in the older person, whilst the pharmacodynamics of heparin in the elderly remain largely unchanged. Older people are vulnerable to adverse effects from psychotropic drugs and may experience delirium, jerky movements and tremor, arrhythmias and postural hypotension. Diazepam, even at lower doses, has an increased sedation effect and postural sway may be seen.

The nurse prescriber will increasingly prescribe for the older age group. The significance of age-related physiological changes must therefore be part of every prescriber's assessment and prescribing decision.

Activity 19.1

When prescribing for any adult, regardless of age, what principles of good prescribing practice do we need to consider and why? Take a few moments to reflect and make some notes.

You should have noted the following, as well as many more factors that you would like to, and should, consider. Figure 19.1 is by no means an exhaustive list.

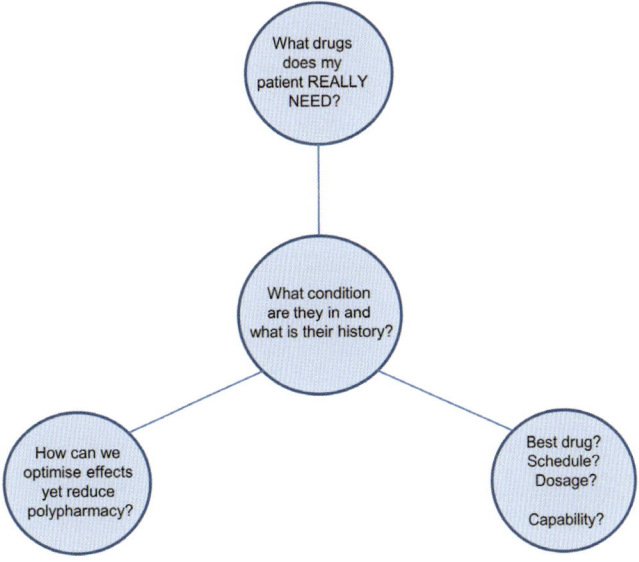

Figure 19.1: Principles of prescribing practice.

Prescribing for complex health needs and particular groups of patients can clearly be particularly challenging and time-consuming and therefore requires a high level of knowledge and expertise. This chapter should provide food for thought on these issues.

Case study: Complex health needs

This case study investigates the management of a 68-year-old woman with complex health needs, who has been referred for assessment and management of her conditions.

Martha has a history of vascular disease, having undergone a coronary bypass at the age of 53. Her past medical history includes type 2 diabetes (diagnosed 10 years ago), hyperlipidaemia, hypertension and atrial fibrillation. She is also a known asthma sufferer, with a history of multiple accident and emergency (A&E) admissions and therapy with prednisolone. Previously reported arthritic knee pain resulted in her reluctant retirement three years ago from her job as a PE teacher. She often feels breathless and has a moderate amount of ankle swelling, which she says is almost always present regardless of the time of day. Martha has also suffered from moderately lengthy depressive episodes in the past few years, since her husband died suddenly and her only daughter migrated to Australia. She has now presented for assessment and management.

The rest of this chapter will therefore consider the management of Martha's drug regime for physical illness as well as for her mental health problems. These mental health issues can be significant as age increases and life-changing events become more frequent and often much more difficult to handle.

Martha now lives alone and has just moved into sheltered accommodation. She has just changed her GP after 35 years and has visited the GP practice only once. Martha's daughter has noted that her mother seems to have become more agitated recently when she calls her, and that she is reporting palpitations, large fluctuations in her blood sugar readings and some shortness of breath on exertion. Martha also suffered a particularly painful fall. Her daughter begins to wonder what is happening with Martha's medication, as she seems to be taking a lot of drugs now, some of which appear to be new. Martha also regularly uses herbal medicine and her daughter has noted that this includes St John's Wort.

Previously, Martha has been treated with a selection of drugs, which included amitriptyline, at times alongside drugs to manage agitation such as temazepam and nitrazepam. Other regular medication includes metformin, aspirin, digoxin, simvastatin, amlodipine, furosemide and telmisartan, with tramadol and diclofenac for arthritic pain and GTN spray and salbutamol inhaler as required (PRN) medications. Martha denies taking alcohol, has never smoked, and has no known allergies.

> ### Activity 19.2
> Consider some factors that may affect the prescriber's decisions on drug dosages in the elderly. Make a note on cause and effect before progressing.

Medication used by older adults

Older people often present at hospital for a variety of reasons. When followed up correctly, these presentations may be attributed to incorrect prescribing. Furthermore, it is widely recognised that hospital admissions due to polypharmacy could be reduced and that such admissions carry with them a risk for vulnerable groups.

As we get older, our bodies change and caution therefore has to be exercised when prescribing, bearing in mind the changing pharmacokinetics and dynamics of the ageing system. Unfortunately many drug trials do not include elderly participants. In the event of drug approval, it follows that the dosage embarked upon may not be suitable for this population group.

From the pharmacodynamic perspective, increasing age may result in an increased sensitivity to the effects of certain drugs, including benzodiazepines and opioids. Martha is taking a variety of drugs, many of them interacting with each other and increasing her risk of suffering drug-related adverse reactions and harmful side effects. Amongst the many drugs that Martha has been prescribed are not one but two benzodiazepines that should be avoided in the elderly, due to the increased risk of confusion and gait problems caused by their hypnotic action, leading to falls and injuries.

> ### Activity 19.3
> Revisit the case study above, and make use of the BNF to note the problems associated with each drug that Martha takes. Look at Appendix I in the BNF and review some of the drug interactions caused by inappropriate prescribing and polypharmacy in Martha's case. Can you see how the interactions are causing some of the problems that she presents with?

Polypharmacy

Polypharmacy is the use of multiple medications by an individual patient. The number of medications used to define 'polypharmacy' varies, but generally runs between five and ten, with some of those medicines being unnecessary. Polypharmacy is usually discussed in relation to prescribed medications but use of over-the-counter (OTC) and herbal therapies should also be considered.

Of particular concern is the fact that older people, when compared to younger individuals, tend to have more conditions for which medicines are prescribed and polypharmacy can then ensue (Rochon, Schmader & Sokol 2020).

The greater the number of drugs used, the greater the risk of adverse events, irrespective of age. However, this issue is of particular concern in the frail elderly (Steinman & Hanlon 2010). Older people are especially affected by polypharmacy for several reasons, such as:

- Use of multiple medications can be worsened by visual or cognitive compromise in many older adults.
- The potential for drug-to-drug interactions rises.
- Metabolic changes in older people, as well as decreased drug clearance, increase the risks, which are worsened by the growing numbers of drugs used.

Polypharmacy increases the possibility of a 'prescribing cascade', which can develop when an adverse drug event is misinterpreted as a new medical condition. This may then lead to additional and misplaced drug prescribing.

Polypharmacy itself has previously been described as an independent risk factor for hip fractures in older adults, although the number of drugs may have been an indicator of a higher exposure to specific types of drugs associated with falls (e.g. central nervous system active drugs) (Perez-Ros et al. 2013).

As a result, prescribers need to strive to strike a balance between over- and under-prescribing when managing the complex health needs of an older person. This may be challenging, and management should be in line with up-to-date clinical guidelines. This will involve the prescriber in a rigorous and systematic overview of need, condition and patient goals when drawing up a care plan. The aim is to avoid as many pitfalls as possible, whilst still providing optimum care. Consequently, some drugs may need to be removed altogether or substituted.

Herbal and dietary supplements

Herbal remedies and historic treatments, as well as OTC remedies, remain popular in this group of patients. It is commonly believed that because the treatments are herbal, they are natural and can do no harm so they are deemed to be completely safe. Yet some of these treatments may lead to serious side effects and interactions with conventional treatments. In a population that is scrutinised for polypharmacy and potential drug-to-drug interactions, the use of herbal remedies, most commonly, gingko biloba, garlic and ginseng, requires consideration by the prescriber (De Souza Silva, Santos Souza, C.A., et al. 2014). A dangerous practice may be almost overlooked when prescribing for a client who does not think to mention this aspect of their regimen. As part of each patient's assessment, all prescribers are therefore obliged to ask about the use of OTC medicines, drugs bought from the Internet, taking medicines prescribed for others, and herbal and alternative medicines.

Inappropriate medications and depression

The prevalence and risks of polypharmacy have been recognised for many years. Martha has been prescribed a selection of drugs over time, some of which may not have been appropriate, and she has now presented for further consideration.

Many conditions may lead to the older person asking for healthcare, including biological needs and illnesses, varying types of pain and mental health conditions. It is recognised that older people suffer increasing loneliness following personal losses (WHO 2017) and this can exacerbate, or be a causative factor in, depression. Martha has been prescribed amitriptyline for depression, which she claims made her feel worse rather than better.

Activity 19.4

Consider Martha's physical assessment results (below) and offer potential explanations for the findings.

Case study (continued)

Martha's physical assessment results are:
- Oedema (pitting) to lower extremities despite furosemide
- BP 168/80 despite medication
- BMI 38, clinically obese
- Capillary blood glucose raised, 12.8mmol/l, despite medication
- Hypokalaemia 3.1mmol/l
- Total cholesterol 5.9, HDL 1, LDL 2.5mmol/l – high LDL despite medication
- Chronic pain – poor walking ability
- No evidence of atrial fibrillation
- Shortness of breath – no wheeze audible
- Liver function normal but digoxin levels are moderately high.

Complexity of need

It is prudent to formulate a systematic evaluation method, along with interventions for a patient's pharmacotherapy, which should ideally be based on the following questions:
- What do you consider to be reasonable outcomes for the patient?
- Based on current guidelines and literature, pharmacology and pathophysiology, what therapeutic endpoints would be needed to achieve these outcomes?

- What potential medication-related problems may prevent achievement of outcomes?
- What will the patient need to achieve in terms of behavioural control to address the problems? What patient education interventions are needed to aid success?
- What needs to be monitored to verify achievement of goals and to detect side effects and toxicity? How often?

In Martha's case, these points are all particularly pertinent and may also be compounded by her history of depression. She also has numerous physical problems and age-related changes to be taken into account. If the goal is to offer Martha the best care, it is vital to look at the whole picture as well as patient expectations, as these are not always congruent. It may turn out that the patient's greatest concern does not correlate with that of the prescriber. For example, Martha may be tired of hospital admissions being caused by her ineffectual asthma management, or it may be the chronic pain of her arthritis that is stopping her sleeping and thus becomes a priority. Meanwhile, the healthcare professional's priority may be the diabetic control.

Thus it becomes evident that there is a need to build on drug therapy and to manage the therapy in steps, taking into account patient compliance along the way. Each disease process and drug that is prescribed can cause a domino effect, which will impinge on the patient's experience and quality of life if not managed well. The patient has to be at the forefront of this process.

Before management is altered, it is necessary to consider the desired therapeutic goals for the patient. This should ensure optimum compliance, patient satisfaction and the maximum potential for symptom and disease control.

Finally, a plan can be co-created by patient and prescriber, which details and considers patient preference, urgency, risk and potential for success. This plan should be ongoing, dynamic, reviewable and achievable.

Activity 19.5

Tabulate Martha's problems that you wish to address pharmacologically. What should you consider?

Monitoring

When developing a plan for monitoring the side effects of the drugs that have been prescribed, you will need to look at side effects, interactions, toxicity issues and patient response (see answers to Activity 19.3, p. 398). Consider the parameters you will use for evidence of effectiveness, and the timeframes for these. You will not be able to monitor all the side effects for every drug with equal diligence and your selection will largely depend on the patient's expressed priorities as well as those issues of toxicity and side effects that are most relevant to their safety.

Summary

It is clear, from Martha's case, that prescribers will be increasingly required to consider a growing number of multi-factorial cases involving very complex needs, histories and age-related conditions. In an ageing population, there is a growing need for expert knowledge in this field.

Answers to activities

Activity 19.1

When prescribing for any adult, regardless of age, what principles of good prescribing do we need to consider and why? Take a few moments to reflect and make some notes.

The British Pharmacological Society has developed 'Ten Principles of Good Prescribing':
1. Be clear about the reasons for prescribing
2. Take into account the patient's medication history before prescribing
3. Take into account other factors that may alter the benefits and risks of treatment
4. Take into account the patient's ideas, concerns and expectations
5. Select effective, safe and cost-effective medicines individualised for the patient
6. Adhere to national guidelines and local formularies where appropriate
7. Write unambiguous legal prescriptions using the correct documentation
8. Monitor the beneficial and adverse effects of medicines
9. Communicate and document prescribing decisions and the reasons for them
10. Prescribe within the limitations of your knowledge, skills and experience.

(Source: The British Pharmacological Society 2020)

Activity 19.2

Consider some factors that may affect the prescriber's decision as to drug dosages in older people. Make a note on cause and effect before progressing.

Cause	Effect on the person
Increase in proportion of fat to skeletal muscle mass	Increased distribution of volume for lipophilic drugs causing drug reservoirs
Larger drug reservoirs	A build-up of the drug, increased plasma concentrations and half-lives and possible toxicity
Natural decline in renal function	Decreased drug clearance
Decreased drug clearance	Increased plasma concentrations
Decreased clearance	Prolonged half-lives

Pharmacology case studies for nurse prescribers

Activity 19.3

Revisit the case study on p. 392, and make use of the BNF to note the problems associated with each drug that Martha takes. Look at Appendix 1 in the BNF and review some of the drug interactions caused by inappropriate prescribing and polypharmacy in Martha's case. Can you see how the interactions are causing some of the problems that she presents with?

Interactions: (BNF app or BNF Online)
*Potentially serious interaction and concomitant use should be avoided or only used with appropriate caution and monitoring.

Amitriptyline (tricyclic antidepressant)	Increased risk of CNS toxicity with *tramadol; sedative effects possibly increased with opioid analgesics		Increased risk of postural hypotension with diuretics	Increased sedative effect with anxiolytics and hypnotics				
Amlodipine (calcium channel blocker)	Enhanced hypotensive effect with angiotensin-II receptor antagonists	Plasma concentration possibly reduced by St John's Wort	Enhanced hypotensive effect with diuretics	Possible increased effect of simvastatin	Hypotensive effect antagonised by NSAIDs	Enhanced hypotensive effect with nitrates	Enhanced hypotensive effect with anxiolytics and hypnotics	
Aspirin	Avoid concomitant use with *NSAIDs due to increased side effects	Possible increased risk of toxicity in high doses with loop diuretic						
Diclofenac (NSAID)	Avoid concomitant use with *aspirin as increased side effects	Increased risk of renal impairment with angiotensin-II receptor antagonists	Antagonise hypotensive effect of calcium channel blockers	Possibly increase plasma concentration of cardiac glycosides; also possible exacerbation of heart failure and reduction of renal function	Risk of nephro-toxicity increased by diuretics and antagonism of diuretic effect	Antagonise hypotensive effect of nitrates		
Digoxin (cardiac glycoside)	Plasma concentrations possibly increased by NSAIDs; also possible exacerbation of heart failure and reduction of renal function	Plasma concentration reduced by *St John's Wort	Increased cardiac toxicity if hypokalaemia occurs with *loop diuretics	Plasma concentrations possibly reduced by salbutamol				

Furosemide (loop diuretic)	Possible reduced effect with aspirin	Enhanced hypotensive effect with *angiotensin-II receptor antagonists	Increased risk of postural hypotension with tricyclic anti-depressants	Antagonise hypoglycaemic effect of anti-diabetics	Enhance hypotensive effect with calcium channel blocker	Hypokalaemia and increased cardiac toxicity with *cardiac glycosides	Enhance hypotensive effect with nitrates	Enhance hypotensive effect with anxiolytics and hypnotics	
GTN spray	Hypotensive effect antagonised by NSAIDs	Enhanced hypotensive effect with angiotensin-II receptor antagonists	Enhanced hypotensive effect with calcium channel blockers	Enhanced hypotensive effect with diuretics	Enhanced hypotensive effect with anxiolytics and hypnotics				
Metformin (oral anti-diabetic)	Hypoglycaemic effect possibly antagonised by loop diuretics								
Nitrazepam (long-acting benzodiazepine) anxiolytics and hypnotics	Increased sedative effect with opioid analgesia	Enhanced hypotensive effect with angiotensin-II receptor antagonists	Increased sedative effect with tricyclic anti-depressants	Enhanced hypotensive effect with calcium channel blockers	Enhanced hypotensive effect with diuretics	Enhanced hypotensive effect with nitrates			
Telmisartan (angiotensin-II receptor antagonist/blocker)	Increased risk of renal impairment and hypotensive effect antagonised with NSAIDs	Enhanced hypotensive effect with anxiolytics and hypnotics	Enhanced hypotensive effect with calcium channel blockers	Enhanced hypotensive effect with diuretics	Enhanced hypotensive effect with nitrates				
Temazepam (short-acting benzodiazepine)	See Nitrazepam								
Tramadol (opioid analgesic)	Increased risk of CNS toxicity and sedative effect possibly increased with tricyclic antidepressants	Increased sedative effect with anxiolytics and hypnotics							
Salbutamol (sympathomimetic Beta-2)	Possibly reduces plasma concentrations of digoxin	Increased risk of hypokalaemia in high doses given with loop diuretics							

Simvastatin (statin)	Plasma concentration reduced by St John's Wort	Possible increased risk of myopathy with *amlodipine						
St John's Wort (herbal remedy for depression)	Reduces plasma concentration of amitriptyline	Reduces plasma concentration of simvastatin	Possibly reduces plasma concentration of amlodipine	Reduces plasma concentration of *digoxin				

Activity 19.4

Consider Martha's physical assessment results (p. 395) and offer potential explanations for the findings.

Physical assessment	Possible causes
Oedema (pitting) to lower extremities despite furosemide	Poor venous return compounded by immobility.
Hypertension despite medication	Blood pressure may be raised due to pain or anxiety.
Clinically obese	Weight gain may be compounded by arthritic pain.
Capillary blood glucose is high despite medication	Consider that an adverse effect of prednisolone is hyperglycaemia.
Low potassium	Consider the effects of diuretics on potassium levels, and the use of potassium-sparing diuretics such as spironolactone.
High LDL despite medication	Hypercholesterolaemia can be familial. LDL can be affected by a diet high in saturated fats and low exercise. Irregular medication times may lower the efficacy of the medication.
Chronic pain – poor walking ability	Arthritic changes may need to be reviewed.
No evidence of atrial fibrillation (AF)	Digoxin is controlling the AF.
Shortness of breath – no wheeze audible	This may be cardiac related (in the presence of oedema).

Activity 19.5

Tabulate Martha's problems that you wish to address pharmacologically. What should you consider?

Problem	Treatment considerations
Asthma control	Effects of diclofenac on asthma
Diabetic control	Adverse effects of hyperglycaemia with prednisolone
Hypertension	Consider use of simvastatin in conjunction with amlodipine
Hyperlipidaemia	Consider an alternative statin
Atrial fibrillation	Monitor for digoxin toxicity
Pain	Consider effects of diclofenac and NSAIDs in asthma
Depression	Consider effects of amitriptyline on cardiac function
Lack of sleep	Consider effects of benzodiazepines in falls
Weight gain	Consider this unpleasant side effect of steroids

References and further reading

Abuhelwa, A.Y., Williams, D.B., Upton, R.N. & Foster, D.J.R. (2017). Food, gastrointestinal pH, and models of oral drug absorption. *European Journal of Pharmaceutics and Biopharmaceutics.* **112**, 234–48.

Alldred, D.P., Raynor, D.K., Hughes, C., et al. (2013). Interventions to optimise prescribing for older people in care homes. *Cochrane Database of Systematic Reviews.* **2**, CD009095.

Boyd, C.M., Darer, J., Boult, C. et al. (2005). Clinical practice guidelines and quality of care for older patients with multiple comorbid diseases: implications for pay for performance. *Journal of the American Medical Association.* **294**, 716.

British Pharmacological Society (2020). Ten Principles of Good Prescribing. https://www.bps.ac.uk/education-engagement/teaching-pharmacology/ten-principles-of-good-prescribing (Last accessed 27 November 2020).

Budnitz, O.S., Shehab, N., Kegler, S.R. & Richards, C.L. (2007). Medication use leading to emergency department visits for adverse drug events in older adults. *Annals of Internal Medicine.* **147**, 755.

De Souza Silva, J.E., Santos Souza, C.A., da Silva, T.B., Gomes, I.A., de Carvalho Brito, G., de Souza Aroujo, A.A., de Lyra-Junior, D.P., da Silva, W.B. & da Silva, F.A. (2014). Use of herbal medicines by elderly patients: A systematic review. *Archives of Gerontology and Geriatrics.* **59** (2), 227–33.

Ferner, R.E. & Aronson, J.K. (2006). Communicating information about drug safety. *British Medical Journal.* **333**, 143.

Hanlon, J.T., Schmader, K.E., Boult, C., et al. (2002). Use of inappropriate prescription drugs by older people. *Journal of the American Geriatrics Society.* **50**, 26.

Hirst, B. (5 June 2003). Polypharmacy remains an issue in elderly patients. *British Medical Journal.* **326**, 1251. doi: http://dx.doi.org/10.1136/bmj.326.7401.1251 (Last accessed 20 November 2020).

Holmes, H.M., Hayley, D.C., Alexander, G.C. & Sachs, G.A. (2006). Reconsidering medication appropriateness for patients late in life. *Archives of Internal Medicine.* **166**, 605.

Kaufman, D.W., Kelly, J.P., Rosenberg, L., et al. (2002). Recent patterns of medication use in the ambulatory adult population of the United States: the Slone survey. *Journal of the American Medical Association.* **287**, 337.

Kelly, J.P., Kaufman, D.W., Kelley, K., et al. (2005). Recent trends in use of herbal and other natural products. *Archives of Internal Medicine*. **165**, 281.

Khan, M. & Roberts, M. (2018). Challenges and innovations of drug delivery in older age. *Advanced Drug Delivery Reviews*. **135**. DOI: 10.1016/j.addr.2018.09.003.

Mangoni, A.A. & Jackson, S.H.D. (2004). Age-related pharmacokinetics and pharmacodynamics: basic principles and practical applications. *British Journal of Clinical Pharmacology*. **57** (1), 6–14.

Nahin, R.L., Pecha, M., Welmerink, D.B., et al. (2009). Concomitant use of prescription drugs and dietary supplements in ambulatory elderly people. *Journal of the American Geriatrics Society*. **57**, 1197.

Oato, D.M., Alexander, G.C., Conti, R.M., et al. (2008). Use of prescription and over-the-counter medications and dietary supplements among older adults in the United States. *Journal of the American Medical Association*. **300**, 2867.

Perez-Ros, P., Martínez-Arnuau, F., Navarro-Illana, E., Tormos-Miñana, I. & Tarazona-Santabalbina, F.J. (2013). Relationship between the risk of falling and prescribed medication in community-dwelling elderly subjects. *Advances in Pharmacology and Pharmacy*. **1** (1), 29–36.

Rochon, P., Schmader, K.E. & Sokol, H.N. (2020). Drug prescribing for older adults. http://www.uptodate.com/contents/drug-prescribing-for-older-adults. (Last accessed 20 November 2020).

Spinewine, A., Schmader, K.E., Barber, N., et al. (2007). Appropriate prescribing in elderly people: how well can it be measured and optimised? *Lancet*. **370**, 173.

Steinman, M.A. & Hanlon, J.T. (2010). Managing medications in clinically complex elders: 'There's got to be a happy medium'. *Journal of the American Medical Association*. **304**, 1592.

Stillhart, C., Vučićević, K., Augustijns, P., Basit, A.W., Batchelor, H., Flanagan, T.R., et al. (2020). Impact of gastrointestinal physiology on drug absorption in special populations - -An UNGAP review. *European Journal of Pharmaceutical Sciences*. **147**. DOI: https://doi.org/10.1016/j.ejps.2020.105280

Tinetti, M.E., Bogardus, S.T. Jr & Agostini, J.V. (2004). Potential pitfalls of disease-specific guidelines for patients with multiple conditions. *New England Journal of Medicine*. **351**, 2870.

World Health Organisation (WHO) (2017). Mental health of older adults. Key facts. December 2017. https://www.who.int/en/news-room/fact-sheets/detail/mental-health-of-older-adults (Last accessed 20 November 2020).

20

Pharmacological case studies: Frailty

Dr Melanie Romain
Consultant Physician and Geriatrician, Royal Free NHS Foundation Trust, London

Frailty can be defined as a loss of functional and cognitive resilience, a state of vulnerability which makes it difficult to return to a normal state of health after illness or injury (Young 2013). In other words, a frail person who experiences a stressor such as pneumonia (or even something relatively minor such as constipation) may not recover to their previous level of function or health. This stressor may therefore result in a fall, delirium or reduced mobility and a prolonged hospital stay (British Geriatric Society 2018), which may in turn lead to a loss of independence (Clegg, Young, et al. 2013). In particular, a fall may be a life-altering event and may result in a hip fracture or head injury (Marvin, Ward, et al. 2016).

We know that frailty leads to a higher rate of hospital admissions, care home admissions and death (British Geriatric Society 2018). It is associated with older age and often occurs in people with multiple and complex chronic medical problems but this is not always the case. It is often associated with dementia. Those who are frail tend to have low energy and slow walking speeds and lack strength (British Geriatric Society 2018).

One of the challenges in clinical practice is how best to diagnose and assess frailty. There are several frailty scales which are in clinical use. The Timed Up-and-Go Test is a commonly used measure of functional mobility and can be used as part of the assessment of frailty. The person is asked to sit on a chair of standardised height, stand up and walk a distance of 3 metres at their normal pace, then turn and sit down again, and this is timed (Savva, Donoghue, et al. 2013). Another test in common use is the Rockwood Clinical Frailty Scale (see Figure 20.1). This can be used in a patient who is at their usual level of function and not when they are acutely ill (Rockwood, Song, et al. 2005).

There are some non-pharmacological interventions that can be tried in order to prevent or mitigate frailty. These include increasing physical exercise, limiting alcohol intake, maintaining social contact and ensuring good nutrition (British Geriatric Society 2018; Puts, Toubasi, et al. 2017).

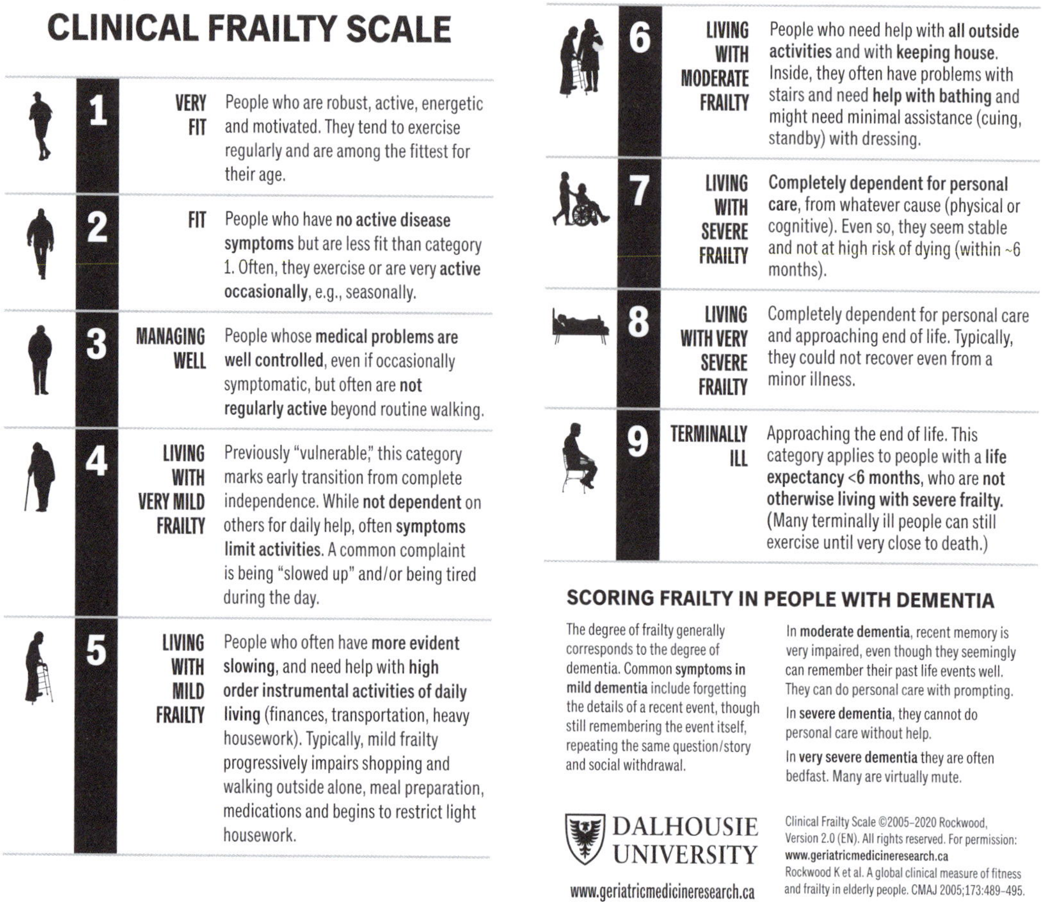

CLINICAL FRAILTY SCALE

1 VERY FIT — People who are robust, active, energetic and motivated. They tend to exercise regularly and are among the fittest for their age.

2 FIT — People who have **no active disease symptoms** but are less fit than category 1. Often, they exercise or are very **active occasionally**, e.g., seasonally.

3 MANAGING WELL — People whose **medical problems are well controlled**, even if occasionally symptomatic, but often are **not regularly active** beyond routine walking.

4 LIVING WITH VERY MILD FRAILTY — Previously "vulnerable," this category marks early transition from complete independence. While **not dependent** on others for daily help, often **symptoms limit activities**. A common complaint is being "slowed up" and/or being tired during the day.

5 LIVING WITH MILD FRAILTY — People who often have **more evident slowing**, and need help with **high order instrumental activities of daily living** (finances, transportation, heavy housework). Typically, mild frailty progressively impairs shopping and walking outside alone, meal preparation, medications and begins to restrict light housework.

6 LIVING WITH MODERATE FRAILTY — People who need help with **all outside activities** and with **keeping house**. Inside, they often have problems with stairs and need **help with bathing** and might need minimal assistance (cuing, standby) with dressing.

7 LIVING WITH SEVERE FRAILTY — **Completely dependent for personal care**, from whatever cause (physical or cognitive). Even so, they seem stable and not at high risk of dying (within ~6 months).

8 LIVING WITH VERY SEVERE FRAILTY — Completely dependent for personal care and approaching end of life. Typically, they could not recover even from a minor illness.

9 TERMINALLY ILL — Approaching the end of life. This category applies to people with a **life expectancy <6 months**, who are **not** otherwise living with severe frailty. (Many terminally ill people can still exercise until very close to death.)

SCORING FRAILTY IN PEOPLE WITH DEMENTIA

The degree of frailty generally corresponds to the degree of dementia. Common **symptoms in mild dementia** include forgetting the details of a recent event, though still remembering the event itself, repeating the same question/story and social withdrawal.

In **moderate dementia**, recent memory is very impaired, even though they seemingly can remember their past life events well. They can do personal care with prompting.

In **severe dementia**, they cannot do personal care without help.

In **very severe dementia** they are often bedfast. Many are virtually mute.

DALHOUSIE UNIVERSITY
www.geriatricmedicineresearch.ca

Clinical Frailty Scale ©2005–2020 Rockwood, Version 2.0 (EN). All rights reserved. For permission: www.geriatricmedicineresearch.ca
Rockwood K et al. A global clinical measure of fitness and frailty in elderly people. CMAJ 2005;173:489–495.

Figure 20.1: Rockwood Clinical Frailty Scale (2005).
Source: Rockwood, K., Song, X., MacKnight, C., et al. (2005). A global clinical measure of fitness and frailty in elderly people. Reproduced with permission.

Drugs

Frail patients often have multiple concurrent conditions and are therefore on several medications. We know that drugs can have a significant effect on frail people in that they may cause or contribute to a deterioration, leading to a fall, delirium or reduced mobility (O'Mahony, O'Sullivan, Byrne, et al. 2015). As a result of changes in drug metabolism in the elderly, drugs which may be well tolerated in a young person may have a more powerful and at times harmful effect on a frail person. In particular, older people clear drugs via the kidneys more slowly and so will be at greater risk when they take nephrotoxic drugs (Joint Formulary Committee 2020). Renal clearance may be reduced further during an acute illness, so these drugs will be even more likely to have adverse effects. Drugs may also have harmful interactions that do not occur to the same extent in non-frail patients.

In view of all these factors, the balance between benefit and harm needs to be weighed up. Drugs that are not providing a clear benefit should be stopped. On the other hand, drugs that could be beneficial should not be withheld simply because of a patient's age (Joint Formulary Committee 2020).

Research evidence shows that around 25% of people over the age of 75 are taking medications they do not need or that may cause them harm (Alhawassi, Alatawi & Alwhaibi 2019). It is recommended that medications are reviewed regularly. When making any changes to frail people's prescriptions, it is important to involve the patient in the decision-making; or, if that is not possible, to consult their family. The healthcare practitioner must check that drugs are being taken as intended and as prescribed. As a general principle, it is worth checking on drugs that are being taken long term and for symptomatic benefit only, such as analgesics or antihistamines. If the patient is not experiencing benefit from these, a plan could be made to either stop or review the drug.

Certain drugs may have particularly deleterious effects on the frail and should therefore be prescribed with caution and with a holistic understanding of the patient. These are:

- Opiates
- Non-steroidal anti-inflammatory drugs (NSAIDs)
- Diuretics.

Opiates

Any drug which acts on the central nervous system may lead to a fall or confusion. These include the commonly prescribed weak opiates (such as codeine phosphate) and stronger opiates, including tramadol and morphine. In a frail patient the safest option is to start with the lowest dose that controls the pain, and then titrate up gradually. When prescribing an opiate, consider the cause of the pain, whether it is neuropathic in origin, and whether it is 'all-over body pain' with no explicable medical cause. An opiate may not be an appropriate choice in some patients, and may in fact cause harm with no clear benefit. Healthcare practitioners should also prescribe opiates only for a limited time and then arrange a review. For example, if a patient has pain due to a soft tissue injury after a fall, one would expect the pain to resolve after around a week, so an ongoing prescription should not be required.

Non-steroidal anti-inflammatory drugs (NSAIDs)

NSAIDs are commonly prescribed for pain and inflammation. However, they are one of the most common causes of adverse drug reactions in the frail and elderly (Joint Formulary Committee 2020). They are associated with an increased risk of gastrointestinal ulceration as well as renal and cardiac toxicity. It is important to be aware of the risk of prescribing them concurrently with anticoagulants (such as warfarin) or anti-platelet drugs (such as aspirin and clopidogrel), as this will further increase the risk of gastrointestinal haemorrhage. The safest approach is to avoid prescribing these drugs altogether in the frail population and it is always best to explore non-drug options first. If prescribing a non-steroidal anti-inflammatory drug is unavoidable, check first for any contraindications and drug interactions, and aim to prescribe the lowest possible dose for the shortest possible time.

Diuretics

Diuretics are frequently used and often overprescribed in the frail elderly. The risk is that they may contribute to hypotension and subsequent falls. They may also lead to electrolyte abnormalities (such as low sodium levels) which may in turn cause confusion and falls or reduced mobility. They are often beneficial in those with cardiac failure but the dose should be kept to the lowest that is effective and reviewed regularly.

Case study: Adjusting a frail patient's medication

An 85-year-old woman is brought to the Accident and Emergency Department by her daughter. Her daughter explains that her mother has seemed vaguer and more confused over the last week. She attended the GP practice 2 weeks ago with swollen ankles and her doctor commenced furosemide 40mg daily. She had a fall 8 days ago but did not sustain any injuries.

Social history: She lives alone in a bungalow, walks with a Zimmer frame and has carers twice a day, to assist with washing and dressing. She does not leave home unaccompanied.

Past medical history: Alzheimer's, dementia, hypertension and osteoarthritis of the knees.

Drug history:

- Furosemide 40mg od
- Bendroflumethiazide 2.5mg od
- Codeine phosphate 60mg qd

On examination:

- The patient looks well.
- BP 110/60mmHg
- Heart rate 70
- Respiratory rate 18
- Chest clear
- Mild ankle oedema.

Activity 20.1 (Case study)

1. What changes would you consider making to her medications?
2. Briefly outline your rationale for making these changes.

Answers to activities to 20.1

1. What changes would you consider making to her medications?

Try reducing the Codeine phosphate to 30mg qds and review in 1–2 weeks. If the patient's knee pain is no worse, try reducing the dose even further and aim to stop it altogether if possible. Initiate regular paracetomol at 1g qds.

2. Briefly outline your rationale for making these changes.

The combination of two diuretics has contributed to a blood pressure which is probably too low for a frail, elderly person. She probably does not require the furosemide for ankle swelling. Advise her to stop this and to try elevating her legs while seated. Request blood tests to check her electrolytes.

References and further reading

Alhawassi, T.M., Alatawi, W. & Alwhaibi, M. (2019). Prevalence of potentially inappropriate medications use among older adults and risk factors using the 2015 American Geriatrics Society Beers criteria. *BMC Geriatrics.* **19**, 154. https://doi.org/10.1186/s12877-019-1168-1 (Last accessed 23 November 2020).

British Geriatric Society (2018). *Frailty: What's it all about?* https://www.bgs.org.uk/resources/frailty-what%E2%80%99s-it-all-about (Last accessed 23 November 2020).

Clegg, A., Young, J., Iliffe, S., Rikkert, M.O. & Rockwood, K. (2013). Frailty in elderly people. *The Lancet.* **381** (9868), 752–76. https://doi.org/10.1016/S0140-6736(12)62167-9 (Last accessed 23 November 2020).

Gallagher, P., Ryan, C., Byrne, S., Kennedy, J. & O'Mahony, D. (2008). STOPP (Screening Tool of Older Persons' Prescriptions) and START (Screening Tool to Alert Doctors to Right Treatment): Consensus Validation. *International Journal of Clinical Pharmacological Therapy.* **46** (2), 72–83.

Joint Formulary Committee (2020). British National Formulary (online). London: BMJ Group and Pharmaceutical Press. https://bnf.nice.org.uk/guidance/prescribing-in-the-elderly.html (Last accessed 23 November 2020).

Marvin, V., Ward, E., Poots, A.J., Heard, K., Rajagopalan, A. & Jubraj, B. (2016). Deprescribing medicines in the acute setting to reduce the risk of falls. *European Journal of Hospital Pharmacy.* **24** (1), 10–15. https://doi:10.1136/ejhpharm-2016-001003 (Last accessed 23 November 2020).

National Institute for Health and Care Excellence (NICE) (2016) [NG56]. Multimorbidity: clinical assessment and management (NICE Guideline No. 56). https://www.nice.org.uk/guidance/ng56/chapter/Recommendations#how-to-assess-frailty (Last accessed 23 November 2020).

O'Mahony, D., O'Sullivan, D., Byrne, S., *et al.* (2015). STOPP/START criteria for potentially inappropriate prescribing in older people: version 2. *Age and Ageing.* **44** (2), 213–18.

Puts, M.T.E., Toubasi, S., Andrew, M.K., *et al.* (2017). Interventions to prevent or reduce the level of frailty in community-dwelling older adults: a scoping review of the literature and international policies. *Age and Ageing.* **46** (3), 383–92. https://doi:10.1093/ageing/afw247 (Last accessed 23 November 2020).

Rockwood, K., Song, X., MacKnight, C., *et al.* (2005). A global clinical measure of fitness and frailty in elderly people. *Canadian Medical Association Journal.* **173** (5), 489–95. https://doi:10.1503/cmaj.050051 (Last accessed 23 November 2020).

Savva, G.M., Donoghue, O.A., Horgan, F., *et al.* (2013). Using Timed Up-and-Go to identify frail members of the older population, *The Journals of Gerontology: Series A.* **68** (4), 441–46. https://doi.org/10.1093/gerona/gls190 (Last accessed 23 November 2020).

Young, J. (2013). NHS England Blog. Frailty – what it means and how to keep well over the winter months. https://www.england.nhs.uk/blog/frailty/ (Last accessed 23 November 2020).

21

Pharmacological case studies: Palliative care

Jo Wilson
PhD, BSc (Hons) Dip HSM, RGN, BA (Hons)
Macmillan Consultant Nurse Palliative Care, Royal Free Hospital, London.

Kirstie Dye
MSc, Bsc (Hons), RN; Clinical Nurse Palliative Care;
Senior Lecturer, Health and Education, Middlesex University, London.

This chapter:
- Gives an insight into how pain is perceived, including discussion of gate control and other pain perception theories
- Develops knowledge and understanding of the pharmacology of the key drugs used to manage symptoms in palliative care
- Offers an approach to managing symptoms in palliative care.

Introduction

This chapter focuses on prescribing for patients with conditions that require palliative care. This area of medicine is large. In 2019, there were 530,841 deaths registered in England and Wales. The leading causes of death were ischaemic heart disease in males (accounting for 13.1% of all male deaths) and dementia and Alzheimer's disease in females (accounting for 16.1% of all female deaths) (ONS 2020). Palliative care refers to the 'holistic care of people with advanced progressive illness' (NICE 2020) and interventions for aspects such as complex symptom management, whilst 'end of life care' relates to the care and support provided in the last year, months and weeks of life and involves, for example, advance care planning in the event of a deterioration in the patient's condition (NICE 2019). These terms are often used interchangeably, which can lead to confusion as not all dying patients require referral to palliative care, and not all patients referred to palliative care are dying.

This chapter focuses on two palliative care case studies, both involving patients with a life-limiting diagnosis and multiple care and symptom control needs. The first patient has a malignant gastric tumour and the second patient has motor neurone disease. The case studies were selected to reflect the varying diagnoses, and ages, of patients requiring palliative care.

> ### Activity 21.1
> Suggest four or five different types of diagnosis for which a patient may receive palliative care.

Patients with long-term conditions may have been living with their symptoms for a long time. They can also have other, unrelated conditions (such as diabetes) and may therefore take a wide range of medications. Patients who have been newly diagnosed with a condition such as cancer may have little experience of the management of their condition. All these factors will affect the needs of these different groups of patients.

Prescribing in palliative care requires an accurate holistic and multidisciplinary assessment of the patient so that the key symptoms affecting the patient's quality of life can be identified and appropriate medications prescribed to manage the symptoms. It is important to try to limit drug administration for patients, as taking any medicine may be an effort and inconvenient. It is therefore necessary to identify the most effective and appropriate medications. It is also important to note concurrent comorbidities, which may prevent usually recommended drugs being administered. For example, metoclopramide would not be administered for nausea to a patient with Parkinson's disease.

> ### Activity 21.2
> Some medications may be prescribed off licence or by unlicensed routes in palliative care. Can you think of reasons why this might happen and identify any examples of this kind of medication?

Symptom management in palliative care requires the identification and management of current symptoms as well as prevention of potential symptoms. There are some core symptoms that most patients receiving palliative care may experience. Pain is a common symptom at the end of life, for which a wide range of medications and interventions may be given. Patients may experience anxiety, nausea and vomiting, breathlessness, increased secretions, oral candida, loss of appetite, constipation, weight loss and agitation. This wide range of symptoms may be complex to manage, and can result in the prescribing of multiple medications. It is important to seek specialist advice when first-line measures are ineffective.

Table 21.1: Common medications used by nurse prescribers in palliative care

Note: Palliative care prescribing relies on impeccable assessment and diagnosis of the cause of the symptom and careful choice of the appropriate class of medication. It also requires due regard to non-pharmacological and nursing intervention.

Symptom	Medication groups	Medication options	Medication route
Pain	Non-opioids	Paracetamol Non-steroidal anti-inflammatory drugs, e.g. Ibuprofen	Oral and intravenous (IV) oral
	Weak opioids	Codeine phosphate	Oral
	Strong opioids	Morphine sulphate	Oral and subcutaneous (SC)
	Adjuvants analgesics (for circumstance specific pain)	Oxycodone hydrochloride	Oral and SC
		Fentanyl	Transdermal
		Buprenorphine	Transdermal
		Antidepressants, e.g. Amitryptilline	Oral
		Anti-epileptics, e.g. Gabapentin	Oral
		Steroids, e.g. Dexamethasone	Oral and IV and SC
Nausea and vomiting	Peripherally acting prokinetic anti-emetic	Domperidone	Oral and per rectum (PR)
	Centrally acting and prokinetic anti-emetic	Metoclopramide	Oral and IV and SC
	Centrally acting receptor specific anti-emetic	Haloperidol	Oral and SC
		Cyclizine	Oral and SC
		Ondansetron	Oral and IV
	Broad-spectrum anti-emetic	Levomepromazine	Oral and SC
Excessive secretions	Anti-cholinergic medication	Hyoscine	Oral and SC
		Butylbromide Glycopyrronium	SC and PEG
		Hyoscine Hydrobromide	Transdermal

(table continued overleaf)

Table 21.1 continued

Symptom	Medication groups	Medication options	Medication route
Agitation	Antipsychotics Benzodiazepines	Haloperidol Midazolam	Oral and SC Buccal and SC
Anxiety	Benzodiazepines	Lorazepam Diazepam Midazolam	Sublingual Oral SC
Breathlessness	Opioid Benzodiazepine	Morphine sulphate Lorazepam	Oral or SC Sublingual
Constipation	Macrogol Softener Stimulant	Polyethylene glycol Docusate sodium Senna	Oral Oral Oral
Oral candida	Antifungal	Nystatin Fluconazole	Oral Oral

In the next two sections we will specifically consider the key symptoms of pain and nausea and vomiting. We will discuss the physiology and the pharmacology of these symptoms, before considering interventions to promote the patient's comfort.

Pain

Pain is a complex phenomenon, which is difficult to define. However, a useful and practical definition is the one by McCaffery (1968), who stated that 'Pain is whatever the experiencing person says it is, existing whenever he says it does'. This definition reminds the practitioner that pain does not necessarily have to have an identifiable physical cause, and that pain is real to that individual patient regardless of the cause. Indeed, almost all pain results from a total body response to a combination of physical and mental elements.

Transmission and perception of pain: gate control theory

Pain is due to damage to tissues, which in the periphery are richly supplied with pain receptors (nociceptors) that detect pain. The small-diameter unmyelinated C fibre and A delta myelinated fibres are responsible for transmitting painful stimuli from the periphery to the dorsal horn of the spinal cord, where they synapse and terminate. The pain impulses then travel along pain pathways (spinothalamic and spinoreticular tract) and synapse in the other parts of the brain, such as the thalamus and somatosensory cortex, where pain is perceived.

Melzack and Wall (1968) first proposed that a gating mechanism existed within the dorsal horn of the spinal cord, which modifies or blocks the transmission of pain impulses to the level of conscious awareness in the pain centres of the brain. It is thought that gating mechanisms occur at each level of the spinal cord and several sites within the brain (e.g. thalamus, reticular formation). Modulation or inhibition of pain transmission in the spinal cord will reduce or prevent pain transmission along the spinothalamic tract and thus perception in the higher centres of the brain.

There are many different types of neurotransmitters located in the dorsal horn of the spinal cord, and the gate is thought to be opened by the release from synapses of excitatory neurotransmitters and closed by inhibitory neurotransmitters. From a clinical perspective, closing of the gate forms the basis of pain relief. The passage of nerve impulses through this gate can be modified or inhibited by opioid peptides such as endorphins, descending fibres from the cortex which synapse in the spinal cord, or by stimulation (for example, by touch such as massage of large-diameter nerve fibres, known as A beta fibres, from the periphery).

The value of this model of pain perception and inhibition is that it helps, to some extent, to explain how pain relief strategies work. However, it should be emphasised that pain perception in the central nervous system is a complex process that is still not fully understood.

Activity 21.3

Having reviewed the gate control theory, can you speculate as to which type of afferent nerve fibres are stimulated by transcutaneous electrical nerve stimulation (TENs) to reduce pain transmission?

Opioids

Opioids are related to morphine, the most important of the alkaloids extracted from the latex of the opium poppy (*Papaver somniferum*). The term 'opioid' means 'acting like opium' but they are also known as opiates (derived from opium) or narcotic analgesics, because high doses produce narcosis (a state of drowsiness or stupor).

Opioid receptors are widely distributed in the central nervous system and periphery. Endogenous (natural substance) opioids, such as endorphins, and exogenous (drug) opioids both produce their effects by attaching to specific opioid receptors within the central nervous system and in peripheral tissues. The main subtype of opioid receptor is the mu receptor. Others include kappa, delta and sigma receptors. Opioids can be classified as agonists (e.g. morphine, diamorphine), partial agonists (e.g. buprenorphine) and antagonists (e.g. naloxone). (See Chapter 2 for an explanation of these terms.)

The mu receptor agonists

These are the most widely used opioids to control pain and are the main drugs used in the management of moderate and severe cancer pain. It is therefore essential that healthcare professionals have an understanding of their therapeutic and adverse effects, as patients need to be monitored for both.

Activity 21.4

Review the therapeutic and adverse effects of opioids in one of the pharmacology texts listed in the further reading list on p. 432, then complete Table 21.2 below by:
- Inserting the correct words in the blank spaces in columns 1 and 2 (Hint: Pain relief and sedation, respiratory depression, cough suppression, nausea and vomiting, miosis, hypotension and bradycardia)
- Identifying the effects that are therapeutic and those that are adverse.

Table 21.2.
Central agonist effects of stimulating opioid receptors (mu)

Patient's experience	Action of opiate	Therapeutic or adverse effect?
	Reduction in pain perception	
Reduced respiratory rate, ineffective oxygenation		
	Depression of the cough centre→dampens cough reflex	
Affect near vision (blurred vision)	Stimulation of occulomotor centre, causing pupil constriction this is known as —	
	Stimulates the vagus nerve	
	Stimulation of the medullar chemoreceptor trigger zone (CTZ)	

Activity 21.5

Complete Table 21.3 opposite by:
- Stating the effects on the patient of activating mu receptors outside the central nervous system. (Hint: urine retention, bronchospasm, flushing and hypotension, constipation)
- Identifying the effects that are therapeutic and those that are adverse.

Table 21.3:
Peripheral agonist effects of stimulating opioid receptors (mu)

Patient's experience	Action of opiate	Therapeutic or adverse effect
	Increases smooth muscle tone in gut and decreases peristalsis	
	Increases smooth muscle tone of the detrusor muscle of the bladder	
	Increases smooth muscle tone of the detrusor muscle of the bladder Stimulates the release of histamine from mast cells, which causes contraction of smooth muscles of bronchioles; flushing and hypotension	

Naloxone

Naloxone reversibly blocks access to opioid receptors and is indicated for reversal of opioid-induced respiratory depression and acute opioid overdose. It has an onset of action of 1–2 minutes when given IV and 2–5 minutes when given SC or IM. It has a half-life of 1 hour (Palliative Care Formulary 2020).

Please note that 'traditional doses' of Naloxone (400 micrograms IV stat) are recommended only in immediately life-threatening situations where patients are unconscious with minimal respiratory effort. In other circumstances, lower doses of Naloxone (e.g. 20–100 micrograms) are recommended to prevent a severe withdrawal crisis (Palliative Care Formulary 2020).

'For patients receiving opioids for pain relief Naloxone is not recommended for drowsiness or delirium which is not life threatening because of the danger of reversing the opioid analgesia. Instead omit or reduce the next dose and then subsequently continue at a reduced dose' (PCF 2017, p. 460).

Nausea and vomiting

Nausea is defined as a feeling of sickness with an inclination to vomit. Vomiting is the forceful ejection of stomach contents through the mouth. People can have one symptom without the other and it is vital that a comprehensive assessment is undertaken.

Koch (2018, p. 3) describes two general mechanisms of nausea and vomiting:

Neurological
- Stimulation of the area postrema [in the brain], which 'senses' noxious chemical agents, e.g. chemotherapy agents, and subsequently stimulates the vagal nuclei, which evokes nausea and co-ordinates the emesis reflex.

- CNS diseases, such as infections or brain tumours, which stimulate CNS structures and elicit nausea and vomiting, ultimately through vagal pathways

Peripheral
- Diseases that originate from the GI tract, which stimulate vagal or spinal afferent nerves that connect with the vagal sensory and vagal efferent motor nuclei. Ultimately cortical centres where nausea is perceived and the efferent pathways that mediate vomiting are stimulated.
- Tumors, infections and drugs in the periphery cause local dysfunction in a variety of organ systems that is sensed as nausea and severe nausea eventually provokes vomiting.

There are likely to be multiple causes of symptoms of nausea and vomiting.

Potential causes include:
- Post-operative side effects
- Side effects of radiotherapy, chemotherapy
- Gastrointestinal obstruction, either internally from a tumour or externally from ascites, and/or constipation
- Raised intracranial pressure, e.g. subsequent to a brain metastasis
- Cough
- Infection
- Fluid and electrolyte imbalance, e.g. hypercalcaemia, renal failure, metabolic disturbances
- Anxiety.

Assessment should include (Rosenberg 2015):
- Experience of nausea
- Frequency of vomit, as well as colour and volume
- Assessment of volume depletion
- Oral mucosa/dental examination
- Abdominal examination
- Neurological assessment
- An assessment of bowel actions and stool consistency
- The impact of the symptoms on the patient's ability to carry on with their activities of daily living.

As mentioned previously, it is also important to assess other comorbidities which may restrict the use of certain classes of anti-emetic. For instance, metoclopramide and haloperidol would not be administered for nausea and vomiting in a patient who had Parkinson's disease. Provided the oral route could be tolerated, then domperidone, which does not cross the blood–brain barrier, could be the anti-emetic of choice (Palliative Care Formulary 2020). However, domperidone should be used at the lowest dose and for the shortest time due to a risk of increased cardiac side effects (MHRA 2014). Assessment of the drug of choice is crucial. It is also important to assess the level of renal and hepatic failure, as these conditions may restrict both the class and dose of drug. For instance, in renal patients with a GFR of <10 mL/min, specialist advice should be sought and most anti-emetics would be started cautiously and in line with guidance (Ashley & Dunleavy 2019).

Anti-emetics are a functionally diverse group of drugs acting on one of more of the sites implicated in nausea and/or vomiting. There is little randomised controlled trial evidence to guide drug selection in palliative care (Palliative Care Formulary 2020) and choice of anti-emetic is therefore guided by the likely mechanism by which the drug acts. NICE guidance exists on the use of anti-emetics at end of life (NICE 2020).

Table 21.4: First-line anti-emetics

Cause of nausea and vomiting in palliative care	First line anti-emetic
For vestibular irritation or raised intra cranial pressure	Cyclizine
For chemical causes of vomiting e.g. morphine, renal failure	Haloperidol
For gastritis or gastric stasis	Domperidone or metoclopramide

Second- and third-line anti-emetics

If symptoms persist, an alternative first-line anti-emetic, or a switch to a broader-spectrum drug (e.g. Levomepromazine) should be considered. If patients have symptoms that are resistant to both first-line and second-line intervention, they should be referred to palliative care for specialist assessment and advice and consideration of third-line anti-emetics.

The use of third-line anti-emetics is very dependent on individual assessment, cause and consideration of other treatments. Third-line anti-emetics can include dexamethasone, benzodiazepines and ondansetron.

If patients are very symptomatic, consider administering the medications via routes other than oral. Very often a 24-hour continuous subcutaneous infusion (CSCI) to administer the medication subcutaneously via a syringe pump (sometimes called a syringe driver) is indicated and this allows assessment of the efficacy of the pharmacological intervention.

Medication routes in palliative care

Symptom management for patients accessing palliative care is likely to be complex and may require a combination of medications to achieve the desired result. For instance, patients with pain may be prescribed morphine as an immediate-release (e.g. Oramorph®) or modified-release preparation – for example, morphine sulphate MR tablets or fentanyl patches (Joint Formulary Committee 2020).

Pharmacology case studies for nurse prescribers

The pharmacokinetics of the various opioids differ in a number of areas. For example, immediate-release oral morphine is reasonably well absorbed, reaching peak effect within approximately 30 minutes, and lasting about 4 hours. It has a high first-pass effect, as up to 75% is broken down after a single dose. It is metabolised in the liver and mostly excreted by the kidneys. Transdermal patches (fentanyl), although more potent than morphine, have a slower onset of action, taking up to 12 hours to reach an effective therapeutic level. Hence an alternative drug should be administered until the therapeutic level is effective and a steady state is attained. Unlike immediate-release morphine, which is suitable for acute pain, transdermal fentanyl is ideal for long-term pain release because the drug is released into body fat, then slowly released into the bloodstream.

Medication administration in palliative care may be by various routes.

Activity 21.6

Review the routes of medication administration listed in Table 21.5 below. Suggest what problems may arise with individual administration routes for palliative care patients and outline any pharmacokinetic considerations.

Table 21.5:
Routes of administration of medicines in palliative care patients

Route	Palliative patient care considerations	Pharmacokinetic considerations
Oral		
Rectal		
Topical		
Transdermal		
Subcutaneous		
Intravenous		

Palliative care medication in practice

Whilst patients may receive medication orally, for patients who have dry mouth, oral candida, disease processes affecting swallowing or causing nausea and vomiting or reduced consciousness level, it may not be appropriate to consider oral administration. The alternate routes may be by subcutaneous injection or infusion with a syringe pump. These are preferable to an intravenous route, as they do not restrict the patient's mobility, can be easily cared for and repositioned, and may be more comfortable than an intravenous cannula.

Where administration is through a continuous subcutaneous infusion via syringe pump, it is common practice to combine medications into one continuous infusion. Nurses should be alert to guidance (DH 2010) regarding the mixing of medicines and administration of the resulting unlicensed medicines. The primary opiate of choice for analgesia delivered by a syringe pump is morphine sulphate (NICE 2012). This is because it is low cost and it mixes well with many other medications, which is useful in reducing the number of syringe pumps the patient may have. Advice on drug compatibility is available – for instance, from the Palliative Care Formulary (PCF7 2020), the Syringe Driver Survey Database (SDSD 2019) and Dickman & Schneider (2016).

The route of administration and other factors (such as lipid solubility of the drug, surface area available for absorption, as well as the concentration gradient) will affect the rate of absorption of drugs taken orally or subcutaneously, as illustrated in the earlier discussion about oral morphine and transdermal fentanyl.

Activity 21.7

Identify the medications that may be combined with morphine sulphate for administration in a syringe pump.

Case study: Gastric cancer

Jane Adams is a 42-year-old woman diagnosed with a gastric tumour three months ago. At the point of diagnosis, Jane has metastatic spread of the disease. Jane has been treated with chemotherapy to shrink the tumour, with the aim of reducing some of the gastric symptoms she has been suffering. On referral to the palliative care service, Jane is complaining of persistent pain in her epigastric/upper abdominal region, which is waking her at night and troubles her intermittently during the day. The pain is thought to be from the primary tumour. The pain is restricting Jane's ability to mobilise and, as a result, Jane does not feel able to 'get out and about'. Jane lives with her husband and her children, who are aged 14 and 12.

Jane's husband feels his wife's reluctance to continue normal activities due to the pain is causing her to feel low and is impacting on their children, as Jane no longer takes them to school or collects them. Jane has been taking morphine sulphate (5mg every 4 hours) for pain relief. Initially this intervention was effective but now this only relieves the pain for 2 hours or less. Jane continues to complain of feeling nauseated and has poor appetite; she finds that preparing food makes her symptoms of nausea worse.

On initial assessment of Jane, you note:

- She is tender in her abdominal area at all times
- She frequently burps and hiccups
- She is underweight
- She tells you she feels sick all the time and cannot eat
- She complains of feeling weak and tired
- During the assessment Jane starts to cry and tells you she feels very down and fearful of the future
- When you examine Jane's mouth you note the presence of oral candida.

Case study: Motor neurone disease

Jim Taylor is a 68-year-old man with motor neurone disease, diagnosed eight years ago. Prior to his diagnosis, Jim smoked 10 cigarettes a day from the age of 16. Jim had previously been diagnosed with chronic obstructive pulmonary disease (COPD) at the age of 54. Although Jim has significantly reduced his smoking to four cigarettes a day, he continues to smoke. Recently Jim's mobility has rapidly deteriorated and he has become unable to walk. He also experiences limited movement of his upper limbs. Jim's speech is deteriorating and he is finding it increasingly difficult to swallow and communicate. As a result, he is unable to swallow his saliva and is constantly drooling, which he finds distressing. Jim feels embarrassed to go out (due to the drooling) and no longer attends the games club he used to go to daily. His interaction with friends is therefore limited. Jim is fully conscious and has had a percutaneous endoscopic gastrostomy (PEG) tube inserted for assisted nutrition. Jim's prognosis may be measured in months. Jim's General Practitioner has asked for prescribing advice on managing the symptom of drooling.

On initial assessment of Jim, you note:
- His slow, slurred speech
- He is constantly trying to wipe his mouth and has a bib on
- He is wheelchair bound
- He tells you he misses his friends, is getting very bored at home and feels there is 'no point in going on'
- He is breathless at rest.

Activity 21.8 (Case studies)

Using the information from Jane's and Jim's assessments, identify all the symptoms they have which may be addressed by pharmacological intervention.

Patients accessing palliative care may have multiple symptom control issues as a result of advancing disease, which may be compounded by other pre-existing diagnoses and depression.

Activity 21.9 (Case studies)

Identify the category of medication that would be an appropriate intervention to address each of Jane's and Jim's symptoms, and describe the pharmacological action of each medication. When considering the medications, think about limiting the number of different prescriptions. For example, are there medications that would address multiple symptoms? It will also be necessary to consider any side effects of your medication choices.

Although Activity 21.9 focuses on the pharmacological management of these symptoms, it is important that other non-pharmacological approaches should also be considered as part of the management. Furthermore, any underlying cause should be addressed, such as depression, anxiety, genitourinary, gastrointestinal, odours or medications. In addition, the views of the patient and carer about such things as eating habits and body image should be taken into consideration, as psychological factors can be extremely important.

When choosing pharmacological interventions for palliative care patients, it is necessary to balance the benefit a medication may achieve in alleviating a symptom with any side effects, and to assess whether the benefit outweighs the potential side effects.

Activity 21.10

For the medication groups identified in Activity 21.9, what would be the issues and side effects to consider with each medication choice?

Activity 21.11 (Case studies)

1. What anti-cholinergic medication and route would you consider to help manage Jim's drooling?
2. How would you review Jane's analgesic regime? What type of issues would you need to consider and what would you recommend?

Activity 21.12 (Case study)

In Jane's case, what would be the advantage of using an immediate-release form of morphine in addition to a modified-release form such as morphine sulphate modified release capsule (MXL)?

Activity 21.13

Identify patients for whom prescription of oral morphine sulphate should be avoided or used with caution.

Activity 21.14 (Case study)

If Jane is found to have a degree of renal impairment, what alternative actions and medications would you consider?

The case studies used in this chapter are representative of patients with cancer (Jane) and other long-term conditions (Jim). Both patients' symptoms are common to many patients accessing palliative care. Completing the activities will demonstrate the wide range of pharmacological interventions available for both malignant and neurological diagnoses, and how good prescribing practice can significantly improve the quality of the patient's life.

Summary

Patients receiving end of life or palliative care will experience diverse and often challenging symptoms, which may be managed using pharmacological and non-pharmacological interventions. Patients may be prescribed many different drugs, with differing modes of action and always with a risk of interactions and adverse side effects. The practitioner prescribing for patients receiving palliative care needs to work in a multi-professional way, with the patient and carers at the centre of all decisions, to ensure that prescribing is safe, ethical and effective.

Answers to activities

Activity 21.1
Suggest four or five different types of diagnosis for which a patient may receive palliative care.
- Malignant tumours: solid (e.g. breast cancer) and non-solid (e.g. leukaemia)
- Neurological conditions (e.g. stroke, motor neurone disease, benign brain tumour, multiple sclerosis)
- Long term conditions (e.g. heart failure, chronic respiratory diseases, chronic kidney disease)
- Genetic disorders (e.g. cystic fibrosis, Huntington's chorea and muscular dystrophy).

Activity 21.2
Some medications may be prescribed off licence or by unlicensed routes in palliative care. Can you think of reasons why this might happen and identify any examples of this kind of medication?

Prescribing unlicensed medicines outside the recommendations of the marketing authorisation (MA) alters (and increases) the professional's responsibility and liability (BNF 74). The prescriber must be able to justify and feel competent to use the medication and inform the patient that the medicine is unlicensed. A good source of advice in palliative care is the *Palliative Care Formulary* (PCF7 2020). The PCF editors prefer the term 'off label' use for the use of a medicinal product beyond its MA. An example would be the mixing of medicines in one syringe pump. This must be carried out in line with best advised practice such as that found on the PCF website under the syringe driver formulary (Syringe Driver Survey Database 2019) or Dickman & Schneider (2016).

Activity 21.3
Having reviewed the gate control theory, can you speculate as to which type of afferent nerve fibres are stimulated by transcutaneous electrical nerve stimulation (TENs) to reduce pain transmission?

A beta fibres.

Activity 21.4

Review the therapeutic and adverse effects of opioids in one of the pharmacology texts listed in the further reading list on p. 432, then complete Table 21.2 below by:
- Inserting the correct words in the blank spaces in columns 1 and 2 (Hint: Pain relief and sedation, respiratory depression, cough suppression, nausea and vomiting, miosis, hypotension and bradycardia)
- Identifying the effects that are therapeutic and those that are adverse.

Table 21.2. Central agonist effects of stimulating opioid receptors (mu)

Patient's experience	Action of opiate	Therapeutic or adverse effect?
Pain relief and sedation	Reduction in pain perception	Therapeutic
Reduced respiratory rate, ineffective oxygenation	Depresses respiration but only when administered in doses larger than needed to control pain or if renal function is impaired (PCF5 2017)	Adverse
Cough suppression	Depression of the cough centre → dampens cough reflex	• Therapeutic and adverse • Suppresses dry persistent irritating cough, but reduces the protective effect of cough reflex
Affect near vision (blurred vision)	Stimulation of occulomotor centre, causing pupil constriction; this is known as miosis	Adverse
Hypotension and bradycardia	Stimulates the vagus nerve	Adverse
Nausea and vomiting in some patients	Stimulation of the medullar chemoreceptor trigger zone (CTZ)	Adverse

Activity 21.5

Complete Table 21.3 below by:
- Stating the effects on the patient of activating mu receptors outside the central nervous system. (Hint: urine retention, bronchospasm, flushing and hypotension, constipation)
- Identifying the effects that are therapeutic and those that are adverse.

Table 21.3: Peripheral agonist effects of stimulating opioid receptors (mu)

Patient's experience	Action of opiate	Therapeutic or adverse effect
Constipation	Increases smooth muscle tone in gut and decreases peristalsis	Adverse effect in treatment of palliative care patients. Requires effective use of laxatives
Urine retention	Increases smooth muscle tone of the detrusor muscle of the bladder	Adverse
Bronchospasm, flushing and hypotension	Stimulates the release of histamine from mast cells, which causes contraction of smooth muscles of bronchioles; flushing and hypotension	Adverse

Activity 21.6

Review the routes of medication administration listed in Table 21.5 below. Suggest what problems may arise with individual administration routes for palliative care patients and outline any pharmacokinetic considerations.

Table 21.5: Routes of administration of medicines in palliative care patients

Route	Palliative care considerations	Pharmacokinetic considerations
Oral	• Dry mouth • Swallowing difficulty • Nausea and vomiting • Gastric tumours • Head and neck tumours causing obstruction • Bowel obstruction • Residing in any care setting or at home	• Easy and convenient for self-administration • Non-invasive • Sublingual administration of appropriate drugs can give rapid absorption • Gastric absorption with varied speed and bioavailability

Route		
Rectal	• Bowel tumours • Patients do not usually prefer this route • Residing in any care setting or at home	• Avoid first-pass effect and destruction by intestinal enzymes or by low pH in the stomach • Used for patients who are vomiting when drug administration by other routes is unavailable • For local and systemic actions
Topical	• Skin irritation • Cachexia • Residing in any care setting or at home	• Easy for self-administration • Used for local actions
Transdermal	• Skin irritation • Non-hairy skin • Residing in any care setting or at home	• Drug is absorbed through layers of the skin into the bloodstream; first-pass hepatic metabolism is avoided and it lasts a long time; therefore replacement is infrequent, e.g. fentanyl patches last for up to 72 hours. • Useful in mobile patients who cannot tolerate taking drugs orally or who do not wish to use a CSCI. • Systemic use • Absorption can also be variable, due to such factors as sweating, so close monitoring of its effect is needed. • Time taken to peak effect so other appropriate medicines will be needed (as required) until the patch achieves its effect
Subcutaneous	• When the oral route is not available • Availability of subcutaneous fat or excessive oedema • Residing in any care setting or home	• Not subject to first-pass metabolism • Used in unconscious cases or patients who are unable to swallow • Used for drugs that are poorly absorbed or unstable in the GI tract • Absorbed relatively slowly

Intravenous	<ul><li>Restricts patient mobility</li><li>Risk of extravasation</li><li>Need to reposition cannula</li><li>Patient comfort</li><li>Highly invasive</li><li>Requires in-patient setting (usually hospital)</li></ul>	<ul><li>Not subject to first-pass metabolism</li><li>Used in unconscious cases</li><li>Used for drugs that are poorly absorbed or unstable in the GI tract</li><li>Rapid action</li><li>Directly delivered into systematic circulation (bioavailability is 100%)</li><li>Easy dose control</li></ul>

Activity 21.7

Identify the medications that may be combined with morphine sulphate for administration in a syringe pump.

The following drugs are separately compatible with morphine sulphate in a syringe pump (diluted with water for injection): cyclizine, haloperidol, hyoscine butylbromide, levomepromazine, metoclopramide, midazolam. Other combinations of drugs are also used in clinical practice – refer to specialist reference sources, e.g. the Palliative Care Formulary (PCF7 2020) and the Syringe Driver Survey Database (SDSD 2019) and Dickman & Schneider (2016).

Activity 21.8

Using the information from Jane's and Jim's assessments, identify all the symptoms they have which may be addressed by pharmacological intervention.

You should have noted the following issues for Jim and Jane; self-assess the ones you identified against the following list:

Jane	Jim
<ul><li>Epigastric pain</li><li>Nausea</li><li>Appetite and weight loss</li><li>Tiredness</li><li>Fearful about the future and may be depressed</li><li>Hiccup</li><li>Oral candida</li></ul>	<ul><li>Drooling</li><li>Breathlessness</li><li>Reduced mobility – prevention of constipation</li><li>Fearful about the future and may be depressed</li></ul>

Activity 21.9 (Case studies)

Identify the type of medication that would be an appropriate intervention to address each of Jane's and Jim's symptoms, and describe the pharmacological action of each medication. When considering the medications, think about limiting the number of different prescriptions. For example, are there medications that would address multiple symptoms? It will also be necessary to consider any side effects of your medication choices.

Jim	Medication type	Pharmacological/physiological action
Drooling	• Antimuscarinics should be considered carefully. Jim may tolerate a hyoscine hydrobromide patch that is replaced every 3 days. Absorption is best when it is placed on hairless skin behind the ear. However, if he suffers undesirable side effects (e.g. delirium or a skin reaction), glycopyrronium via the PEG may be a better option.	• Block acetylcholine on cholinergic receptors, reducing saliva production
Breathlessness – rule out all treatable causes, e.g. fluid overload or asthmatic component	• Opioids, e.g. morphine sulphate (first line) • Benzodiazepines, e.g. lorazepam (second line); useful in reducing breathlessness associated with anxiety	• Opioids reduce the work of breathing (Barnes, McDonald, et al. 2016) • Bind to GABA receptors in the brain, reducing anxiety
Reduced mobility – prevention of constipation	• Stool softeners, e.g. docusate sodium • Stimulant laxatives, e.g. senna	• Increase water content of the bowel • Increase peristalsis
Depression	• Antidepressants, e.g. citalopram	• Block serotonin uptake

Jane	Medication type	Pharmacological/physiological action
Epigastric pain	• Analgesics, e.g. morphine sulphate	• Bind to opioid receptors in the gastrointestinal tract

Nausea	• Anti-emetics, e.g. metoclopramide	• Metoclopramide is a D2 antagonist which acts on chemoreceptor trigger zone (CTZ) and peripherally in the GI tract, where it blocks the dopamine brake on gastric emptying induced by stress, anxiety and nausea (PCF 2017)
Appetite loss	• Steroids, e.g. dexamethasone	• Reduces swelling around the tumour, thereby increasing the space at the gastric outlet so food can pass through into the small bowel
Depression	• Antidepressants, e.g. citalopram	• Block the reuptake of serotonin
Hiccups	• Antacids or prokinetics, metoclopramide	• Metoclopramide (see above) • Antacids have a neutralisation effect, thus reducing acidity in the stomach
Oral candida	• Antifungals, e.g. fluconazole	• Binds to the fungus and disrupts the cell wall which is vital to its survival

Activity 21.10

For the medication groups identified in Activity 21.9, what would be the issues and side effects to consider with each medication choice?

Jim's symptoms	Medication	Issues to consider
Drooling	Glycopyrronium Hyoscine hydrobromide patch	Pros: Easy administration via PEG; no central effects Pros: Easy administration via patch; small dose of drug required and therefore low risk of central effects Cons: If patient sweats, the patch may not adhere properly **Side effects of anticholinergics** *Peripheral effects:* • Cardiovascular, e.g. palpitations • Gastro-intestinal, e.g. constipation • Urinary, e.g. retention of urine • Visual, e.g. blurred vision *Central effects:* • Drowsiness • Delirium • Agitation

Breathlessness	Morphine sulphate	• Manual dexterity required to self-administer liquid morphine sulphate when breathless • Opiates cause constipation and require laxative prescription
Prevention of constipation	Docusate sodium	• Is it inappropriate to prescribe a laxative as a preventative measure? Does he already have very loose stools? • Can the medicine be administered via a PEG?
Depression	Citalopram	• Whether psychological support is preferable? • Time lag before therapeutic effect? • Acceptableness to patient?

Jane's symptoms	Medication	Issues to consider
Epigastric pain	Opioids	• Can she tolerate an oral dose, given gastric symptoms? • Would a syringe pump be a preferable route of administration to titrate up the analgesia in a prompt fashion before converting to another route of administration, e.g. transdermal or long-acting opiate? • How should breakthrough doses of analgesia be administered? • Consider laxatives
Burping and hiccups	Metoclopramide	Metoclopramide: • Likely to benefit from the prokinetic effect, but metoclopramide is contraindicated if there is a complete obstruction. • Timing of administration – are the hiccups constant or post-prandial? • Would a syringe pump be an effective way of ensuring the medication is not vomited and there is constant administration?

	Dexamethasone	Dexamethasone: • Steroids have serious side effects. • Is there gastric cover through a proton pump inhibitor? • What dose of steroids and for how long? • Remember BNF advice for the patient on taking steroids.
Nausea	Anti-emetics (see above)	• See above
Tiredness	Steroids, e.g. megestrol acetate	• Research shows varying efficacy of the medications for patients experiencing fatigue.
Oral candida	• Antifungals, e.g. local nystatin, or systemic fluconazole	• Patient education for appropriate administration; should be held in the mouth for up to 1 minute or more (longer contact time more effective), before swallowing. • Dentures are a source of reinfection and patients should be advised to clean thoroughly or soak in chlorhexidine mouthwash overnight. Chewing pineapple chunks is also used in palliative care to stimulate saliva production in order to cleanse the mouth.

Activity 21.11 (Case studies)

1 What anti-cholinergic medication and route would you consider to help manage Jim's drooling?

You should consider in your response the side effects of hyoscine hydrobromide. As this medication is easily absorbed across membranes such as the gut and the blood–brain barrier (BBB), it can cause sedation and confusion. Whilst this is rare when a patch is used, it would be a significant disadvantage for Jim, as he remains alert and was previously able to attend social activities. The side effects could impact on Jim's quality of life in an adverse way, despite controlling the symptom. It may therefore be more appropriate to consider glycopyrronium, as this medication has larger molecules than hyoscine hydrobromide. Glycopyrronium does not cross the BBB or gut easily and it is excreted largely unchanged in urine, thus lessening the side effects. It can be administered three times a day via the PEG.

2 How would you review Jane's analgesic regime? What type of issues would you need to consider and what would you recommend?

You should consider a complete pain assessment, as well as the dose, frequency and effectiveness of the analgesia Jane is already taking. You should also consider how Jane can maintain her activities of daily living and those things that bring meaning to her life. For instance, it may be particularly important to Jane that she can continue to do activities with her children and the 'school run' has already been raised as an issue by Jane's husband. This will give a clue to the importance of the activity to the family. A syringe pump may be a temporary measure to gain control of the symptoms before switching to either a transdermal patch or long-acting oral medicines. Care will need to be taken with dose conversions of oral opiates to subcutaneous routes. If necessary, seek specialist advice.

Activity 21.12 (Case study)

In Jane's case, what would be the advantage of using an immediate-release form of morphine rather than a modified-release form such as MST®?

For Jane, an immediate-release form would allow easier adjustment of dosage to achieve optimum pain relief. This would also allow doses to be timed to fit in with Jane's peaks of activity, such as the school run or after-school playtime. An immediate-release form is also absorbed more quickly and provides quicker pain relief. In some circumstances, use of a modified-release preparation may provide more consistent pain relief. However, this should always be prescribed alongside appropriate immediate-release rescue therapy for breakthrough pain.

Activity 21.13 (Case study)

Identify patients for whom prescription of oral morphine should be avoided or used with caution.

Patients with reduced renal function and renal disease should be prescribed morphine sulphate cautiously or not at all. The kidneys are the main organs of excretion for morphine and its more potent active metabolite morphine-6-glucuronide. In patients with renal impairment, the effects of morphine will therefore be prolonged, with potential for toxicity. The BNF recommends reducing the dosage or avoiding use in renal impairment. The side effects of morphine are also poorly tolerated by patients with renal impairment. Always seek specialist advice.

Activity 21.14 (Case study)

If Jane is found to have a degree of renal impairment, what alternative actions and medications would you consider?

Dose reduction should be considered if the medication is controlling Jane's pain and optimising her quality of life. Alternative medications (such as fentanyl transdermal patch or oxycodone) could also be considered, as both are metabolised in the liver and are less dependent on renal excretion.

References and further reading

Ashley, C. & Dunleavy, A. (2019). *The Renal Drug Handbook: The ultimate prescribing guide for renal practitioners*. 5th edn. Boca Raton, Florida: CRC Press.

Barnes, H., McDonald, J., Smallwood, N. & Manser, R. (2016). Opioids for the palliation of refractory breathlessness in adults with advanced disease and terminal illness. *Cochrane Review*. https://www.cochranelibrary.com/cdsr/doi/10.1002/14651858.CD011008.pub2/full (Last accessed 2 December 2020).

Department of Health (DH) (2010). Mixing of medicines prior to administration in clinical practice: Medical non-medical prescribing. London: HMSO.

Dickman, A. & Schneider, J. (2016). *The Syringe Driver: Continuous Subcutaneous Infusions in Palliative Care.* 4th edn. Oxford: Oxford University Press.

Joint Formulary Committee (2020). *British National Formulary.* London: BMJ Group and Pharmaceutical Press.

Koch, K.L. (2018). BMJ Best practice. Assessment of nausea and vomiting, adults. Available at https://bestpractice.bmj.com/topics/en-gb/631/pdf/631.pdf (Accessed: 21 August 2019).

McCaffery, M. (1968). *Nursing Practice Theories Related to Cognition, Bodily Pain, and Man-Environment Interactions.* Los Angeles: University of California at LA Students Store.

Melzack, R. & Wall, P.D. (1965). Pain mechanisms: a new theory. *Science.* **150** (3699), 971–79.

Medicines and Healthcare Products Authority (MHRA) (2014). Domperidone: risks of cardiac side effects. https://www.gov.uk/drug-safety-update/domperidone-risks-of-cardiac-side-effects (Last accessed 19 November 2020).

National Institute for Health and Care Excellence (NICE) (2012). Palliative care for adults: strong opioids for pain relief. Clinical guideline [CG140] Available online: https://www.nice.org.uk/guidance/cg140 (Last accessed 12 February 2021).

National Institute for Health and Care Excellence (NICE) (2019). End of Life Care for Adults: Service delivery. https://www.nice.org.uk/guidance/ng142 (Last accessed 29 November 2020).

National Institute for Health and Care Excellence (NICE) (2020). Palliative Care: General Issues. https://cks.nice.org.uk/topics/palliative-care-general-issues/?_escaped_fragment_=scenario#:~:text=The%20National%20Institute%20for%20Health,and%20spiritual%20support%20is%20paramount (Last accessed 29 November 2020).

NICE Clinical Knowledge Summaries (CKS) (2020). Palliative care - nausea and vomiting: scenario: end of life [online]. Available at: https://cks.nice.org.uk/topics/palliative-care-nausea-vomiting/management/end-of-life/ (Accessed 12 February 2020).

Office for National Statistics (2020). Deaths registered in England and Wales 2019. https://www.ons.gov.uk/peoplepopulationandcommunity/birthsdeathsandmarriages/deaths/bulletins/deathsregistrationsummarytables/2019 (Last accessed 29 November 2020).

Palliative Care Formulary (2017). 6th edn. Edited by Twycross, R., Wilcock, A. and Howard, P., UK: Pharmaceutical Press.

Palliative Care Formulary (2020). 7th edn. Edited by Wilcock, A., Howard, P. & Charlesworth, S. UK: Pharmaceutical Press.

Ridgeway, V. (2011). 'Caring for the older person'. Chapter 6 in M.A. Baldwin & J. Woodhouse (eds). *Key Concepts in Palliative Care.* London: Sage Publications.

Rosenberg, J. (2015). Assessing nausea and vomiting. Available at: https://www.ausmed.com/cpd/articles/assessing-nausea-and-vomiting (Accessed: 21 August 2019).

Royal Pharmaceutical Society (RPS) and Royal College of Nursing (RCN) (2019). Professional Guidance on the Administration of Medicines in Healthcare Settings. https://www.rpharms.com/Portals/0/RPS%20document%20library/Open%20access/Professional%20standards/SSHM%20and%20Admin/Admin%20of%20Meds%20prof%20guidance.pdf?ver=2019-01-23-145026-567 (Last accessed 19 November 2020).

Scholefield, D.M. (2006). *Pharmacology for Nursing Practice.* BMS2004 (Course Text). Middlesex University. Unpublished.

Syringe Driver Survey Database (SDSD) (2019). Palliativedrugs.com *Essential independent drug information for palliative and hospice care.* https://www.palliativedrugs.com/syringe-driver-database-introduction.html
(Last accessed 29 November 2020).

22

Insights into professional prescribing

Alison Harris
Senior Lecturer, Health and Education, Middlesex University, London.
Community practitioner nurse prescriber

This chapter:

- Reflects on the accountability imposed by the RPS Competency Framework
- Considers the impact of the changes to non-medical prescribing programmes
- Sets out the challenges for nurse and midwife prescribers.

Introduction

Non-medical prescribing in the UK is now well established, and the growth in the numbers of nurse and midwife prescribers is visibly linked to the development of their roles as well as being intrinsic to the clinical commissioning programme and to workforce development (NHS 2019, NHS Scotland 2017). Healthcare services are being transformed by advanced clinical practitioners, who are non-medical prescribers (NMPs), and who are driving enhanced patient services, working across traditional professional boundaries and providing innovative models of care (Health Education England 2017).

Studies show that outcomes of non-medical prescribing are similar to those of medical prescribing and NMPs offer service user satisfaction (Weeks, George, et al. 2016; Courtenay, Carey, et al. 2011; Latter, Blenkinsopp, et al. 2010). Nurse-led services continue to develop in diagnostics, preventative health and in the acute and primary care sectors. Non-medical prescribing offers the service user continuity of care and more efficient access to medicines and increases the capacity of the healthcare workforce to meet healthcare expectations (Welsh Government 2017). Non-medical prescribing plays a central part in these services being effective and meeting the demands of a larger, older and more diverse population.

Medical and non-medical prescribing

Since the first edition of this book was published in 2015, a lot of changes have been made, which have affected the programme of study needed to attain the non-medical prescribing qualification as well as the professional accountability of the non-medical prescriber. In 2016 the Royal Pharmaceutical Society published the long-anticipated *Competency Framework for all Prescribers* (RPS 2016). This coincided with the archiving of the 2006 Nursing and Midwifery Council (NMC) *Standards of Proficiency for Nurse and Midwife Prescribers* (NMC 2006). The RPS Framework now sets the minimum benchmark for the accountability, professional practice and clinical governance expected of all prescribers.

The NMC has adopted this Framework and any prescribing programmes must assess all students as having met the RPS competencies, in full, before they can qualify as non-medical prescribers (NMC 2018b). All trainee and qualified non-medical prescribers must be familiar with these RPS competencies to support accountable prescribing practice. In addition, nurses and midwives are reminded by their regulatory body that, where there are any issues of professionalism that are not made clear by the RPS Framework, the NMC Code takes precedence (NMC 2018a).

As professional boundaries are blurred and new roles created, the Framework enables prescribers to consistently understand what is expected of both medical and non-medical prescribers. The generic Framework enables all prescribers across the wider inter-professional team (both medical and non-medical) to adhere to the same level of competency and accountability; and this consistent understanding becomes incredibly important in team prescribing.

Nurse and midwife prescribing

The *NMC Standards for Prescribing Programmes* came into effect in January 2019. These standards set out the requirements for entry on to a prescribing programme. Any nurse or midwife wishing to undertake the independent or supplementary nurse or midwife programme, leading to the V300 qualification, must be qualified for a minimum of one year. There is no minimum period of registration required for access to the community practitioner nurse or midwife prescribing programme, which leads to the V150 qualification (NMC 2018b). The NMC is therefore clearly stating that there is now a professional expectation that newly registered nurses will readily advance to take on a prescribing role. (Guidance on midwives is still awaited as this book goes to press.)

Challenges remain in the possible further evolution of nurse and midwife prescribing. Under the 2018 *NMC Standards for Prescribing Practice*, there is no longer any guidance to higher education institutions on the number of days the programme of study needs to take. With greater coverage of pharmacology and medicines safety in the pre-registration nursing curriculum (NMC 2018c), it is possible that the NMP trainee will access a significantly shorter prescribing programme.

Alternatively, a single prescribing programme (for independent, supplementary and community practitioners) may emerge from the drive to speed up the advancement of new registrants.

Studies have highlighted the need for the Nurse Prescribers' Formulary (NPF) to be updated to reflect the prescribing requirements of community nursing and midwifery prescribers (Courtenay, Carey, et al. 2018). In October 2020, the NPF in the back pages of the BNF, was digitalised to allow community nurse prescribers to benefit from access to the monographs and drug interactions via the BNF app and online.

Activity 22.1
Bearing in mind your professional status and accountability, how will you ensure that you are a safe prescriber?

The cost of prescriptions

The cost of medicines remains central to ethical and accountable prescribing practice. The overall gross cost of medicines, in 2017/18, for NHS secondary and primary care in England, was £18.2 million. This represented an increase of 39.6% from 2010/11 (NHS Digital 2018). Every prescriber recognises their responsibility to prescribe effectively and to avoid polypharmacy and unnecessary prescribing. As staff resources are strained, so non-medical prescribers are making greater use of prescribing aids such as the online BNF and the BNF app, thus ensuring that their prescribing decisions are guided by the most up-to-date evidence. Electronic prescribing, which currently delivers 67% of all general practice prescriptions, offers greater efficiency and saves time and money (NHS 2019).

Guidance for service users

We now have clearer guidance for service users on the prescribing of over-the-counter medicines, to support the prescriber's decision not to prescribe for certain minor illnesses (NHS England 2018). Non-medical prescribers are at the forefront of guiding best practice in patient-centred prescribing, reassessment and de-prescribing. Assessment tools, like the STOPP/START medication review for frail, older people (O'Mahony, O'Sullivan, et al. 2015), allows non-medical prescribers to assess for over-prescribing and polypharmacy, inappropriate drugs and drug avoidance (NHS England 2017).

Answers to activities

Activity 22.1

Bearing in mind your professional status and accountability, how will you ensure that you are a safe prescriber?

Safe prescribing can be ensured by having prescribing supervised, and by continuous professional development (CPD) in the form of attending prescribing groups, updates and conferences that include prescribing for a particular clinical area of practice. Prescriptions can also be audited, with data being scrutinised to check rationale and cost of prescribing decisions.

References and further reading

Courtenay, M., Carey, N., Stenner, K., Lawton, S., & Peters, J. (2011). Patients' views of nurse prescribing: effects on care, concordance and medicine taking. *British Journal of Dermatology*. **164** (2), 396–401. https://doi.org/10.1111/j.1365-2133.2010.10119.x (Last accessed 25 November 2020).

Health Education England (HEE) (2017). Multi-professional framework for advanced clinical practice in England. https://www.hee.nhs.uk/ (Last accessed 25 November 2020).

Latter, S., Blenkinsopp, A., Smith, A., Chapman, S., Tinelli, M., Gerard, L., Little, P., Celino, N., Granby, T., Nicholls, P. & Dorer, G. (2010). *Evaluation of nurse and pharmacist independent prescribing*. University of Southampton and University of Keele on behalf of the DoH, Southampton.

NHS (2019). *The NHS Long Term Plan*. https://www.longtermplan.nhs.uk/ (Last accessed 25 November 2020).

NHS Digital. (2018). Prescribing costs in the hospital and community, England 2017/18. https://digital.nhs.uk/data-and-information/publications/statistical/prescribing-costs-in-hospitals-and-the-community/2017-18#key-facts (Last accessed 26 November 2020).

NHS England (2017). *Toolkit for general practice in supporting older people living with frailty*. https://www.england.nhs.uk/publication/toolkit-for-general-practice-in-supporting-older-people-living-with-frailty/ (Last accessed 25 November 2020).

NHS England (2018). *Prescribing of over the counter medicines is changing: patient leaflets*. https://www.england.nhs.uk/publication/prescribing-of-over-the-counter-medicines-is-changing/ (Last accessed 25 November 2020).

NHS Scotland (2017). *Everyone matters: 2020 workforce vision implementation plan 2018-20*. https://www.gov.scot/publications/everyone-matters-2020-workforce-vision-implementation-plan-2018-20/pages/8/ (Last accessed 25 November 2020).

Nursing and Midwifery Council (NMC) (2006). The standards of proficiency for nurse and midwife prescribers (2006). https://www.nmc.org.uk/standards/standards-for-post-registration/standards-for-prescribers/ (Last accessed 26 November 2020).

Nursing and Midwifery Council (NMC) (2018a). *The Code. Professional standards of practice and behaviour for nurses, midwives and nursing associates*. https://www.nmc.org.uk/standards/code/ (Last accessed 25 November 2020).

Nursing and Midwifery Council (NMC) (2018b). Standards for prescribing programmes. https://www.nmc.org.uk/globalassets/sitedocuments/education-standards/programme-standards-prescribing.pdf (Last accessed 25 November 2020).

Nursing and Midwifery Council (NMC) (2018c). *Standards for pre-registration nursing programmes*. https://www.nmc.org.uk/globalassets/sitedocuments/standards-of-proficiency/standards-for-pre-registration-nursing-programmes/programme-standards-nursing.pdf (Last accessed 25 November 2020).

Nursing and Midwifery Council (NMC) (2019). *Standards for prescribing programmes*. https://www.nmc.org.uk/standards/standards-for-post-registration/standards-for-prescribers/standards-for-prescribing-programmes/ (Last accessed 25 November 2020).

O'Mahony, D., O'Sullivan, D., Byrne, S., O'Connor, M.N., Ryan, C., & Gallagher, P. (2015). STOPP/START criteria for potentially inappropriate prescribing in older people: version 2. *Age and Ageing*. **44**, 213–18.

Royal Pharmaceutical Society (RPS) (2016). *A Competency Framework for all Prescribers*. https://www.rpharms.com/Portals/0/RPS%20document%20library/Open%20access/Professional%20standards/Prescribing%20competency%20framework/prescribing-competency-framework.pdf (Last accessed 25 November 2020).

Weeks, G., George, J., Maclure, K. & Stewart, D. (2016). Non-medical prescribing versus medical prescribing for acute and chronic disease management in primary and secondary care. *Cochrane Database Systematic Review.* 11, CD011227.

Welsh Government (2017). *Non-medical prescribing in Wales guidance.* https://gov.wales/non-medical-prescribing-wales-whc2017035 (Last accessed 25 November 2020).

Glossary

absorption In a pharmaceutical context, the process by which a drug crosses biological membranes from its administration site to reach the systemic circulation.

active transport An energy-dependent process involving the movement of substances across a cell membrane against a concentration gradient, from a low concentration to a high concentration. This process is often facilitated by the binding of the substance to a carrier protein in the cell membrane.

adherence In a healthcare context, adherence is the extent to which an individual's behaviour, when taking medication, following dietary advice or other lifestyle changes, corresponds to that recommended by a healthcare provider.

agonist A substance that, when combined with a receptor, initiates a physiological response.

angiotensin converting enzyme inhibitor Medication that slows (inhibits) the activity of the enzyme ACE, which decreases the production of angiotensin II.

angiotensin receptor blocker Medication that blocks the action of angiotensin II by preventing angiotensin II from binding to angiotensin II receptors on the muscles surrounding blood vessels.

angiotensin receptor/neprilysin inhibitors A combination medicine that contains both an angiotensin receptor blocker and a neprilysin inhibitor.

antagonist A substance that interferes with, or blocks, a physiological response. This is usually achieved by blocking the binding of an agonist to a receptor.

anticholinergic A substance that inhibits the physiological effects of acetylcholine; also used to describe the type or nature of effect(s) observed when this occurs.

antimuscarinic A substance that inhibits the physiological effects of muscarine or similar substances on the parasympathetic nervous system.

atrial fibrillation An abnormal heart rhythm (arrhythmia) characterised by rapid and irregular beating of the atrial chambers of the heart.

beta-blocker A drug that inhibits beta-adrenoceptors in the autonomic nervous system; also referred to as a beta-adrenoceptor antagonist.

bioavailability A pharmacokinetic term used to describe both the rate and extent of absorption of a drug into the systemic circulation. In practice, it is usually expressed as a percentage of administered drug that reaches the systemic circulation.

bioequivalence A pharmacokinetic term used to describe the anticipated in vivo behaviour of two or more different formulations of the same drug. Bioequivalent products are essentially expected to behave in the same manner.

biotransformation The chemical transformation of a substance, often a drug, that occurs within the body; also referred to as metabolism.

blood–brain barrier A term used to describe the tight packing of cells lining the capillaries of the brain. In effect, this is a natural defence mechanism that reduces the free passage of drugs and other substances from the blood into the brain. This means that highly water-soluble drugs or substances do not freely pass into the brain, in contrast to highly lipid-soluble drugs or substances, which do so more easily.

British National Formulary A United Kingdom (UK) pharmaceutical reference book.

canthus Either the inner (inner/medial canthus) or outer (lateral canthus) corner of the eye; the location where the upper and lower eyelids meet.

cardiac output The amount of blood the heart pumps through the circulatory system in a minute.

catecholamine An endogenous hormone/neurotransmitter derived from the amino acid tyrosine. Examples include noradrenaline, dopamine and serotonin.

chelation A term used to describe the chemical binding of a metal ion to a chemical compound.

Cmax A pharmacokinetic term – the maximum drug concentration reached after complete absorption of a drug or substance.

coenzyme An organic, non-protein substance that binds to an enzyme to enhance its activity.

competency framework The competency framework issued by the Royal Pharmaceutical Society, designed to ensure that prescribers assess patients they prescribe for holistically. All prescribers should work within this framework to prescribe safely.

compliance In a healthcare context, the extent to which a patient acts in accordance with a prescribed medication regimen in terms of timing, dosage and frequency.

conjugation In relation to drug metabolism, the binding together of a drug with an endogenous chemical compound that generally results in either the formation of a less active compound, or one that can be eliminated more easily. Note that in some cases the drug-conjugate may be more active than the drug alone.

contraindication In relation to drug therapy, the presence of a condition or factor that provides sufficient cause to withhold a particular drug or treatment.

controlled release In relation to drug therapy, a formulation designed to release a drug over a prolonged period of time in an attempt to prolong the duration of action of the drug; also referred to as extended, slow or sustained release.

degradative In relation to drug therapy, describing the breakdown of a drug.

distribution volume See volume of distribution.

dopamine A substance present in the body that acts as a neurotransmitter and is also a precursor of other compounds such as adrenaline and noradrenaline.

dyslipidaemia An abnormal amount of lipids (fat) in the blood; namely high levels of triglycerides, total cholesterol, or low-density lipoprotein (LDL) cholesterol, and/or low levels of high-density lipoprotein (HDL) cholesterol.

ejection fraction A measurement, expressed as a percentage, of how much blood the left ventricle pumps out with each contraction.

elimination rate constant A pharmacokinetic term used to describe the rate at which a drug is removed from the body. It is expressed as the fraction of drug eliminated per unit of time.

endocytosis The incorporation of a substance or material into a living cell by invagination of the cell membrane around it.

endorphin A group of endogenous peptides (short chain proteins) present in the brain and nervous system that act as morphine-like substances, binding to opiate receptors and resulting in a raised pain threshold or analgesic effects.

enteral Within or by way of the intestine.

enteric coating A pharmaceutical formulation technique that coats tablets, capsules or drug particles with an impervious layer or coating that is resistant to gastric acid. The layer breaks up at alkaline pH, allowing the drug to be released after it has passed through the stomach. This is used either to protect the stomach from direct irritant effects of a drug (e.g. non-steroidal anti-inflammatory drugs such as diclofenac and aspirin) or to protect the drug from being broken down and deactivated by gastric acid (e.g. proton-pump inhibitors such as omeprazole and lansoprazole). The technique can also be used as a method of targeting release of a drug to the small intestine for increased local effects (e.g. aminosalicylates such as mesalazine in the treatment of inflammatory bowel disease).

extrapyramidal side effects (EPSEs) A range of drug-induced movement disorders; physical symptoms resulting from adverse effects of dopamine antagonist agents (principally antipsychotic drugs) blocking dopamine transmission in the nervous system. EPSEs include dystonia, akathisia, parkinsonism and tardive dyskinesia.

facilitated diffusion The passive (non-energy-requiring) movement of a substance bound to a specific membrane-bound transport or carrier molecule across a cell membrane from an area of low concentration to an area of high concentration. This is also referred to as facilitated transport.

first-pass effect The metabolism of a drug by the liver after its absorption from the gastrointestinal tract through the hepatic portal vein, prior to the drug reaching the systemic circulation.

frailty 'A progressive, long term health condition characterised by a loss of physical and/or cognitive resilience' (NHS England 2014). This condition mainly relates to the elderly, as physical and cognitive functions often decline due to the ageing process. In this population group, minor events or illnesses can cause significant and unexpected deterioration. Frail individuals have an increased risk of adverse events such as falls, hospital admissions and disability.

genetic polymorphism The existence of two or more variants of an expressed gene. In relation to drug metabolism, this may result in a lesser or greater degree of enzyme-related drug metabolism, which in turn influences the inter-individual variability of response to a drug.

glomerular filtration The process by which fluid in the blood is filtered across the glomerulus of the kidney into the urinary space.

glomerular filtration rate A description of the flow rate of filtered fluid through the kidney glomerulus which is used as a measure of kidney function.

glutamate hypothesis of schizophrenia The glutamate theory suggests that hypofunction of the neurotransmitter glutamate and antagonism of N-methyl-D-aspartate (NMDA) receptors in the brain could contribute to the positive and negative psychotic symptoms reported in schizophrenia.

half-life A pharmacokinetic term describing the time taken for 50% of the drug in a body to be removed. This is equal to the time taken for the plasma concentration of a drug to fall by 50% as a result of its elimination from the system.

heart failure This is when the pumping heart fails to such an extent that it is unable to meet the metabolic requirement of the tissues.

heart failure with reduced ejection fraction Heart failure due to left ventricular systolic dysfunction, which is associated with reduced left ventricular ejection fraction.

heart failure with preserved ejection fraction Heart failure in which the ejection fraction is normal and is characterised by abnormal diastolic function.

histamine A substance released as part of the inflammatory response resulting from an allergy or injury. This results in contraction of smooth muscle and dilation of capillaries. Also regulates gastric function and acts as a neurotransmitter.

hydrolysis A chemical process involving the breakdown of a compound by reaction with water. This is a common process in drug metabolism.

hydrophobic In a pharmaceutical context, a compound that is relatively poorly water-soluble; such compounds are also termed lipophilic, i.e. compounds that are highly fat-soluble. Hydrophobic/lipophilic drugs cross cell membranes relatively easily.

hydroxylation A chemical process resulting in the introduction of a hydroxyl functional group, made up of one hydrogen and one oxygen atom, into a compound. In biological systems, this is catalysed by enzymes known as hydroxylases. This is a common process in drug metabolism.

intravenous infusion The slow administration, often over several hours, of a fluid that may or may not include a drug, directly into a vein.

ionised A chemical state in which a molecule carries an electrical charge. In the pharmaceutical context, ionised drugs tend to be polar or hydrophilic (i.e. water-soluble) and do not readily cross membranes.

isoenzymes A group of related but chemically distinct enzymes that catalyse the same reaction.

isozyme A synonym for isoenzyme.

lipophilic In a pharmaceutical context, describing a compound that is relatively fat-soluble; such compounds are also termed hydrophobic (i.e. poorly water-soluble). Hydrophobic/lipophilic drugs cross cell membranes relatively easily.

left ventricular failure (LVF) (can be used interchangeably with LVSD) Impaired left ventricular performance.

left ventricular systolic dysfunction (LVSD) An impairment of left ventricular performance.

log10 dose-response curve A dose-response curve plots the concentration of a drug (X axis) against an observed response (Y-axis). As dose-response experiments often use 10-fold serial increments (i.e. 1 unit, 10 units, 100 units of a drug), a logarithmic scale on the X-axis is used so that the dose increments are shown equally spaced.

medicine optimisation Involves collaboration between the patient and the prescriber to ensure that the right medicine is prescribed to improve the patient's health.

metabolic syndrome Also known as syndrome X or dysmetabolic syndrome; a cluster of conditions which, when combined, increase the risk of cardiovascular disease, stroke and heart attack. The defining medical conditions in metabolic syndrome are: abdominal obesity, high blood pressure, high glucose levels and dyslipidaemia.

metabolite A substance produced as a result of metabolism; a substance that is itself metabolised.

mineralocorticoid receptor antagonist Class of drugs which block the effects of aldosterone.

mydriatic A drug or substance that causes mydriasis or dilation of the pupil.

narcosis A drug-induced state characterised by stupor, drowsiness or unconsciousness.

National Institute for Health and Care Excellence (NICE) Provides national guidance and advice to improve health and social care.

non-steroidal anti-inflammatory drugs (NSAIDs) Medicines that are widely used to relieve pain, reduce inflammation, and bring down a high temperature.

NYHA New York Heart Association classification system that provides a simple way of identifying the extent of heart failure, based on the patient's symptoms and functional capacity.

non-compliance When a patient does not act in accordance with a prescribed medication regimen in terms of timing, dosage and frequency.

off-label In relation to the prescribing or administration of a drug, either for a particular condition, or at a different dose, to those for which it has been formally approved for use by the relevant licensing authority.

oxidation A chemical process involving the reaction of a substance with oxygen, resulting in either the addition of oxygen, or loss of either hydrogen or electrons. This is a common process in drug metabolism.

parenteral Administered or otherwise occurring outside the mouth and gastrointestinal tract.

partial agonist A drug or substance that stimulates a receptor but produces a submaximal response.

passive diffusion The free movement of a substance across a biological membrane, from an area of high concentration to one of a lower concentration.

peptidoglycan A polymer consisting of sugars and amino acids which forms the cell wall surrounding most bacteria.

pH Potential of hydrogen; a scale used to measure acidity or alkalinity on a scale of 0–14. Less than 7 indicates acidity and more than 7 indicates alkalinity.

pharmacodynamics The study of the action of drugs on different organs, tissues and biological systems.

pharmacokinetics The study of the effects of the body on a drug, in terms of the processes of absorption, distribution, metabolism and excretion.

physicochemical Relates to the physical and chemical properties of the drug. The ability of the drug to produce a therapeutic effect depends on the physicochemical properties of the drug and the molecules it interacts with. These include factors such as how soluble, permeable and stable the drug is, and these aspects are in turn related to factors such as pH, molecular size, temperature, bonds, oxidation, reduction and hydrolysis reactions; barriers to absorption.

polarity In a pharmaceutical context, a chemical property that means a compound has relatively high water-solubility and poor fat-solubility. Polar compounds do not readily cross cell membranes.

prodrug An inactive (or less active) drug that is administered and subsequently metabolised in the body to an active (or more active) drug. A prodrug may have certain properties, such as better absorption than the active form of the drug.

punctum Lacrimal punctum or puncta (plural); two small holes seen on the inner upper and lower margins of the eyelids that lead to the lacrimal sac (drain tears from the surface of the eyes). Tears enter the lacrimal sac via the puncta.

renin-angiotensin-aldosterone-system A hormone system that regulates blood pressure and fluid and electrolyte balance, as well as systemic vascular resistance.

right ventricular systolic dysfunction Impairment of right ventricular performance.

serotonin A monoamine neurotransmitter, considered a natural mood stabiliser; serotonin helps in sleeping, eating, mood regulation and digestive processes.

stroke volume The amount of blood put out by the left ventricle of the heart in one contraction.

sublingual Under the tongue; a route of administration that may have certain advantages such as rapid onset of effect or avoidance of first-pass metabolism.

teratogenic Potential to cause birth defects.

therapeutic window The gap between the minimum effective plasma level and the minimum toxic plasma level of a drug. A drug with a narrow therapeutic window is one where the effects of dosing, drug metabolism and clearance, and the administration of interacting drugs, are much more critical than normal in ensuring efficacy with minimum potential for toxicity. Also referred to as the therapeutic range or therapeutic index.

Tmax A pharmacokinetic term meaning the time taken to reach maximum drug concentration after complete absorption of a drug or substance.

transdermal Across the skin; a method of drug administration whereby the drug is applied to the skin to allow absorption into the blood and thus a systemic effect.

tri-cycle In relation to oral contraceptive use, the taking of three packs or strips of tablets continuously (omitting the placebo tablets in 'every day' preparations), before a seven-day pill-free interval to induce a withdrawal bleed. This pattern is then repeated.

venous thromboembolism A condition where a blood clot forms, most commonly in a deep vein of the leg.

volume of distribution A pharmacokinetic term referring to the theoretical volume that would contain the total amount of drug present in the body, at the same concentration as it is in blood. This is used as an indicator of the extent of drug distribution into tissues.

xenobiotic A chemical compound, including a drug or pesticide, that is foreign to a living organism.

List of abbreviations

5-HMT 5-hydroxymethyltolterodine
5-HT 5-hydroxytryptamine
ABG arterial blood gas
ABPM ambulatory blood pressure monitoring
ACEI angiotensin-converting enzyme inhibitor
ACh acetylcholine
ACS acute coronary syndrome
ADME absorption, distribution, metabolism, excretion
ADRs adverse drug reactions
AED anti-epileptic drug
AF atrial fibrillation
ALT alanine aminotransferase

ANS autonomic nervous system
ARB angiotensin receptor blocker
ARNI angiotensin receptor/neprilysin inhibitor
ART anti-retroviral therapy
AST aspartate aminotransferase
ATP adenosine triphosphate
BBB blood–brain barrier
BD bipolar disorder
BDNF brain-derived neurotrophic factor
BMI body mass index
BNF British National Formulary
BNFC British National Formulary for Children
BNP B-type natriuretic peptide
BP blood pressure
bpm beats per minute
cAMP cyclic adenosine monophosphate
CAP community-acquired pneumonia
CAT COPD assessment test
CCBs calcium channel blockers
CCF congestive cardiac failure
CHC combined hormonal contraception
CHD coronary heart disease
Cl systemic clearance of drug from the body
Cmax maximum drug concentration after absorption
CNS central nervous system
CO cardiac output
COC combined oral contraceptive
COMT cathechol-O-methyl transferase
COPD chronic obstructive pulmonary disease
COX cyclooxygenase
CTPA computer tomography pulmonary angiogram
CTZ chemoreceptor trigger zone

CVD cardiovascular disease

CXR chest X-ray

CYP cytochrome P450

DA dopamine

DNA deoxyribonucleic acid

DoTS dose-related, time-related and susceptibility factors

DPP-4 dipeptidyl peptidase-4

ECG electrocardiogram

EEG electroencephalogram

EF ejection fraction

eGFR estimated glomerular filtration rate

EPSE extrapyramidal side effects

ESM early systolic murmur

F bioavailability of a drug

FEV1 forced expiratory volume in 1 second

FGA first-generation antipsychotic

FSH follicle stimulating hormone

FVC forced vital capacity

GABA gamma amino butyric acid

GI gastrointestinal

GIP glucose-dependent insulinotrophic peptide

GIT gastrointestinal tract

GLP-1 glucagon-like peptide-1

GORD gastro-oesophageal reflux disease

GPCRs G-protein coupled receptors

GTN glyceryl trinitrate

GUM genitourinary medicine

HBPM home blood pressure monitoring

HCl hydrochloric acid

HDL high density lipoprotein

HF heart failure

HFpEF heart failure with preserved ejection fraction

HRrEF heart failure with reduced ejection fraction
HR heart rate
HRCT high resonant computer tomography
IBS irritable bowel syndrome
ICS inhaled corticosteroid
IFG impaired fasting glycaemia
IGT impaired glucose tolerance
IM intramuscular
INR international normalised ratio
IR immediate release
IV intravenous
JVP jugular venous pressure
Ke drug elimination rate constant
LABA long-acting beta-2 agonist
LAMA long-acting muscarinic antagonist
LAD left anterior descending artery
LDL low density lipoprotein
LH luteinising hormone
LVF left ventricular failure (can be used interchangeably with LVSD)
LVSD left ventricular systolic dysfunction
LVH left ventricular hypertrophy
MAOI monoamine oxidase inhibitor
MC&S microscopy, culture and sensitivity
MDD major depressive disorder
MDI metered dose inhaler
MEL minimum effective level
MHRA Medicines and Healthcare Products Regulatory Authority
MI myocardial infarction
MRA mineralocorticoid receptor antagonist
MTC minimum toxic concentration
NICE National Institute for Health and Care Excellence
NRT nicotine replacement therapy

NSAID non-steroidal anti-inflammatory drug
OAB overactive bladder
OGTT oral glucose tolerance test
OTC over the counter
PCI percutaneous coronary intervention
PD Parkinson's disease
PEP post-exposure prophylaxis
PEPSE post-exposure prophylaxis after sexual intercourse
pH potential of hydrogen
PO per oral (by mouth)
POC progestogen-only contraception
POP progestogen-only pill
PPI proton pump inhibitor
PR pulmonary rehabilitation
PrEP pre-exposure prophylaxis
PRN pro re nata (Latin), meaning 'as required'
PVR peripheral vascular resistance
RAAS renin-angiotensin-aldosterone-system
RACPC rapid access chest pain clinic
RCT randomised controlled trial
RIMA reversible inhibitor of monoamine oxidase A
RPS Royal Pharmaceutical Society
RVSD right ventricular systolic dysfunction
SABA short-acting beta-2 agonist
SAMA short-acting muscarinic antagonist
SE side effect
SGA second-generation antipsychotic
SGL2 sodium glucose co-transporter 2
SNRI serotonin and noradrenaline reuptake inhibitor
SOB shortness of breath
SPC Summary of Product Characteristics
SSRI selective serotonin reuptake inhibitor

STEMI ST segment elevation myocardial infarction
SUI stress urinary incontinence
$t^{1/2}$ half-life (of a drug)
TCA tricyclic antidepressant
TENS transcutaneous electrical nerve stimulation
TI therapeutic index
TLE temporal lobe epilepsy
Tmax time needed to achieve maximum drug concentration
TZD thiazolidinedione
UKPDS United Kingdom Prospective Diabetes Study
UTI urinary tract infection
UUI urge urinary incontinence
Vd volume of distribution
WHO World Health Organisation

Index

abdominal pain 274
absorption, distribution, metabolism and excretion (ADME) 2
Acanthamoeba keratitis 379
acarbose 319
ACE-inhibitors, adverse effects of 191, 203
acetylcholine 285
active transport 5
acute angle closure glaucoma (AACG) 376
acute coronary syndrome 153
acute pain management 274
adherence 81–94, 187, 381
adherence, characteristics that inhibit 86
adherence, characteristics that support 83
advance care planning 411
adverse drug reactions 45–60, 394, 407
adverse drug reactions and interactions 45–60, 191
adverse drug reactions, classification of 46, 47
adverse drug reactions, definition of 46
adverse drug reactions, identification of 50
adverse drug reactions, reporting of 50, 51
affinity 35, 38
age and adherence 87
age and immaturity, influence on medication 120
age-related pharmacokinetic and pharmacodynamic changes 389, 406
age-related physiological changes 391
agonists 32, 33
airflow obstruction criteria in COPD 223
alpha 2 antagonist 347
alpha-1 adrenoreceptor antagonists 183
analgesia, prescribing for children 121
analgesic drugs, categories 121, 122
analgesic ladder 122
anaphylaxis 49
angina, management of 154
angina, patient education and 155
angina, stable 151–172
angina, unstable 152, 153
angiotensin-converting enzyme inhibitors (ACEis) 28, 180, 202, 204
angiotensin receptor blockers (ARBs) 180, 203
angiotensin receptors/neprilysin inhibitors (ARNIs) 206
antacids 264, 265
antacids, drug interactions 265
antagonists 32, 33, 34
antibiotic stewardship 88
antibiotics in COPD exacerbations 229
antibiotics in gastric treatment 267

antidepressants 343, 349
antidepressants, mechanisms of action of 344
anti-diabetic medication 314
anti-diarrhoea drugs 271
anti-emetics 106, 419
anti-epileptic drugs 241–44
anti-epileptic drugs, adverse effects of 245
anti-hypertensive drug, choice of 184
anti-hypertensive treatment, management of 187
antimicrobials and drug resistance 143
antimuscarinic drugs 285, 290, 291
anti-platelets 164
antipsychotic medications, management of people taking 338
antipsychotics 329
antipsychotics, mechanism of action of 330
antipsychotics, side effects of 330, 331, 332
antiretroviral drugs 144, 145
appendicitis 268
aqueous humour 363, 364
arterial atheroma, complications of 154
artificial tear products 371
aspirin use in CVD 164
atherosclerosis 152

back pain during pregnancy 108
bacterial vaginosis 144
benzodiazepines in the elderly 393
beta-agonists 28
beta-blockers 183, 204, 205
beta-blockers, contraindications 205
beta-blockers in angina 161
binding of drug to receptor site 35
bioavailability 8
bioequivalence 8
bladder dysfunction, drugs that can cause or exacerbate 295
bladder retraining 290
bladder-sphincter dyssynergia 285
blepharitis 372, 373
blood–brain barrier 10
blood drug concentration 2, 18
blood pressure, factors determining 176, 177
blood pressure monitoring 174, 178
blood pressure targets 178
BNF abbreviations 75, 76
BNF, accessing the 62
BNF drug monographs 73–75
BNF medicines guidance section 68–71
BNF platforms 63
BNF pricing 76

BNF, searching 67
BNF symbols 75, 76
BNF tables 71
BNFs, information types 65
breast cancer 140
breastfeeding 111–18
breastfeeding mothers, principles of prescription in 112
breathlessness 221, 226, 230
British National Formulary (see also BNF), use of 61–80
bronchiectasis 234
bronchodilators, short-acting 229

calcium antagonists 28
calcium channel blockers (CCBs) 182, 191
calcium channel blockers in angina 162
cardiac output 198, 199
cardiovascular disease 151
cervical cancer 140
chest pain 165
child, definition of 120
children 119–32
cholesterol 162
chronic obstructive pulmonary disease, see COPD
clopidogrel 164
clozapine 352
codeine 126
combined hormonal contraception (CHC) 134
combined hormonal contraception, risks associated with 139
competencies, RPS 438
complex health needs 389–401
compliance 81
concordance 82
conjunctivitis 380
conjunctivitis, bacterial 379
conjunctivitis, neonatal 379, 380
constipation 267, 268
constipation and peptic ulcer 269
constipation in pregnancy 107
contact lens hypersensitivity 372
continence assessment 288
continence physiology 284
contraception 103, 133–50
contraception, storing and administering 142
contraceptive methods, categories of 134
contraceptive pills, generations of 139
contraceptive vaginal ring 142
COPD 221–38
COPD assessment test (CAT) 223, 224
COPD exacerbations 226, 228, 229
COPD, comorbidities in 223
COPD, diagnosis of 222
COPD, pathophysiology of 222

COPD, prevalence of 222
COPD, treatment options 225, 226, 227
cornea 362
coronary artery disease 199
coronary artery disease, atypical presentation of 156, 157
coronary artery occlusion 153
coronary heart disease 151
coronary heart disease, classification of 152
corticosteroids in COPD 229
corticosteroids in IBD 274
cost of prescriptions 439
Crohn's disease 272
cyclic adenosine monophosphate (cAMP) system 40
cyclooxygenase 262
cytochrome P450 12

darifenacin 294
depression 339, 342, 349
depression, diagnosis of 340
depression, inappropriate medications and 395
depression, monoamine theory of 341
depression, treatment of 340
diabetes 305–25
diabetes diagnosis and classification 306, 307, 308, 309, 310
diabetes in pregnancy 108, 115
diabetes mellitus 27
diabetes prevalence 305
diabetes, complications of 310, 311
diabetic nephropathy 311
diabetic neuropathies 311
diarrhoea 271
dietary supplements 394
digoxin 28, 209
digoxin, adverse effects of 209
dipeptidylpeptidase-4 (DPP-4) inhibitors (gliptins) 317
disease, definition of 27
distribution volume (Vd) 8
diuretics 182, 206, 207
diuretics in frail patients 408
dopamine 330
dopamine pathways 329
dopamine-receptor agonists 248
dose-response curve 37, 38
drug absorption 3, 6
drug absorption in the eye 365
drug activities 33
drug distribution 8, 9
drug effects in frail patients 406, 407
drug excretion 15
drug formulations and administration routes 3
drug interactions 51, 52, 66, 382, 398–400, 407
drug interactions, anti-epileptic drugs 246

Index

drug metabolism 11
drug monitoring 18
drug–food interactions 54
drug–herb interactions 55, 56
drug–receptor interactions 29
dual bronchodilator 225
duloxetine 289
dyspepsia in pregnancy 107
eclampsia 110
efficacy 35, 37, 38
embryonic stage 97
end of life care 411
endocytosis 5
endophthalmitis, bacterial 379
enteric system 258
enzyme-inducing drugs 136, 137
enzyme-inhibiting drugs 136
epilepsy 239–46
ethnicity and adherence 86
evaluation, systematic 395
eye anatomy 362, 363
eye infections 379
eye medication, topical 365
eye problems 361–88

factors affecting drug absorption and drug bioavailability 5, 6
factors affecting drug excretion 16, 17
factors affecting drug metabolism 13, 14
fesoterodine fumarate 293
first messenger 41
first-pass drug metabolism in older people 390
first-pass effect 7, 23
foetal development 96, 97
foetal stage 97
folic acid 104
frailty 405–9
frailty scales 405, 406
Frank-Starling curve 199
fungal infection of the cornea 379

gastric acid production 264
gastric cancer 421
gastric secretion, drugs that reduce 266
gastrointestinal conditions affecting drug absorption 275
gastrointestinal conditions, drugs acting on 259
gastrointestinal conditions 257–82
gastrointestinal tract (GIT), structure of 257, 258, 259
gate control theory of pain 414
gender and adherence 88
genetic polymorphism 137
gestational diabetes 109, 309
glaucoma 363, 374, 375, 376, 378

glaucoma medications 376
glomerular filtration 15
glucagon-like peptide (GLP-1) receptor agonists 316
glucose monitoring 336
glucose regulation impairment 309
glyceryl trinitrate 159
gonorrhoea 143
G-protein coupled receptors (GPCRs) 30, 31
guidance for service users 439

haemorrhoids in pregnancy 108
half-life of a drug 18
heart failure 197–219
heart failure, definition of 199
heart failure, drug treatment of 201, 202, 210
heart failure, types of 200, 201
heart, function of 198
herbal remedies 394
herpes simplex keratitis 379
histamine H2 receptor antagonists 266
history taking 369
hormonal contraception, interactions with 138
hormonal contraception, pharmacokinetics of 135
hormones, prescribing 134
human immunodeficiency virus (HIV) 144
hydralazine 208
hyperglycaemia 310
hyperkalaemia 205
hypersensitivity reactions 48, 49
hypertension 173–96, 199
hypertension, classification of 175
hypertension, definition of 174
hypertension, drugs used in treatment of 178–84
hypertension in pregnancy 110, 111, 117
hypertension, lifestyle changes and 173
hypertension, prevalence of 173, 176
hypoglycaemia 318, 322

ibuprofen in children 124, 125
immunosuppressant drugs in IBD 274
incontinence assessment 288
incretin 316
infant, definition of 120
inflammatory bowel disease 272
inflammatory bowel disease, drugs used in 273
instillation of eye medications 370, 382
insulin production 306
insulin resistance 306
insulin, use in pregnancy 109
intestinal and biliary excretion 16
iris 362
iron 104

ischaemic stroke 140
isosorbide dinitrate and mononitrate 160
ivabradine 208

ketoacidosis 315
kinase-linked receptors 31

laxatives 267, 269
left ventricular failure 201
lens 363
levodopa 248
licensing of medicines for children 120
ligand 29
ligand-gated ion channel receptors 30
lipid monitoring 337
lipid-lowering drugs 163
loading dose 22
long-term medication and adherence 88
lubricants 371

macula 364
maintenance dose 22
mechanisms of drug action 28
medication event monitoring systems (MEMS) 83
medication management 332
medication review 407
medication-taking behaviour 81
Medicines Information Services 61
medicines optimisation 64
medicines optimisation, principles of 82
meglitinides 319
menstrual cycle, endocrine control of the 135
mental health disorders in pregnancy 111
mental illness 327–60
mental illness, causes of 328
mental illness, definition of 328
metformin 314, 315
methotrexate and pregnancy 103
midwife prescribers 95
midwife prescribing 438
midwives' exemptions 96
migraine 140
mineralocorticoid receptor antagonists (MRAs) 205
mirabegron 294
mixed urinary incontinence 287, 296
monitoring the side effects of drugs 396
morphine 126, 127
motor neurone disease 422
mu receptor agonists 415
Myerson's sign 247, 252
myocardial infarction (MI) 140, 152
naloxone 417

nausea 417
nausea and vomiting in early pregnancy 105
need, complexity of 395
neonate, definition of 120
neurological problems 239–55
neurotransmitters 285
nicotinic acetylcholine receptor 29
nitrates 159, 160, 161
nitrates, adverse effects of 161
non-adherence, scale of 85
non-adherent behaviour patterns 84
non-medical prescribers (NMPs) 437, 438
non-specific abdominal pain (NSAP) 275
non-ST segment elevation myocardial infarction (NSTEMI) 153
non-steroidal anti-inflammatory drugs (NSAIDs) 28
non-steroidal anti-inflammatory drugs (NSAIDs) in frail patients 407
noradrenaline 33
NSAIDs and peptic ulcer disease 261, 262
NSAIDs in children 124
NSAIDs side effects 263
nuclear receptors 32
nurse prescribing 438
nutritional supplements and pregnancy 104

ocular structure and physiology 362, 363
oedema, peripheral 212
oestrogen in urinary incontinence 295
oestrogen 134
off-label prescribing 121, 141
ophthalmic medications, administration of 380
ophthalmic medications, classification of 367, 368, 369
ophthalmic pharmacodynamics and pharmacokinetics 364
opiates in frail patients 407
opioid analgesia in children 126
opioids 415
oral rehydration therapy 271
OTC remedies 394
overactive bladder 287
overactive bladder (OAB) symptoms, pharmacological management of 290
oxybutynin hydrochloride 291, 292

P450 cytochrome enzymes and hormonal contraception 136
pain 414–17
pain tools 121
pain, transmission and perception of 414
palliative care 411–35
palliative care, common medications in 413
palliative care, medication routes in 419, 420, 421
palliative care, symptom management in 412
paracetamol dosing in children 123

paracetamol hepatotoxicity 122
paracetamol in children 122, 123, 124
Parkinson's disease (PD) 246–50
Parkinson's disease, drug therapy for 247, 249
partial agonists 32, 33, 34
passive diffusion 5
paternal exposure 103
pelvic floor exercises 289, 290
peptic ulcer symptoms 261
peptic ulcers, drugs used to treat 260
pharmacodynamic drug interactions 52
pharmacodynamics 1, 27–44
pharmacokinetic drug interactions 53
pharmacokinetic parameters 2, 3
pharmacokinetics 1¬–25
pharmacokinetics, anti-epileptic drugs 245, 246
Phase I metabolism 12
Phase II metabolism 12, 13
placenta, properties of drugs crossing the 102
plasma protein binding 10, 11
polypharmacy 87, 389–401, 439
polypharmacy, definition of 393
polypharmacy in the elderly 394
post-exposure prophylaxis 146
potency 37
pre-conception 102
pre-eclampsia 110
pre-embryonic stage 96
pre-exposure prophylaxis 146
pregnancy 95–111
pregnancy, management of common symptoms in 105
pregnancy, physiological and pharmacokinetic changes in 100, 101
pregnancy planning 102
pregnancy prevention programme 103
pregnancy testing 103
prescribing practice, principles of 391, 397
preservatives and active ingredients 371
pre-systemic metabolism 7
primary open angle glaucoma (POAG) 375
Prinzmetal's angina 153
prodrug 215
professional accountability of the non-medical prescriber 438
progesterone 134
propiverine hydrochloride 294
protease inhibitors 146
proton pump inhibitors (PPIs) 266, 267
psychotropic medications 327

receptor down regulation 41
receptor locations within a cell 29
receptor subtypes 35, 36
receptor up regulation 41
receptors 29
renal excretion 15
renal impairment and morphine 434
renin-aldosterone-angiotensin system 181, 204
retina 364
retinopathy 311
reverse transcriptase inhibitors 145

schizophrenia, dopamine theory of 329
schizophrenia, glutamate hypothesis of 329
second-generation antipsychotics (SGAs) 332
second messenger systems 40, 41
seizure 240, 241
selective serotonin reuptake inhibitors (SSRIs) 348
serotonin and noradrenaline reuptake inhibitors (SNRIs) 347
sexual health 133–50
sexually transmitted infections 143
short-term medication and adherence 88
side effects, definition of 46
small doses, prescribing 120
smoking 222, 231
smoking cessation 236
sodium glucose co-transporter 2 (SGLT2) inhibitors 315
sodium valproate 244
sodium valproate teratogenicity 103
solifenacin succinate 294
SSRIs, side effects 348
ST segment elevation myocardial infarction (STEMI) 153
stable angina, drugs used in 157, 158
Starling's law 198
statins 162, 163
steady state concentration 19, 20, 21, 22
stress urinary incontinence (SUI) 286
stress urinary incontinence, pharmacological management of 289
stroke 151
sublingual route 7
sulfonylureas 318
sympathetic nervous system 192
synapses, processes in 341
systemic diseases and drug interactions 369

temporal lobe epilepsy 240
teratogenic drugs 138
teratogenic effects caused by specific drugs or agents 99, 100
teratogenicity 98, 99
thalidomide 98
therapeutic equivalence 8
therapeutic index and ADRs 48
therapeutic range 21, 22
thiazolidinediones (glitazones) 318

Todd's Palsy 241, 251
tolerance 160, 168
tolterodine tartrate 293
transportation of drugs 5
treatment summary (BNF) 65
tricyclic antidepressants 28, 345
trospium chloride 293
Type 1 diabetes mellitus (T1D) 309
Type 2 diabetes (T2D) 309
Type 2 diabetes, management of 312

UK Teratology Information Service (UKTIS) 104
ulcerative colitis 272
ulcers 260
unlicensed prescribing 120
urgency urinary incontinence 287
urinary incontinence, approach to management 283, 284
urinary incontinence in adults 283–304
urinary tract infection 288
urinary tract, innervation of the lower 285

vaginal discharge in pregnancy 108
varicose veins in pregnancy 108
venous thromboembolism 139
vitamin A 105
vitamin D 105
vomiting 417

warfarin 11
warfarin–amiodarone interaction 57
weight gain monitoring with antipsychotic medication 335
weight loss in T2D 313

Yellow Card Scheme 50